Algorithms for Intelligent Systems

This book series publishes research on the analysis and development of algorithms for intelligent systems with their applications to various real world problems. It covers research related to autonomous agents, multi-agent systems, behavioral modeling, reinforcement learning, game theory, mechanism design, machine learning, meta-heuristic search, optimization, planning and scheduling, artificial neural networks, evolutionary computation, swarm intelligence and other algorithms for intelligent systems.

The book series includes recent advancements, modification and applications of the artificial neural networks, evolutionary computation, swarm intelligence, artificial immune systems, fuzzy system, autonomous and multi agent systems, machine learning and other intelligent systems related areas. The material will be beneficial for the graduate students, post-graduate students as well as the researchers who want a broader view of advances in algorithms for intelligent systems. The contents will also be useful to the researchers from other fields who have no knowledge of the power of intelligent systems, e.g. the researchers in the field of bioinformatics, biochemists, mechanical and chemical engineers, economists, musicians and medical practitioners.

The series publishes monographs, edited volumes, advanced textbooks and selected proceedings.

More information about this series at http://www.springer.com/series/16171

M. Niranjanamurthy · Siddhartha Bhattacharyya ·
Neeraj Kumar
Editors

Intelligent Data Analysis for COVID-19 Pandemic

Springer

Editors
M. Niranjanamurthy
Department of MCA
M. S. Ramaiah Institute of Technology
Bengaluru, Karnataka, India

Siddhartha Bhattacharyya
Rajnagar Mahavidyalaya
Birbhum, West Bengal, India

Neeraj Kumar
Department of Information Technology
Babasaheb Bhimrao Ambedkar University
(A Central University)
Lucknow, Uttar Pradesh, India

ISSN 2524-7565 ISSN 2524-7573 (electronic)
Algorithms for Intelligent Systems
ISBN 978-981-16-1573-3 ISBN 978-981-16-1574-0 (eBook)
https://doi.org/10.1007/978-981-16-1574-0

This Springer imprint is published by the registered company Springer Nature Singapore Pte Ltd.
The registered company address is: 152 Beach Road, #21-01/04 Gateway East, Singapore 189721, Singapore

Niranjanamurthy would like to dedicate this book to his Teachers, who changed his life, especially Dr. Hemant Yadav from Government Polytechnic, Budaun, for Diploma Engineering and Prof. (Dr.) Shirshu Varma, Prof. Shekhar Varma, and Prof. R. C. Tripathi for IIITA, M.Tech. (IT), and without whose inspiration, this task could not have been accomplished.

Siddhartha Bhattacharyya would like to dedicate this book to the frontline COVID-19 warriors all across the world.

Neeraj Kumar would like to dedicate this book to his students, researchers, and readers, for their enthusiasm in disseminating the best of their intelligent data analysis practice, research, and education.

Preface

Coronavirus disease or COVID-19 or SARS-CoV-2 infection is the latest pandemic that has affected humans globally. Intelligent data analysis (IDA) is one of the intense issues in the field of artificial intelligence and information. As the goal of intelligent data analysis is to extract useful knowledge, the process demands a combination of extraction, analysis, conversion, classification, organization, reasoning, and so on for solving the problems.

The book is dedicated to addressing the major challenges in fighting the COVID-19 pandemic using intelligent data analysis. The authors present the latest theoretical developments, real-world applications, and future perspectives on this topic. The book brings together a broad multidisciplinary community, aiming to integrate ideas, theories, models, and techniques from across different disciplines on intelligent solutions/systems.

The book comprises fifteen well-versed self-contained chapters focused on the survey and applications of intelligent tools and techniques for analysis, diagnosis, and prediction of COVID-19.

Chapter "Machine Learning-Based Ensemble Approach for Predicting the Mortality Risk of COVID-19 Patients: A Case Study" illustrates the application of two different machine learning-based ensembling approaches in the form of boosting and bagging on COVID-19 data set obtained from Kaggle (https://www.kaggle.com/) and GitHub (https://github.com/datasets/covid-19). The chapter discusses a comparative study to evaluate how the implemented ensemble method helps in classifying significant predictors and their effects on COVID-19 patients' mortality. The outcomes of the experiments indicate all classifiers exhibit satisfactory performance in intercepting the mortality risk of the patients.

Chapter "Role of Internet of Health Things (IoHTs) and Innovative Internet of 5G Medical Robotic Things (IIo-5GMRTs) in COVID-19 Global Health Risk Management and Logistics Planning" presents cost-effective healthcare technologies for hospital disinfection routine operations and remote access monitoring using Internet of Things Medical Robotics to lower the risk of hospital-acquired infection in the ongoing COVID-19 pandemic.

The crisis of COVID-19 has traumatized the world. The advancement and sophistication of digital technologies, viz. mobile applications, artificial intelligence, Internet of Things (IoT), big data analytics, and social media tools, have the potential to curb the spread of virus. Chapter "Battling COVID-19 with Process Model of Integrated Digital Technology: An Analysis of Qualitative Data" attempts to develop an integrated model of digital technology by utilizing the resources available in the literature.

The COVID-19 pandemic situation has made the development of low-cost ventilators urgent around the world. These ventilators must include functionality to meet the needs of patients with severe respiratory disease, where lung compliance and patient breathing cycles are highly dynamic, and require precise, controllable ventilator design with high levels of integration. A low-cost ventilator design is presented in chapter "High-Fidelity Intelligence Ventilator to Help Infect with COVID-19 Based on Artificial Intelligence" using essential pressure and volumetric control ventilation modes for critical patients while being cost-effective compared to all other options.

Chapter "Boon of Artificial Intelligence in Diagnosis of COVID-19" presents a survey of intelligent analytics to curb the spread of COVID-19. In this context, artificial intelligence (AI) is gaining importance for the diagnosis of COVID-19. For confirmation of this infection, real-time reverse transcriptase-polymerase chain reaction (RT-PCR) is considered as the gold standard. For the diagnosis of COVID-19, imaging analysis techniques such as computed tomography (CT) and chest X-ray can also be exploited. Chest X-ray of COVID-19 patients shows bilateral infiltrates in the early stage of the disease. For quick diagnosis, Infervision (a start-up) is being used as a deep learning medical imaging platform. Additionally, according to China National Health Commission, nasopharyngeal and oropharyngeal swab testing is considered as the standard test for its diagnosis. Besides, a new AI-authorized face detection, temperature detection, and dual sensing via infrared cameras have been used for its detection in early stages. Thus, for the diagnosis and better management of COVID-19, AI and big data seem to have tremendous potential in the future.

In December 2019, the initially infected patient of the novel coronavirus disease (COVID-19) was discovered in China. Globally, the pandemic has disseminated in almost 216 countries and considerably influenced all aspects of life. The numbers of confirmed cases and deaths are 24,854,140 million and 838,924 thousand, respectively, until August 31, 2020, and yet growing with no sign of control. Techniques for artificial intelligence (AI) and big data could contribute significantly in addressing the COVID-19 pandemic via various attracting solutions, ranging from monitoring the outbreak, detecting the viral infection to diagnosing and managing. Chapter "Artificial Intelligence and Big Data Solutions for COVID-19" focuses on the significant applications of AI and big data in responding to the coronavirus pandemic where it describes AI and big data, applications, limitations, and recommendations to control the COVID-19. This chapter provides novel perspectives on how AI and big data have enhanced responding to the COVID-19.

Chapter "Emerging Trends in Higher Education During Pandemic Covid-19: An Impact Study from West Bengal" concerns with the COVID-19 pandemic impact on Higher Educational Institutes (HEIs) predominantly. The pandemic impact has frozen educational institutes and their works. It has also made HEIs all over the world clueless to enhance safety environment for teaching–learning. The pandemic lockdown has masqueraded numerous challenges to Higher Educational Institutes (HEI), particularly to West Bengal. This study has been conducted with a predetermined size of 143 Higher Educational Institutes as sample organizations from the populations of 200 from West Bengal. The data have been collected and computed for analysis and discussion. HEIs have also used artificial intelligence components to enhanced machine learning interventions to meet the demands of the students and stakeholders. It has been observed further that HEIs in West Bengal have used computational intelligence to bridge the learning outcomes through computer programming and data structure. Thus, this chapter explores newer technological solutions to bridge the learning gap and help the students to be innovative through computational intelligence and digital platforms and become merely a student-centered approach.

Chapter "COVID-19: Virology, Epidemiology, Diagnostics and Predictive Modeling" provides an interim insight into virology, origin of SARS-CoV-2, epidemiology of COVID-19, diagnostics, and treatment based on the literature. A detailed summary of articles reported on the virology of SARS-CoV-2 is reported in the chapter. This chapter also reports developments in vaccines and therapeutics to cure COVID-19 briefly. The differences between the demography and contact structure of India, USA, and Spain have been studied. A mathematical model is also constituted for predicting COVID-19 spread in India.

Logistic regression model is so far the most widely used model for the analysis of binary response data. In chapter "Improved Estimation in Logistic Regression Through Quadratic Bootstrap Approach: An Application in Indian Agricultural E-learning System During COVID-19 Pandemic," logistic regression modeling has been used for classification purposes with a view to investigate the discomfort of Indian agricultural students in e-learning during the COVID-19 pandemic. A total of 1370 responses has been received through Google form from the agricultural students all over India. Out of these responses, 1096 responses have been selected randomly for the training purpose, whereas the rest 274 responses have been retained as test data set. The presence or absence of discomfort of Indian agricultural students in e-learning has been considered as the response variable. Subsequently, a quadratic bootstrap estimation procedure has been used for improved estimation under logistic regression setup with the most influential explanatory variable (Internet speed) for classification. The performance of quadratic bootstrap-based estimator has been found to be better in terms of both width of the confidence interval of the parameter estimates and classificatory ability of the model.

Chapter "COVID-19 and Stock Markets: Deaths and Strict Policies" investigates the effects of the pandemic on the stock markets in G7 and E7 countries. First, the cross-section dependency between the series and the stationarity of the variables are investigated. After determining that variables are stationary, fixed effects and random effects models, for G7 and E7 countries, respectively, are used for coefficient estimation. The analysis reveals that the rise in deaths caused by COVID-19 has had no effect on stock markets in G7 and E7 countries, but the strict measures taken to prevent the spread of the virus have had some negative effects.

Chapter "Artificial Intelligence Techniques in Medical Imaging for Detection of Coronavirus (COVID-19/SARS-COV-2): A Brief Survey" aims to review different kinds of machine learning techniques, including deep learning, transfer learning, and deep convolution neural network models, namely ResNet-50, VGG-19, InceptionV3, MobileNet, and Inception-ResNetV2, for image recognition and image classification and their performance analysis for detection of COVID-19 using a large open-access data set of real-time chest X-ray images that are publicly available and open source.

An improved scheduling for the disinfection process of the new coronavirus (COVID-19) is introduced in chapter "A Travelling Disinfection-Man Problem (TDP) for COVID-19: A Nonlinear Binary Constrained Gaining-Sharing Knowledge-Based Optimization Algorithm". The scheduling aims at achieving the best utilization of the available day time, which is calculated as the total disinfection time minus the total loss traveling time. In this regard, a new application problem is presented, which is called a traveling disinfection-man problem (TDP).

A survey has been presented in chapter "COVID-19 Lock Down Impact on Mental Health: A Cross-Sectional Online Survey from Kerala, India" to investigate the impact of COVID-19 lockdown on the emotional and mental status of individuals in the state of Kerala, India. A questionnaire was circulated to collect information from individuals who belonged to categories like professionals, engineering, medical students, and others. The response from 9852 individuals was collected, segregated, and tabulated. Analysis was done on the collected data, and charts were plotted to provide a visual representation of the segregated data. It was observed that a significant impact is there on the mental health of individuals during lockdown due to this pandemic. It is suggested that international organizations like the World Health Organization (WHO) and the governments can play a vital role in addressing the mental and psychological issues caused due to a lockdown and make people comfortable to face the pandemic.

The huge measure of COVID-19 treatment information in overall medical clinics requires AI techniques to be propelled for examining customized restorative impacts for assessing new patients, for example, hospitalization forecast, which can give better mind to every patient as well as add to neighborhood emergency clinic game plan and activity. Chapter "Analysis, Modelling and Prediction of COVID-19 Outbreaks Using Machine Learning Algorithms" focuses on a target approach while anticipating the continuation of the COVID-19 utilizing a straightforward, however, amazing technique to do as such. Accepting that the information utilized is solid and that the future will keep on following the previous example of the infection, the chapter recommends a proceeding with increment in the confirmed COVID-19 cases with sizable-related vulnerability.

Tracking and analysis of corona disease are very important to avoid the spread of COVID-19. Collecting data and information from WHO and other medical department sectors, using AI techniques, the system can track and predict the corona disease. Computer-based intelligence can be utilized to follow (counting nowcasting) and to anticipate how the COVID-19 sickness will spread over the long run. Chapter "Tracking and Analysis of Corona Disease Using Intelligent Data Analysis" discusses the tracking and analysis of corona disease using intelligent data analysis.

Bengaluru, India M. Niranjanamurthy
Birbhum, India Siddhartha Bhattacharyya
Lucknow, India Neeraj Kumar
January 2021

Contents

Editors and Contributors

About the Editors

Dr. M. Niranjanamurthy is Assistant Professor, Department of Computer Applications, M S Ramaiah Institute of Technology, Bangalore, Karnataka, India. He completed Ph.D. in Computer Science at JJTU, Rajasthan (2016); M.Phil. in Computer Science at VMU, Salem (2009); Masters in Computer Applications at Visvesvaraiah Technological University, Belgaum, Karnataka (2007); BCA from Kuvempu University 2004 with University 5th Rank. He has 10 years of teaching experience and 2 years of industry experience as Software Engineer. He has published books in Scholars Press Germany and CRC Press. He also published 56 research papers and filed 12 patents. Currently, he is guiding four Ph.D. research scholars in the areas of data science, edge computing, ML, and networking. He is Reviewer of 22 international journals and Series Editor in CRC Press and Scrivener Publishing. He has received best research journal reviewer and researcher awards. He is a member of IEEE, CSTA, IAENG, and INSC. His areas of interest are data science, ML, edge computing, software engineering, web services, cloud computing, and networking.

Dr. Siddhartha Bhattacharyya [LFOSI, LFISRD, FIET (UK), FIETE, FIE(I), SMIEEE, SMIETI, SMACM, LMCRSI, LMCSI, LMISTE, LMIUPRAI, LMCEGR, LMICCI, LMALI, MIRSS, MIAENG, MCSTA, MIAASSE, MIDES, MISSIP, MSDIWC] is currently serving as the Principal at Rajnagar Mahavidyalaya, Birbhum, India. He is Co-Author of 6 books and Co-Editor of 75 books and has more than 300 research publications in international journals and conference proceedings to his credit. He has got two PCTs to his credit. He is Associate Editor of several reputed journals including *Applied Soft Computing*, *IEEE Access*, *Evolutionary Intelligence*, and *IET Quantum Communications*. He is Editor of *International Journal of Pattern Recognition Research* and Founding Editor-in-Chief of *International Journal of Hybrid Intelligence, Inderscience*. His research interests include hybrid intelligence, pattern recognition, multimedia data processing, social networks, and quantum computing.

Dr. Neeraj Kumar is currently engaged with the Department of Information Technology, Babasaheb Bhimrao Ambedkar University (A Central University), Lucknow (India). He has completed his Doctorate in Information Technology from BBAU, Lucknow, in March 2020. He has completed his basic education from Government Polytechnic, Budaun, and then graduation and PG from UPTU, Lucknow, and IIIT Allahabad in the year 2005 and 2010, respectively. After graduation, he was appointed as Lecturer in BSACET, Mathura, while after PG, appointed as Assistant Professor in various institutes of RTU and UPTU. He has published more than two dozen research articles in reputed international journals and conferences. He has published few patents related to computer science and disaster management. He has published few authored and edited books with the publishers of national repute. He has research interests in topics related to real-life problem, including disaster management, IoT, big data, soft computing, cyber security, and quantum cryptography.

Contributors

Umar Abdu Adamu Polymer Technology Department, Hussaini Adamu Federal Polytechnic, Kazaure, Nigeria

Prachi Agrawal Department of Mathematics and Scientific Computing, National Institute of Technology Hamirpur, Hamirpur, Himachal Pradesh, India

V. Ajantha Devi Research Head, Chennai, India

Ali Altiner Recep Tayyip Erdoğan University, Rize, Turkey

Onyebuchi Amaonwu Computer Science Department, Hussaini Adamu Federal Polytechnic, Kazaure, Nigeria

M. P. Amulya Department of Computer Science and Engineering, Adichunchanagiri University, Mandya, India

Mourade Azrour Moulay Ismail University, Department of Computer Science, Faculty of Sciences and Techniques, IDMS Team, Errachidia, Morocco

Bishvajit Bakshi Centre for Management of Health Services, Indian Institute of Management-Ahmedabad, Ahmedabad, Gujarat, India

Anindya Banerjee Department of Electronics and Communication Engineering, Kalyani Government Engineering College, Kalyani, West Bengal, India

Sawan Bharti Invertis University, Bareilly, Uttar Pradesh, India

Simran Bhatia Center for Medical Biotechnology, Amity Institute of Biotechnology, Amity University Uttar Pradesh, Noida, India

Eda Bozkurt Atatürk University, Erzurum, Turkey

Balendra V. S. Chauhan Department of Mechanical Engineering, Invertis University, Bareilly, Uttar Pradesh, India

Nafih Cherappurath Department of Physical Education, University of Calicut, Calicut, Kerala, India

Ravi Deval Invertis University, Bareilly, Uttar Pradesh, India

Driss Dhiba International Water Research Institute IWRI, University Mohammed VI Polytechnic (UM6P), Benguerir, Morocco

Masilamani Elayaraja Department of Physical Education & Sports, Pondicherry University, Pondicherry, India

Talari Ganesh Department of Mathematics and Scientific Computing, National Institute of Technology Hamirpur, Hamirpur, Himachal Pradesh, India

Raj Krishan Ghosh Centre of Excellence in Artificial Intelligence, Indian Institute of Technology Kharagpur, Kharagpur, West Bengal, India

Sneh Gour Invertis University, Bareilly, Uttar Pradesh, India

Yuvraj Goyal Center for Medical Biotechnology, Amity Institute of Biotechnology, Amity University Uttar Pradesh, Noida, India

Dheeraj Gunwant GET Group of Institutions-Faculty of Technology, Bazpur, Uttarakhand, India;
Invertis University, Bareilly, Uttar Pradesh, India

Souad El Hajjaji Laboratory of Spectroscopy, Molecular Modeling, Materials, Nanomaterial, Water and Environment, CERN2D, Faculty of Science, Mohammed V University in Rabat, Agdal, Rabat, Morocco

Ibrahim M. Hassan Computer Science Department, Hussaini Adamu Federal Polytechnic, Kazaure, Nigeria

Said Ali Hassan Department of Operations Research and Decision Support, Faculty of Computers and Artificial Intelligence, Cairo University, Giza, Egypt

Sakeer Hussain Department of Physical Education, University of Calicut, Calicut, Kerala, India

Aminu Abdulahi Kazaure Computer Science Department, Hussaini Adamu Federal Polytechnic, Kazaure, Nigeria

Jazuli S. Kazaure Electrical Electronics Engineering Department, Hussaini Adamu Federal Polytechnic, Kazaure, Nigeria

K. N. Krishnamurthy Department of Agricultural Statistics, Applied Mathematics and Computer Science, University of Agricultural Sciences, Bengaluru, Karnataka, India

Koushal Kumar Department of Computer Applications, Sikh National College, Qadian, Gurdaspur, Punjab, India

Vikas Kumar Invertis University, Bareilly, Uttar Pradesh, India

Jamal Mabrouki Laboratory of Spectroscopy, Molecular Modeling, Materials, Nanomaterial, Water and Environment, CERN2D, Faculty of Science, Mohammed V University in Rabat, Agdal, Rabat, Morocco

Ugochukwu O. Matthew Computer Science Department, Hussaini Adamu Federal Polytechnic, Kazaure, Nigeria

Ali Wagdy Mohamed Operations Research Department, Faculty of Graduate Studies for Statistical Research, Cairo University, Giza, Egypt;
Wireless Intelligent Networks Center (WINC), School of Engineering and Applied Sciences, Nile University, Giza, Egypt

K. Mourlin Xavier Business School (XBS), St. Xavier's University, Kolkata, India

M. Niranjanamurthy Department of Master of Computer Applications, M S Ramaiah Institute of Technology, Bangalore, India

Pramit Pandit Department of Agricultural Statistics, Bidhan Chandra Krishi Viswavidyalaya, Mohanpur, West Bengal, India

C B Rajesh Department of Physical Education, NSS College of Engineering, Palakkad, Kerala, India

G. K. Ravikumar Adichunchanagiri University, Mandya, India

Rehab A. Rayan Department of Epidemiology, High Institute of Public Health, Alexandria University, Alexandria, Egypt

Girish Sharma Center for Medical Biotechnology, Amity Institute of Biotechnology, Amity University Uttar Pradesh, Noida, India;
Amity Center for Cancer Epidemiology and Cancer Research, Amity University Uttar Pradesh, Noida, India

Shakti Sharma Donau- Ries Klinikum, Donauwörth, Germany

N. Sreelekha Department of Applied Psychology, Pondicherry University, Pondicherry, India

Yılmaz Toktaş Amasya University, Amasya, Turkey

Christos Tsagkaris Faculty of Medicine, University of Crete, Heraklion, Greece

Chibueze N. Ubochi Micheal Okpara University of Agriculture Umudike, Umudike, Nigeria

Harshit Upadhyay Invertis University, Bareilly, Uttar Pradesh, India

Ajitanshu Vedrtnam Invertis University, Bareilly, Uttar Pradesh, India;
Universidad de Alcalá, Alcalá, Spain

Aastha Verma South Campus, Ramlal Anand College, University of Delhi, New Delhi, India

Rohit Verma Donau- Ries Klinikum, Donauwörth, Germany

V. Vinod Department of Mechanical Engineering, NSS College of Engineering, Palakkad, Kerala, India

H. K. Yogish Department of Master of Computer Applications, M S Ramaiah Institute of Technology, Bangalore, India

Imran Zafar Department of Bioinformatics and Computational Biology, Virtual University of Pakistan, Lahore, Pakistan

Machine Learning-Based Ensemble Approach for Predicting the Mortality Risk of COVID-19 Patients: A Case Study

Koushal Kumar

1 Introduction

The proliferation of a novel coronavirus disease (COVID-19) pandemic has attracted wide attentions, since "December 2019." COVID-19 has escalated from China, which outbreaks in the Wuhan city and rapidly spreads all around the world. According to data provided by World Health Organization (WHO) Health Emergency Dashboard report till date **(July 29, 2020),** globally 16,737,842 confirmed cases with 659,374 deaths have been reported [1–3]. Data as reported by WHO on COVID-19 indicates that this infectious disease has caused unprecedented morbidity and mortality across the globe. To curb this unusual situation and proliferation of the COVID-19, majority of countries have closed their schools, colleges, offices, borders, airports, and other public places as a precautionary measure. Notwithstanding, the implementations of several rigorous preventive methods worldwide and the spread of this disease have not been curbed till date. COVID-19 infected patients can be separated into mild moderate, serious, and critical stages, based on the severity of the infection. Some usual clinical features of hospitalized patients infected with COVID-19 include fever, shortness of breath, fatigue, diarrhea, dry cough, and respiratory distress. Few other less growing symptoms include body pain, headache, rhinorrhea, sore throat, and vomiting [4–7]. Few recent studies suggest that COVID-19 is much more likely to affect older males and can lead to severe and even fatal respiratory illnesses, thus make males more prone to death as compared to females [8–10]. Epidemiological evidence indicates that older age people with diseases such as cardiovascular disease, severe lung disorder and diabetes put patients' lives at high risk [11, 12]. The major death cause in COVID-19 is due to virus-induced pneumonia, leading to acute respiratory failure also called acute respiratory distress syndrome (ARDS) [13]. According to the World Health Organization, the projected incubation time (period from exposure to the development of

K. Kumar (✉)
Department of Computer Applications, Sikh National College, Qadian, Gurdaspur, Punjab, India

M. Niranjanamurthy et al. (eds.), *Intelligent Data Analysis for COVID-19 Pandemic*, Algorithms for Intelligent Systems, https://doi.org/10.1007/978-981-16-1574-0_1

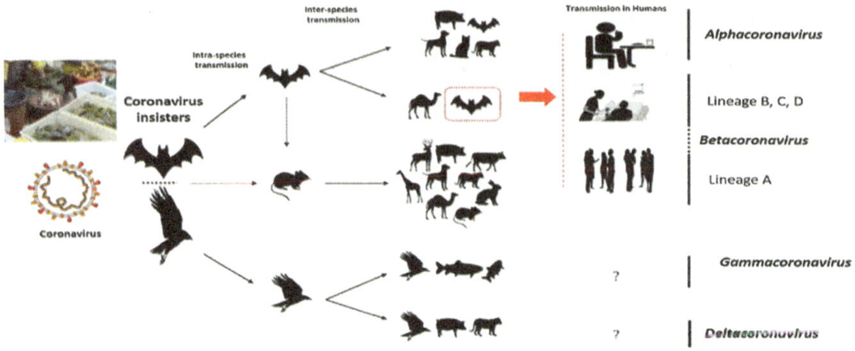

Fig. 1 Vital source sequence of coronaviruses transmission

symptoms) of COVID-19 can be between 2 and 14 days [14, 15]. This COVID-19 pandemic is overspreading around the world and putting enormous pressure on the health system of many developed and developing countries [16, 17]. As the number of cases in these countries rises, their hospitals are continuously reporting shortages of key equipments such as ventilators, personal protective equipment (PPE), gloves, N95 respirator masks, gowns, and hand sanitizer for medical staff.

According to the Center for Disease Control (CDC), when COVID-19 infected people create respiratory droplets by coughing or sneezing or even talking, they can spread the disease and these droplets may fall in the mouths or nose of people who are nearby or likely inhaled into the lungs. The CDC recommends that one should stay at least six feet away from others to minimize the risk of transmission in public places. The transmission process of COVID-19 is outlined below in Fig. 1, which confirms that the use of infected animal in food is a major cause of disease transmission along with close contacts with infected persons. Dotted arrows represent the likelihood of viral transmission via bats, whereas solid black arrow indicates the confirmed spread [18–21].

Generally, an upsurging infectious disease such as COVID-19 jeopardizing the health of numerous people, and thus, needs a quick action to prevent this pandemic spread at the grassroots level [22]. As we know, COVID-19 pandemic relentlessly ravaging the whole world and in response worldwide scientists are working to recognize, curb, and contain its spread. Recently, machine learning-based supervised models have been used in wide range of applications, such as bioinformatics, human–computer interaction, speech recognition, and language translation, and results show considerable accuracy. In the recent times, most widely used applications of machine learning are prediction and classification of the data based upon set of conditions applied. For this research work, I have used the publicly available dataset from Kaggle and GitHub, two online communities of data scientists. As we know, various classification algorithms have different prediction accuracy and error rates, so we opted ensembling technique for prediction and analysis. In machine learning, ensembling is a robust approach for improving the prediction performance of your classifier model, which strategically combines the different models and produces stable and better results as compared to a single model. In this research work, I have applied **boosting and bagging** ensembling approaches to predict and analyze novel risk factors of COVID-19 patients including average time required to hospitalize the infected patient, mortality risk, gender impact, etc. The outcomes of the research could potentially contribute in finding the mortality risk of COVID-19 patients and help the researchers in comprehensive study of the disease. **The key objectives of our case study include the following.**

1. To predict the average recovery time of the COVID-19 hospitalized patients.
2. The significance of age factor in predicting the morality risk of the COVID-19 patients.
3. To find the relationship of mortality rates in both sexes and their comparison.
4. To determine if one model results are more precise and reliable than the others which is done by applying Wilcoxon signed-rank test.

The remaining sections of the paper are organized as follows: Sect. 2 describes the literature review of machine learning used in the context of COVID-19, Sect. 3 comprises the methodology and dataset used in this research work, Sect. 4 presents various ensembling approaches applied in this study, Sect. 5 examines the experiments and results obtained after experimental study, and last Sect. 6, provides the conclusion of the present work.

2 Literature Review

Very less literature reviews are available in literature related to our research problem but, and we have tried best to collect all in a single paper. As we know machine learning is an artificial intelligence subfield and is effective for a broad range of real-life problems. Therefore, this literature review contains work related to COVID-19 disease and its prediction using machine learning.

Yan et al. [23] draw our attention on a novel approach and proposed a prognostic machine learning-based predictive model using XGBoost algorithm, which can precisely identify critical patients from their epidemiological and clinical data facts. They used clinical data of 2799 patients collected from Tongji hospital in Wuhan and shortlisted three key clinical features, i.e., lym-phocyte, lactic dehydrogenase (LDH), and high-sensitivity C-reactive protein from a set of 300 features. Their proposed approach predicts the survival rates of severe and critical patients with more than 90% accuracy, enabling the early diagnosis which results in reduction of mortality in high-risk COVID-19 patients.

Narin et al. [24] proposed three different classification models specified as (ResNet-50, Inception-v3, and Inception–ResNet-v2) based upon convolutional neural networks for the identification of patients infected with coronavirus pneumonia using chest X-ray radiographs. In this study, the authors used radiographic chest images of COVID-19 patients obtained from the open-source GitHub repository. The obtained results revealed that the accuracy of the ResNet-50 model (98%) is the best among other models. This study provides insights into how deep transfer learning methods can be used to detect COVID-19 at an early stage.

Wang et al. [25] formulated a deep learning-based smart model for quick and accurate evaluation of COVID-19 patients. The authors examined 1065 CT images of pathogen-verified 40 COVID cases including those diagnosed recently with typical viral pneumonia. This purpose of this study is to distinguish between COVID-19 and other common viral pneumonia, both of which have similar radiologic properties. The final outcomes of this study show significant prediction accuracy (89.5%) between a normal pneumonia and COVID-19 disease.

Rahman et al. [26] developed a Naïve deep learning model to detect COVID-19 patients in early period of the infection. For this research, authors have used dataset (till March 21, 2020) obtained from data center of Johns Hopkins University for the analysis of epidemiological characteristics. Their model can predict with 90% accuracy, and there are no overfitting and underfitting problems.

Chen et al. [27] constructed a framework using deep learning for detecting COVID-19 pneumonia in the early stage using high resolution computed tomography (CT) images. To validate their model, they processed 46,096 confidential images of 106 patients, including 51 confirmed COVID-19 pneumonia at the Renmin University Hospital in Wuhan. The newly developed deep learning-based model obtained sensitivity of 100%, specificity of 92.55%, and accuracy of 95%. The final validated model performed like an expert radiologist and took less time in diagnosis.

Sethi et al. [28] presented a support vector machine (SVM)-based system for detecting COVID-19 infected patients using X-ray images. They processed X-ray images obtained from GitHub repository and used this dataset for feature extraction focused on deep learning models such as AlexNet, VGG-16, and ResNet-18. The extracted features are classified using SVM and found the best classification model using statistical analysis. Among all classification models, the ResNet-50 plus SVM is statistically superior compared to other eight models, and it gives 95.38% accuracy which is much higher than other models used.

Xu et al. [29] suggested a 3D deep learning model, which will help the doctors in early screening and identifying the COVID-19 infection from Influenza-A viral. For training and validating model, 618 CT scans images samples were obtained, out of which 222 belonged to COVID-19 infection, 221 samples of Influenza-A viral, and 175 CT samples from normal people. The obtained results show that proposed model classifies COVID-19 on chest X-ray with a notable accuracy of 86.7%.

Qi et al. [30] advised a CT radiomics model based on machine learning which helps in predicting patients stay in hospitals who are infected with pneumonia associated with COVID-19 infection. Infected patients CT images were collected from various hospitals laboratories for conducting this study. Infected patients optimal hospital stay was categorized into short period ($\leq$10 days) and long period (>10 days). The features extraction and model building were performed on lung lobe level using the radiomics model, which apply logistic regression and random forest method on the data. The findings obtained from the proposed model indicate that it is appropriate for both training and testing processes in more than 90% cases.

Sarkar et al. [31] analyzed the mortality risk of COVID-19 infected patients by applying supervised machine learning algorithms. For this research work, they used the clinical data of 1085 COVID-19 infected patients collected from Kaggle online portal. Authors have used machine learning-based random forest classification algorithm on the dataset to recognize major predictors and their influence on mortality. After the results, they come up with the conclusion that age was the most significant predictors in mortality prediction preceded by the time difference between onset of the symptom and hospitalization.

Pourhomayoun et al. [32] present a supervised machine learning-based predictive model to diagnose the health risk in early stage and to predict the mortality risk of COVID-19 patients. For their experimental purpose, they used a dataset of more than 117,000 COVID-19 patients across 76 nations. For predicting the morality rate of patients, they applied different machine learning algorithms such as support vector machine, neural networks, decision tree, random forest, logistic regression, and K-nearest neighbor (KNN). The results showed that neural network with tenfold cross-validation performed the best among others.

3 Dataset and Methodology Used

3.1 Dataset Description and Preparation

The COVID-19 dataset from machine learning repositories Kaggle and GitHub was used for this research work. The dataset contains reported cases from the 38 countries across the world out of which we randomly selected 75,000 cases with ten attributes. These selected cases belong to countries that are severely infected with COVID-19 infection, and these shortlisted cases can help in accurate prediction and analysis. The dataset is presented in Table 1.

As shown in above Table 1, we have assigned a unique **Patient ID** to each reported case to distinguish one from another. The attribute **Country** has been assigned a numeric value in the range from 1 to 38 because our dataset contains COVID-19 patients from 38 different countries. Another attribute **Location** has been given unique values in the range from 1 to 130, since our dataset consists of 130 different locations from which patients belongs. Attribute **Gender** is also categorized into two classes, where gender male has given a value 1 and for female patient's value is 0. Attribute **Age** contains value in the range from 2 to 91, which are minimum and maximum values of age present in dataset. Since there are total eight blood groups in human body, so this attribute has range from 1 to 8. **Symptoms Onset** is the date when COVID-19 symptoms firstly appeared in patient. **Diagnosed Date** represents that date when patient test report confirmed COVID-19 positive and patient admitted in hospital for further treatment. **Current Status** describes the latest state

Table 1 Features information of COVID-19 dataset

S. No.	Attributes name	Description	Range of value
1	Patient ID	This attribute represents a unique number assigned to each COVID-19 patient	1–14,000
2	Country	This attribute represents the country patient belongs to	1–38
3	Location	This attribute corresponds to the region patient admitted in such as city or village of patient	1–130
4	Gender	It represents sex of patient, i.e., male or female	0, 1
5	Age	It stands for age of the patient	2 (min) to 91 (max)
6	Blood Group	This attribute denotes blood group of the patient	1–8
7	Symptoms Onset	It shows that date when symptoms first appeared in patients	1/4/2020 to 20/7/2020
8	Diagnosed Date	This attribute represents the date when patient got hospitalized	1/4/2020 to 14/7/2020
9	Current Status	This attribute is used to represent the current status of the patient such as recovered death and hospitalized	0 for recovered 1 for Death 2 for Hospitalized
10	Status_Change_Date	This attribute denotes the date when patients change their status. Example status got changed from infected to recover, infected to death, etc.	10/4/2020 to 14/7/2020

of patient such as recovered or cured, mortality, and hospitalized. The last attribute **Status_Change_Date** denotes the date when patients change their status.

3.2 Data Preprocessing

As we know the machine learning models accuracy largely depends on the quality of data supplied to machine learning algorithm, therefore, it is extremely important to preprocess the dataset, before the final processing of the data, where dirty data is repaired or removed. As we are going to apply ensembling approach for prediction and classification, so we need to convert our dataset in a format where we can apply more than one algorithm on same dataset. Generally, unprocessed and noisy data in the real-world datasets has vital role in potential capability of the learning model as it may directly lead you toward less efficient model if we do not tackle it [33, 34]. The COVID-19 dataset used in this research work has many missing or null values that we have filled using imputation technique. The basic concept of simple imputation technique is to swap each missing value with the average of the observed values or a nominal attribute with the most observed value. For each attribute fi with missing instance values, learn a classifier $C_i(...)$ that takes the values of the other $n - 1$ attributes$\{f_j \mid j \neq i\}$ as an input and returns the value for missed instancef_i [35].

3.3 *Classification and Ensembling Approaches*

Classification is a supervised machine learning approach which is based on predicting a qualitative response by analyzing data and recognizing patterns. Data classification is a two-stage process; the first step is called the learning step, also known as training phase, in which a classification model is built by making the model learn using the training dataset available, and second is a classification phase where the model is used to evaluate the class labels for a separate unseen given dataset called the testing dataset [36]. In this research work, ensemble of individual classifiers has been used to improve the predictions of multiple classifiers (base or weak classifiers). The key concept behind the ensemble is to bring together a group of weak learners to constitute a strong learning model by consolidating their strengths, thus increasing the accuracy of the final model. To carry out this research work, we have applied three different classifiers such as random forest, Naïve Bayes, and support vector machine in conjunction with boosting and bagging ensembling approach for the analysis of COVID-19 datasets. The dataset has been divided into training and a test dataset and individual classifiers trained on training dataset. The performance of the classifier's models is tested with the test sets. The individual classifiers are explained in the next section.

3.3.1 Naïve Bayes

The Naïve Bayes (NB) machine learning classifier is an elementary and robust probabilistic classifier algorithm derived from Bayes theorem. NB is called naive because it claims that each variable is independent also known as class conditional independence [37]. The NB algorithm is often used for analyzing high-dimensional datasets. Let D be our COVID-19 dataset and each tuple in the dataset is defined with n attributes that are represented by: $X = \{a_1, a_2, \ldots, a_n)$. Let there be k classes represented by $C_1, C_2, C_3, \ldots, C_k$. For a given row X, the algorithm predicts that X belongs to that class which has the highest posterior probability. The NB classifier predicts that the tuple X belongs to the class C_i if and only if $P(C_i|X)$ it is maximum among all, i.e.,

$$P(C_i|X) > P\left(C_j|X\right) \quad \text{for} \quad 1 \leq jk,\ j \neq i \tag{1}$$

According to Bayes theorem,

$$P(C_i|X) = \frac{P(X|C_i)P(C_i)}{P(X)} \tag{2}$$

If the attribute values are conditionally independent of one another,

$$(P(X|C_i) = \prod_{k=1}^{n} P(x_k|C_i) \tag{3}$$

where x_k refers to the value of attribute A_k for tuple X. The classifier predicts the class label of X which is the class C_i if and only if

$$P(X|C_i)P(C_i) > P\left(X|C_j\right)P\left(C_j\right) \quad \text{for} \quad 1 \leq j \leq k,\ j \neq i \tag{4}$$

3.3.2 Random Forest

Random forest (RF) machine learning algorithm is also known as a tree-based ensemble learning, which creates a forest of many decision trees. RF ensures that the behaviors of each individual decision tree produced are not too correlated with the behavior of any other decision tree in the model. Since our dataset has 75,000 observations or instances and ten attributes, this algorithm will randomly pick a sample of 15,000 observations and then select five initial attributes randomly to build decision tree model. This process will continue about 5 times, and then algorithm makes a final prediction on each of the observations. This final prediction can simply be the mean of all the observed predictions. Therefore, the different decision trees obtained using RF algorithm are trained using the different parts of the training dataset, which is the reason behind its unbiased nature and superior prediction accuracy. The output of the RF is easy to understand because it resembles more closely to human decision-making processes [38, 39]. The algorithm of RF is shown below in Fig. 2.

3.3.3 Support Vector Machine

As introduced in 1979 by Vapnik and Lerner, support vector machines (SVM) are another supervised machine learning-based classification algorithm widely deals with predictive and regression analysis. The primary goal of SVM algorithm is to search a decision boundary in an N-dimensional feature space which classifies the data points uniquely while maximizing the marginal distance for both classes and minimizing the errors in classification process. For a class, the marginal distance is the distance between the decision hyperplane and its closest instance which is a part of that class. The data points closest to the decision surface (or hyperplane) are referred to as support vectors, and these points help us in constructing SVM. The

Training phase:
Step1: Consider D be a training subset of the original dataset with n instances, p attributes with target attribute.
-B: total number of target attribute classes.
-C: total number of classifiers available in tree forest
Procedure:
For c = 1 to C
Step2: Generate a testing sample $D^{*}_{t,}$ from training part by randomly selecting "k" attributes from total of "p" attributes where k<<m.
Step3: Among selected "**k**" attributes, evaluate the node "**d**" by applying the best split method.
Step4: Apply best split values divide the node into child nodes.
Step 5: Repeat steps 2 to step 4 until stopping rules encountered.
Step6: Built trained classifiers C_b
Testing Phase: Integrate the C trained classifiers by applying simple majority vote approach.
For a test instance x, the predicted class label from classifiers C_b is:
$C_B(x) = \text{argmax}_j \sum_{b=1}^{C} I(C_b(x) = j)$, for j = 1,2, … …K

Fig. 2 RF classifier algorithm

aim of SVM algorithm is to maximize the distance between all the data points and the hyperplane [40]. The loss function which allows us in maximizing the margin is given below.

$$C(x, y(f(x)) = f(x) = \begin{cases} 0, & x < 0 \\ 1 - y * f(x) & \text{else} \end{cases} \quad (5)$$

$$C(x, y(f(x)) = (1 - y * f(x))_{+} \quad (6)$$

The equation of the line in 2D space is $y = a + bx$. By renaming x with x_1 and y with x_2, the equation will change to $ax_1 - x_2 + b = 0$. If we specify $X = (x_1, x_2)$ and $w = (a, -1)$, we get

$$F(x) = w \cdot x + b \quad \text{where} \quad w, x \in R^n \quad \text{and} \quad b \in R \quad (7)$$

Equation (7) is called the equation of the hyperplane, which linearly separates the data.

The hypothesis function h in SVM classifier can be defined as follows:

$$h(x) = \begin{cases} +1 & \text{if} \quad w.x + bx \geq 0 \\ -1 & \text{if} \quad w.x + b < 0 \end{cases} \quad (8)$$

The position above or even on the hyperplane is labeled as class +1, and the position just below hyperplane is labeled as class −1. SVM classifier amounts to minimizing an expression of the form given below.

$$\left[\frac{1}{n}\sum_{i=1}^{n} Max(0, 1 - y_i(w.x_i - b))\right] \tag{9}$$

SVM is very effective in high-dimensional spaces as compared to other classifiers such as K-nearest neighbor and j48, etc. The reason to choose this classifier in this research is its robust nature due to its optimal margin gap between separating hyperplanes and gives a well-defined boundary to classify the data. It can learn efficiently in all kind of environment such as simple linear and very complex nonlinear functions using the "Kernel trick".

4 Ensembling Approaches

Ensembling techniques simulate the human social learning behaviors of seeking opinions from different familiar's persons, before making any crucial decision. Ensembles are machine learning-based computational algorithms which generate a collection of classification models and then predict different points by taking votes of predictions. This is a successful meta-classification method that integrates weak learners or base classifiers with strong learners to improve the poor learner's predictive accuracy [41, 42]. Various studies have been published, which informs us that single individual models have been improved using ensembling technique in diverse application domains, including information security [43, 44], remote sensing [45, 46], image processing [47, 48], medical diagnosis [49, 50], and bioinformatics [51].

The performance of an ensemble system relies on the data supplied to the ensemble model and the variety of the base classifiers making up the ensemble model. The most noteworthy point in the context of ensembling is that combining the diverse classifiers outcomes not always contribute in a classification results, which is assured to be superior than the best classifier in the ensemble. Comparatively, it reduces our chances of choosing a poor classifier, and we would only use best performing classifier as we have prior knowledge of it now. Few recent researches also show that growing popularity of ensemble approach among various fields is due to its capability of reducing variance and bias and enhancing the generalization capabilities of output. A diagrammatic illustration of the variance reduction potential functionality of the ensemble is shown in Fig. 3.

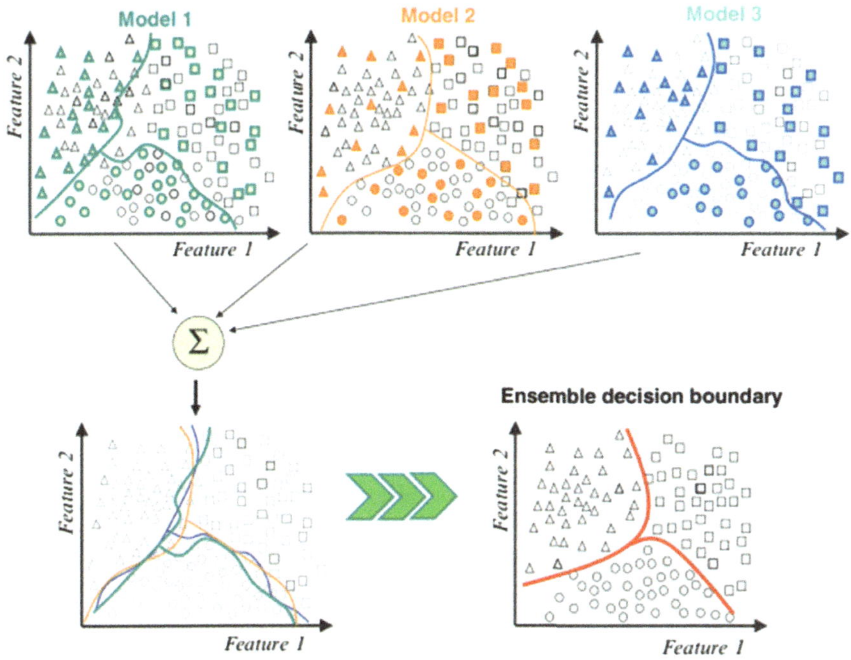

Fig. 3 Variance reduction using ensemble classifiers

4.1 Boosting

Boosting algorithm is an ensembling method that helps to improve model performance and accuracy by combining a group of weak classifiers into a strong machine learner classifier. This is an iterative technique for creating a strong classifier such that the newly generated classifier has low training error and high prediction accuracy. This iterative nature of the boosting algorithm makes it possible to focus on the instances that were incorrectly classified in previous iterative step. The model accuracy is improved by adjusting the inputs weights, which were misclassified in previous iteration [52].

In order to better understand boosting scheme, let us create a hypothesis that our first base learner model 1 is trained on a randomly selected subset of data; the second base learner model 2 is now trained on different subset of the original dataset. We assume half of data is correctly classified by model 1, and another half is incorrectly classified. The next classifier model 3 is then trained with data which were incorrectly classified by model 1 and 2, and this process is applied on each classifier. These "N" classifiers are integrated through N-way majority vote mechanism. Therefore, in this approach, the succeeding models' performance completely dependent on the previous model is demonstrated in Fig. 4.

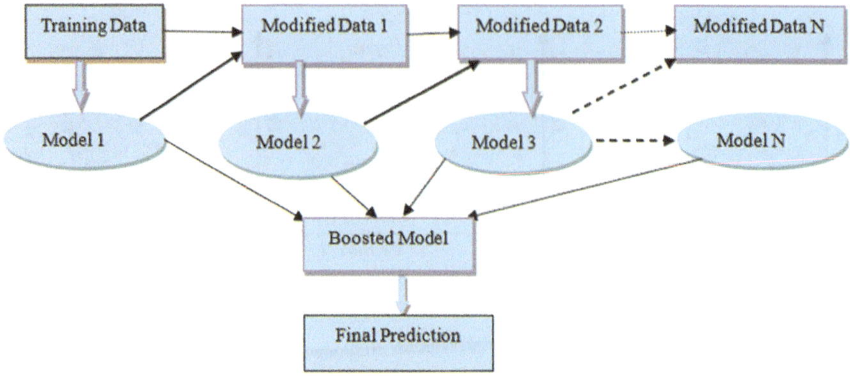

Fig. 4 Illustration of boosting scheme

Weak learner's outputs can be combined in several ways including mean rule, weighted average, product rule, or generalized mean, etc. In mathematical notation, these can be rewritten as Eq. (10) representing mean rule, Eq. (11) representing weighted average and Eq. (12) shows generalized mean rule.

$$u_c(x) = \frac{1}{T}\sum_{t=1}^{T} d_{t,c(x)} \tag{10}$$

$$u_C(x) = \frac{1}{T}\sum_{t=1}^{T} w_{t,C} d_{t,C}(x) \tag{11}$$

$$\mu_C(x) = \left(\frac{1}{T}\sum_{t=1}^{T} \left(d_{t,c}(x)\right)^{\alpha}\right)^{1/\alpha} \tag{12}$$

Here, $w_{t,c}$ is representing the weight of the tth classifier model for classifying w_c class instances. The algorithm of boosting is shown in Fig. 5.

4.2 Bagging

Bagging ensemble approach is one of the oldest yet successful ensemble-based algorithmic approaches. As its name suggests, the bagging ensembling technique constitutes of two ingredients bootstrap and aggregation. In this technique, samples are repeatedly selected from the dataset using uniform probability distribution, and each sample has same size [53]. The newly formed training dataset will have same number of instances set with a few omissions and repetitions as the original training dataset. Bagging approach helps to reduce variances in classifiers and cut down the chances

Step1: Let ={a_1,a_2,a_3, … a_n} are the given subsets of the main dataset A
Let's take E = {}, are the groups of the various Ensemble classifiers with size of each ensemble T
C = {b_1, b_2, b_3, …b_n}, are the set of weak classifiers
X = the training set which is a subset of the dataset A, i.e, X ⊂A
Y = the test set is also a part of dataset i.e, Y ⊂A
Now M = n(A)
Now Let init = 1 (pre condition)
Step2: S(init)=A randomly selected subset of X; S(init) ⊂ X
Q(0) = { }
For j =1 to M do
if j>1
s(j) = Incorrect instances of Q(j-1) + S(j)
Q(j) = Trained classifier using C(i) on S(i)
Step3: E = E ∪ C(j)
end if
next j
for j = 1 to L
R(j) = Y classified by E(j)
next j
Result = Max(R(j): j=1,2,3, …, n)

Fig. 5 Boosting ensembling algorithm

of classifier overfitting, resulting in a more generalized outcome. Figure 6 shown below illustrates the bagging scheme.

In the process of bagging, bootstrap samples are extracted from the dataset, and each classifier is trained on a specific sample. Bagging generally adopts the voting approach for aggregating the base learner outputs. Boosting notable property is that it can be applied for binary as well as multi-class classification problems. Bagging approach works exceptionally well, with unstable base classifiers, and it reduces variances through smoothing effect. The bagging algorithm is shown in Fig. 7.

5 Experiments and Results

To retrieve precise and generalized results from machine learning classifiers, a balanced dataset for both recovered and deceased patients was created. A correlative analysis of three classifiers on the COVID-19 dataset has been implemented, and their findings disclosed that some have good performance accuracy while other performance is unacceptable (poor). An ensemble of individual classifiers has been used to improve the classification performance of the weak classifier's models. To evaluate the classifier prediction performance, the main parametric measurements

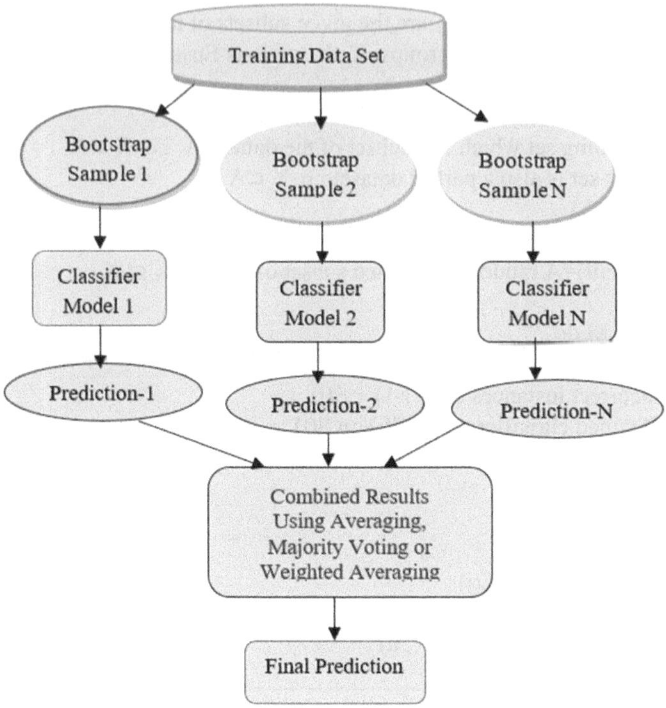

Fig. 6 Bagging ensemble process

Inputs: Training Data Set D; Base Classifier δ; T is the Number of base classifiers and percent P to generate bootstrapped training data

$D = \{(a_1,b_1), (a_2,b_2), \ldots\ldots\ldots\ldots\ldots\ldots (a_m,b_m)\}$;

Process:

For n=1………,N:

Create a bootstrap replica D_{bs}, by randomly fetching P% of dataset D

Label base classifier with D_{bs} and create a new hypothesis classifier (h_t)

$h_t = \delta(D, D_{bs})$ % D_{bs} is the bootstrap distribution end

Ensemble Union: Simple Majority Voting

Output:

$H(x) = \underset{y \in Y}{\operatorname{argmax}} \sum_{t=1}^{T} I(h(x) = y)$ % Class with the highest H(x)

Fig. 7 Bagging ensemble algorithm

used in this study are accuracy, precision, error rate, F-measure, and recall, etc. In classification problems, precision (also called positive predictive value) is the subset of correctly classified instances which are retrieved, while recall represents those relevant instances that have been fetched over total instances. Accuracy of the model can be defined as the ratio of the correctly labeled attributes to the whole pool of variables.

F-measure is weighted average of precision and recall. This work has used two ensembling techniques such as bagging and boosting. In this study, the bagging approach performs an ensemble with the RF, NB, and SVM classifiers, while for boosting AdaBoost algorithm has been used for ensemble. To train our individual classifiers, we split our COVID-19 datasets into two subsets with a train–test split of 75%/25%, respectively.

5.1 Feature Selection of Patient Attributes

Several researches have shown that irrelevant or partially relevant features can negatively impact the prediction performance of your model. Accordingly, before training our model, we have applied correlation-based feature selection process and only selected those features which contribute most in prediction variable. If there is strong correlation between two attributes, then we can derive the value of one from another attribute. One of the mostly used dependency measures is the Pearson correlation coefficient in mathematical notation which is given below.

$$\rho(X, Y) = \frac{\Sigma_i (x_i - \overline{x})(y_i - \overline{y})}{\left[\sum (x_i - \overline{x})^2 (y_i - \overline{y})^2\right]^{1/2}} \tag{13}$$

where X and Y are variables with measurements $\{x_i\}$ and $\{y_i\}$ and mean $\overline{x}$ and $\overline{y}$.

5.2 Performance of Individual Classifiers

Experiment 1 To predict the average recovery time of the COVID-19 patients, we considered only three attributes from the dataset, such as Diagnosed Date, Status_Change_Date, and Current Status, and rest of the attributes are discarded. Before experiment, some of the duplicated patient records such as hospitalization on the same day and recovered on the same day were removed. Our dataset contains 874 instances of recovered patients, and it is classified according to the number of days they remain in hospital (minimum to maximum) "7", "12", "20", "28" days, and 32 days. Figure 8 presents the class distribution which shows number of patients who hospitalized for 7 days (min) to 32 days (Max). It depicts that the number of

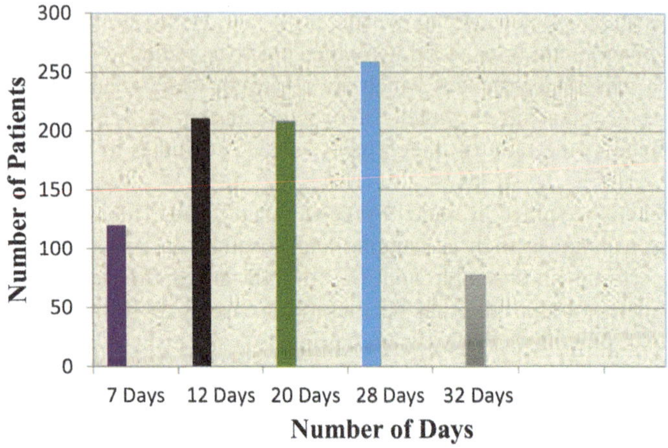

Fig. 8 Class distribution of patients stay in hospital

Table 2 Performance of individual classifiers

Classifiers	Precision	*F*-measure	Recall	MSE	Accuracy
NB	0.878	0.785	0.892	0.952	86.2
RF	0.841	0.812	0.828	0.762	83.6
SVM	0.781	0.673	0.727	0.892	77.6

patients who hospitalized for "7 days" is 120, 12 days are 210, 20 days are 208, 28 days are 259, and for 32 days are 77.

We applied NB, SVM, and RF algorithms to estimate average hospitalized period of a COVID-19 patient. In this experimental work, firstly all classifiers are trained on training dataset and then evaluated on testing dataset. Only optimal attributes were fed into the classifiers before training and testing of classifiers. The results of Table 2 clearly show that NB results in maximum accuracy among RF and SVM classifiers.

The NB classifier model exhibits accuracy of 86.2%, whereas RF and SVM classifiers show 83.6% and 77.6%, respectively. One of the important parameters in these results is mean square error (MSE), i.e., the average square difference between the outputs and expected and RF gives least resultant error. Studies show that few classifiers can work directly with noisy data, but they repeatedly lead to significant classification errors that can negatively impact the prediction performance of model. To improve the performance of these individual classifiers, we applied bagging ensemble technique. In this experiment, we have integrated bagging and feature selection to improve classification with incomplete data. Since in bagging technique, each base classifier is trained using different emulated training set constructed using resampling.

However, generally resampled datasets contain irrelevant features which need to be eliminate. To obtain maximum prediction accuracy from our trained model,

Table 3 Performance of individual classifiers with bagging

Classifiers	Precision	*F*-measure	Recall	MSE	Accuracy
NB	0.918	0.645	0.913	0.752	91.20
RF	0.832	0.743	0.863	0.862	87.30
SVM	0.807	0.671	0.782	0.723	79.30

a wrapper-based feature selection approach has been used to select suitable feature subsets for bagging. We add or delete features from the subset based on the inferences that we observed from the previous model. After the models have been trained on various subsets, final prediction is performed using averaging, majority voting, or weighted averaging.

Table 3 shown below presents that bagging technique significantly improves the accuracy along with other important parameters of RF and NB classifier but does not perform well with SVM.

After comparing the results from Tables 1 and 2, it is clearly seen that bagging approach helps in improving an accuracy of 5% in case of NB, 3.9% for RF but only 1.7% in case of SVM. Figure 9 compares the classification accuracy of individual classifiers without bagging and after applying bagging method.

After seeing the various parametric values in resultant Tables 2 and 3, it is evident that NB algorithm performs best among other two algorithms in both cases, i.e., before bagging and after bagging. NB algorithm exhibits better prediction accuracy for patients, which stayed in the hospital for longer time, i.e., 28 plus days. On the other side, the RF and SVM algorithms correctly classified 87.30% and 79.30% of the patients which stayed in the hospital from 12 to 20 days, respectively. These predicted results were compared with confusion matrix and the attributes supplied in training phase, where two attributes (Attribute 8 & 10) from our datasets were expressed in the form of mean ±SD, median. Finally, the outcome of this experiment is that average

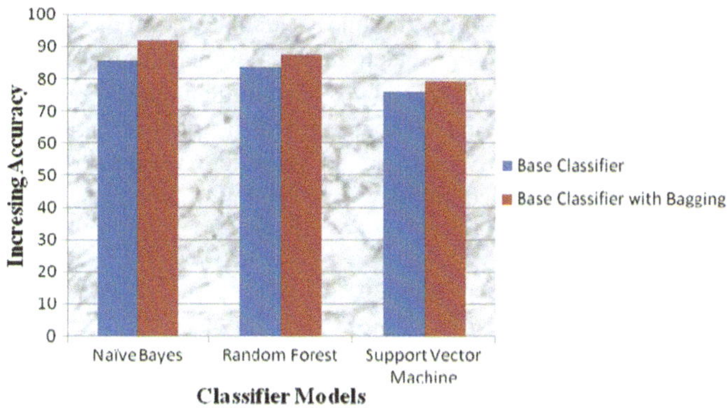

Fig. 9 Comparison of classifiers without and with bagging

hospitalized time of patients is 21 days (approx.), and NB algorithm performs best among other classifiers.

Experiment 2 In this experimental task, we aim to achieve our objective 2 and objective 3 as stated in Sect. 1. In this work, our purpose is to identify the importance of age factor associated with mortality of coronavirus infected persons and to find the mortality rate in male and female.

For better training the machine learning model, we applied feature selection technique in which our system selects an appropriate subset of features from the original features set. The feature ranking-based approach based on information gain algorithm (IG) type of filtering approach has been used in this study. To assign a score to features, an appropriate ranking criterion is used, and a threshold is used to illuminate features below the threshold value. IG analyzes individual feature in isolation, measures its gain of information, and calculates their importance against the target class attribute. Determining the information gain for a feature requires calculating the class entropy and subtracting the conditional entropies for each possible value of that feature. For statistical analysis of the attributes and results, the required attributes were expressed in the form of mean ±SD, median (interquartile range (IQR)). The differences between the two groups are analyzed using mean and percentage values between the attribute's values using paired two-tailed t test. RStudio software was used to conduct statistical analyses test (64-bit version v1.3.947-1) and $P < 0.05$ (two-tailed) considered to be statistically significant. The statistics of the recovered and confirmed death cases is shown in Table 4.

The age of deceased patients both male and female is classified into five classes to predict the age and gender which is more prone to mortality under COVID-19 disease. Figure 10 shown indicates the class distribution of number of deceased patients according to their age and gender. The percentages of older age in the range of 56 years to 75 years were much higher in the deceased group as compared to other age classes. A well-known statistical test known as Chi square (χ^2) is implemented for confirmation, which also clearly indicates that male tends to be more serious than women ($P = 0.046$) and has high mortality chances.

We applied boosting ensembling technique to calculate the predictive performance of the individual algorithms on the selected attributes, and comparative analysis is performed. Boosting ensembling method has been implemented on the dataset with both deaths and recovered patients (excluding still hospitalize patients) using the Weka machine learning software (version 3.8). Since here, we are working on limited set of data; therefore, we applied tenfold cross-validation procedure for resembling

Table 4 Death and confirmed recovery statistics

Attribute	Recovered	Death	Total	p-value
Instances	874	485	1359	
Age	62 ± 13.5	74 ± 16.3	64 ± 12	<0.0001
Gender (M)	430 (31.64)	318 (23.39)	748	0.04
Gender (F)	444 (32.67)	167 (12.29)	611	0.02

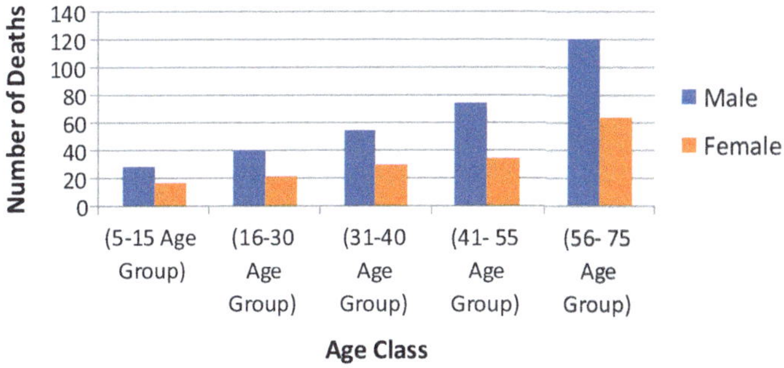

Fig. 10 Statistics relationship between age and mortality

and evaluation of our machine learning models. In this approach, the whole dataset is randomly divided into set of observations of "k" groups, or folds, of approximately same size. The first fold works as validation set, and the model is fit on the remaining $k - 1$ folds for training purposes. The prediction accuracy of the obtained models is measured by evaluating the area under the ROC curve calculated during model validation process.

The area under ROC (AUROC) on the test dataset was found to be 0.8553, which indicates that age, gender, and time difference between the onset of symptoms, and hospitalization is most critical attributes in predicting the mortality of the patient. Therefore, attributes which have high ranking values are selected and leaving remaining attributes with less ranker value using ranking-based attribute selection algorithm. In this experimental work, AdaBoost the most well-known boosting algorithm was used. AdaBoost is an implementation of ensemble methods which generate new and improved base classifiers by manipulating the training dataset iteratively. The comparison of the individual base learner with the strong learners (boosted classifiers) is shown in Table 5. The resultant table reveals that without boosting, NB algorithm performs best with predictive accuracy of 78.23%, SVM classifier comes second in race with predictive accuracy of 74.76, and RF shows accuracy

Table 5 Before and after ensembling comparison of classifiers

	Base-level classifier (before boosting)			Meta-level classifier (after boosting)		
Classifier	NB	RF	SVM	NB	RF	SVM
Accuracy	78.23	70.83	74.76	83.20	73.45	83.67
MAE	0.2834	0.254	0.2482	0.178	0.219	0.165
TP rate	0.746	0.708	0.773	0.832	0.736	0.833
FP rate	0.364	0.305	0.289	0.185	0.245	0.174
Precision	0.785	0.691	0.745	0.83.3	0.739	0.82.8
Recall	0.723	0.708	0.723	0.835	0.712	0.81.6
F-measure	0.625	0.698	0.674	0.543	0.632	0.368

of 70.83%. Ensembling NB with strong classifier models enhances the accuracy by 4.9% (Approx.). Ensembling RF with strong classifier models improves the accuracy by 2.6 and a considerable gain of 9.86% in case of SVM.

Figure 11 shown illustrates and compares the classification accuracy of individual classifiers without boosting and after applying boosting. We can easily conclude that boosting helps in improving the prediction accuracy by 9.86% (max) of SVM and 2.6% (min) for RF algorithm.

Figure 12 shown depicts the confusion matrixes obtained from various classifiers, which is a summary of prediction results on a classification problem. Figure 12a–c describes the correct and incorrect predictions given by SVM, NB, and RB classifier algorithms, respectively.

The line graph in Fig. 12d presents the outcome of this experiment, which shows age and sex-specific probability of dying due to COVID-19 disease. The graph illustrates the mortality rates for males and females at different age groups, and it shows that mortality rate in females is almost half as compared to male's during childhood stage of 5–15 years. From age group of 16 onward up to 30, the probability of dying falls gradually in both sexes. However, mortality risk again increases moderately in male and female at the age group of 30–40 years. At the age slot between 41 and 55 years, males are more susceptible and have greater risk of death as compared to females. In the last age group between 56 and 72 years old, it is found that there is a sudden increase in mortality rate in both gender, but male has almost double mortality chances as compared to females.

There is an interesting outcome of this experiment, which indicates that male's risk of dying due to COVID-19 is higher than females, at all stages of age. To examine if there is a statistical difference among the three classifiers models, we implemented Wilcoxon signed-rank test which is a nonparametric statistical hypothesis test.

To evaluate the model performance on imbalanced data and find the best among other, we have employed two statistical parameters to measure the errors between the predicted and the observed values such as mean absolute error (MAE), root mean square error (RMSE) MAE, and RMSE are statistical parameters, and it expresses the average errors of the model and measures how close your model is predicted to the eventual outcomes. Smaller their values indicate the model closely predicted the

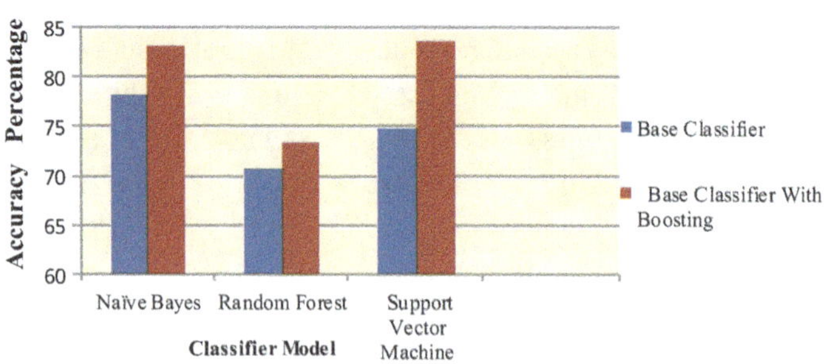

Fig. 11 Comparison of classifiers with accuracies using boosting

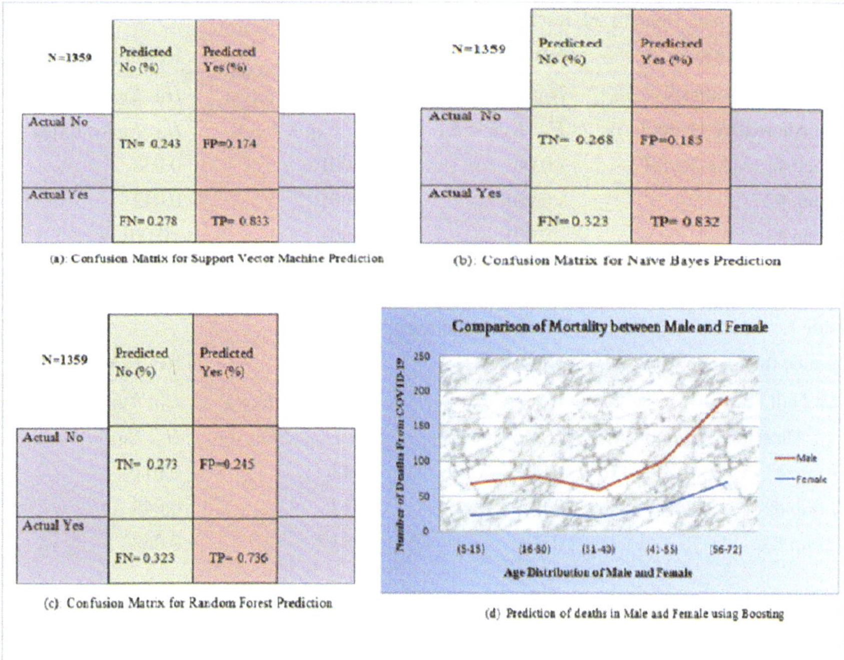

Fig. 12 Confusion matrix of different classifiers

actual values. To evaluate the models, let us suppose Y denote the observed value, and $m1$, $m2$ and $m3$ denote the predicted value of NB and RF and SVM algorithms. The RMSE and MAE of each model can be represented as follows:

$$\text{RMSE} = \sqrt{\sum (y - y2)^2}$$

$$E_1 = |Y - m1|$$

$$E_2 = |Y - m2|$$

$$E3 = |Y - m3|$$

We implemented the single-tailed hypothesis test to determine whether one model predicts more accurately than the others. Our null hypothesis (H_0) works as the two models have the same predictive error ($E1 = E2$). On the other side, alternative hypothesis (H_a) assumes that our first model has a smaller error than the second model ($E1 < E2$).

We chose a significance level of 0.05 in this Wilcoxon signed-rank test. The decision whether to reject or not our null hypothesis is dependent on the resulting p-value. If the p-value is greater than 0.05, the null hypothesis will not be rejected. If the p-value is less than 0.05, the null hypothesis will be rejected at a 95% confidence level.

Table 6 Wilcoxon signed-rank test results (on training data)

p-value (training)	NB-RF	NB-SVM	RF-SVM
H_0: Null Hypothesis	H_0: $E_{\mathrm{NB}} = E_{\mathrm{RF}}$	H_0: $E_{\mathrm{NB}} = E_{\mathrm{SVM}}$	H_0: $E_{\mathrm{RF}} = E_{\mathrm{SVM}}$
H_a: Alternative Hypothesis	H_a: $E_{\mathrm{NB}} < E_{\mathrm{RF}}$	H_a: $E_{\mathrm{NB}} < E_{\mathrm{SVM}}$	H_a: $E_{\mathrm{RF}} < E_{\mathrm{SVM}}$
Group #1 (MAE/RMSE)	<0.001	<0.001	0.038
Group #2	<0.001	<0.001	0.042
Group #3	<0.001	<0.001	<0.001

Table 7 Wilcoxon signed-rank test results (on testing data)

p-value (testing)	NB-RF	NB-SVM	RF-SVM
H_0: Null Hypothesis	H_0: $E_{\mathrm{NB}} = E_{\mathrm{RF}}$	H_0: $E_{\mathrm{NB}} = E_{\mathrm{SVM}}$	H_0: $E_{\mathrm{RF}} = E_{\mathrm{SVM}}$
H_a: Alternative Hypothesis	H_a: $E_{\mathrm{NB}} < E_{\mathrm{RF}}$	H_a: $E_{\mathrm{NB}} < E_{\mathrm{SVM}}$	H_a: $E_{\mathrm{RF}} < E_{\mathrm{SVM}}$
Group #1	0.003	0.043	0.011
Group #2	0.043	0.012	0.045
Group #3	0.02	0.083	0.062

Table 6 shows that in case of training data, the p-values between NB-RF are quite small and less than our threshold value of 0.05. Similarly, the p-values between NB-SVM are less as compared to threshold value. Hence, we can conclude that NB is a statistically better model than both RF and SVM when the classifiers models were trained on training dataset. But still the p-values of RF and SVM are not small enough to dismiss our null hypothesis.

Hence, we cannot claim if there is a statistically significant difference exists in the predictive performance of these two models. However, a statistically significant difference exists among the three models in case of test dataset. As displayed in Table 7, the p-values are all quite less than our selected threshold value of 0.05. Hence, we can dismiss our chosen null hypothesis in favor of the alternative hypothesis.

6 Conclusion

This case study analyzes the predictive accuracy of the patients infected with COVID-19 using ensemble of machine learning classifiers. One significant aspect of this research is that this is the first study comparing machine learning classifiers to predict COVID-19 patient mortality risk. The COVID-19 dataset from the Kaggle and GitHub machine learning repository was used for analysis. For the stage of data cleaning and normalization, we used imputation technique which is widely used for filling missing values in the dataset. Concurrently infected patients gender distribution was taken symmetrical in the survivors and deceased of COVID-19. We employed three classifiers labeled NB, RF, and SVM for analysis, and the ensemble techniques bagging and boosting were utilized for improving the prediction accuracy.

In this study, we identified the average duration of stay in hospital and risk factors associated with mortality of coronavirus infected patients. In the first experiment, we applied NB, RF, and SVM classifiers to predict the average hospitalized period of a COVID-19 patients, and the results of the experiment reveal that NB algorithm performed best among other classifiers. When bagging technique was used on weak classifiers, the accuracy is enhanced by a maximum of 5% in case of Naïve Bayes, 3.9% for RF but only 1.7% in case of SVM classifiers. In second experiment, we worked out to examine the role of age factor associated with mortality of coronavirus infected patients and to identify mortality rate in males and females. In this experiment, we used an ensemble of NB, RF, and SVM with boosting technique.

The results illustrate that incorporation of the boosting algorithm (AdaBoost) in ensemble with weak classifiers provides a significant prediction improvement regarding highly diverse datasets. Results reveal that boosting helps in improving the prediction accuracy by 9.86% (max) of SVM classifier. The most intriguing findings from this experiment are that, at early age, males have almost double mortality risk as compared to females, and male patients aged beyond 55 years have substantially higher chances of death due to COVID-19. The result of this experiment demonstrates that males have high chances of mortality at all stages of age as compare to females.

References

1. World Health Organization Home Page. Retrieved on July 15, 2020, from https://www.who.int/docs/default-source/coronaviruse/situation-reports/20200411-sitrep-82-covid-19.pdf?sfvrsn=74a5d15_2
2. Worlometers [Internet] COVID-19 Coronavirus Pandemic. (2020). https://www.worldometers.info/coronavirus/
3. Sarkar, J., & Chakrabarti, P. (2020). A machine learning model reveals older age and delayed hospitalization as predictors of mortality in patients with COVID-19. medRxiv the preprint server for health sciences (pp. 89–101).
4. Cascella, M., Rajnik, M., Cuomo, A., et al. (2020). Features, evaluation and treatment coronavirus (COVID-19). In StatPearls [Internet]. StatPearls Publishing.
5. Hassan, S., Sheikh, N., Jamal, S., et al. (2020). Coronavirus (COVID-19): A review of clinical features, diagnosis, and treatment. *Cureus, 12*(3).
6. Yixuan, W., Wang, Y., Chen, Y., & Qin, Q. (2020). Unique epidemiological and clinical features of the emerging 2019 novel coronavirus pneumonia (COVID-19) implicate special control measures. *Journal of medical Virology*.
7. Chen, N., Zhou, M., et al. (2020). Epidemiological and clinical characteristics of 99 cases of 2019 novel coronavirus pneumonia in Wuhan, China: A descriptive study (pp. 507–513).
8. Wenham, C., Smith, J., & Morgan, R. (2020, March). COVID-19: The gendered impacts of the outbreak. *The Lancet, 395*(10227), 846–848.
9. Jian-Min, J., Bai, P., et al. (2020, March 05). Gender differences in patients with COVID-19: Focus on severity and mortality. medRxiv The Preprint Server For Health Sciences.
10. Yi, Y., Lagniton, P., Ye, S., Li, et al. (2020). COVID-19: What has been learned and to be learned about the novel coronavirus disease. *International Journal of Biological Sciences, 16*(10), 1753–1766.

11. World Health Organization Home Page. Retrieved on July 10, 2020, from https://www.who.int/docs/default-source/coronaviruse/situation-reports/20200311-sitrep-51-covid19.pdf?sfvrsn=1ba62e57_8
12. Mao, R., & Liang, J. (2020, May). Implications of COVID-19 for patients with pre-existing digestive diseases. *The Lancet Gastroenterology & Hepatology, 5*(5), 426–428.
13. Shi, Y., Wang, Y., Shao, C., et al. (2020). COVID-19 infection: The perspectives on immune responses. *Cell Death & Differentiation.*
14. World Health Organization Home Page. Retrieved on July 18, 2020, from https://www.worldometers.info/coronavirus/coronavirus-incubation-period/.
15. Lauer, S. A., Kyra, H., et al. (2020). The incubation period of coronavirus disease 2019 (COVID-19) from publicly reported confirmed cases: Estimation and application. *Journal of Annals of Internal Medicine.*
16. Ranney, M. L., et al. (2020). Critical supply shortages—The need for ventilators and personal protective equipment during the Covid-19 pandemic. *The New England Journal of Medicine.*
17. The guardian home page. Retrieved on July 21, 2020, from https://www.theguardian.com/world/2020/apr/13/coronavirus-world-map-which-countries-have-the-most-cases-and-deaths#maincontent
18. The center for disease control and prevention home page. https://www.cdc.gov/coronavirus/2019-ncov/prevent-getting-sick/how-covid-spreads.html
19. The center for disease control and prevention home page. https://www.cdc.gov/coronavirus/2019-ncov/prevent-getting-sick/cloth-face-cover.html
20. Kucharski, A. J., Russel, T. W., et al. (2020). *Early dynamics of transmission and control of COVID-19: A mathematical modelling study*. Centre for Mathematical Modelling of Infectious Diseases, London School of Hygiene & Tropical Medicine.
21. Shereen, M., Khan, S., et al. (2020). COVID-19 infection: Origin, transmission, and characteristics of human coronaviruses. *Journal of Advanced Research, 24*, 91–98.
22. Lin., L., McCloud, R. F., et al. (2016). Tuning in and catching on? Examining the relationship between pandemic communication and awareness and knowledge of MERS in the USA. *Journal of Public Health.*
23. Yan, L., Zhang, H.-T., et al. (2020). Prediction of criticality in patients with severe Covid-19 infection using three clinical features: A machine learning-based prognostic model with clinical data in Wuhan. medRxiv preprint.
24. Narin, A., Kaya, C., & Pamuk, Z. (2020). Automatic detection of coronavirus disease (COVID-19) using x-ray images and deep convolutional neural networks (pp. 109–121).
25. Wang, S., Kang, B., et al. (2020). A deep learning algorithm using CT images to screen for Corona Virus Disease (COVID-19). medRxiv preprint.
26. Rahmana, M. S., Uddinb, M. A., et al. (2020). A study on epidemiological characteristics and ML based detection of novel COVID-19.
27. Chen, J., Wu, L., et al. (2020). Deep learning-based model for detecting 2019 novel coronavirus pneumonia on high-resolution computed tomography: A prospective study.
28. Prabira Kumar Sethy, P. B., & Behera, S. K. (2020). Detection of coronavirus disease (COVID-19) based on deep features. Preprints.
29. Xu, X., Jiang, X., et al. (2020). Deep learning system to screen coronavirus disease 2019 Pneumonia (pp. 187–199).
30. Qi, X., Jiang, Z., et al. (2020). Machine learning-based CT radiomics model for predicting hospital stay in patients with pneumonia associated with SARS-CoV-2 infection: A multicenter study. medRxiv preprint.
31. Sarkar, J., & Chakrabarti, P. (2020). A machine learning model reveals older age and delayed hospitalization as predictors of mortality in patients with COVID-19. medRxiv preprint.
32. Pourhomayoun, M., & Shakibi, M. (2020). Predicting mortality risk in patients with COVID-19 using artificial intelligence to help medical decision-making. medRxiv preprint.
33. Mathura Bai, B., Mangathayaru, N., et al. (2015). An approach to find missing values in medical datasets. In *Proceedings of the International Conference on Engineering & MIS*, Istanbul, Turkey (pp. 1–6).

34. Su, X., Greiner, R., et al. (2011). Using classifier-based nominal imputation to improve machine learning. In *Pacific-Asia Conference 2011*, May lecture notes in computer science, Shenzhen, China (Vol. 6634, pp. 124–135). Springer, Berlin, Heidelberg.
35. Madhu, G., & Rajinikanth, T. V. (2012). A novel index measure imputation algorithm for missing data values: A machine learning approach. In *2012 IEEE International Conference on Computational Intelligence and Computing Research*, Coimbatore (pp. 1–7).
36. Narayanan, U., Unnikrishnan, A., et al. (2017). A survey on various supervised classification algorithms. In *2017 International Conference on Energy, Communication, Data Analytics and Soft Computing (ICECDS)*, Chennai (pp. 2118–2124).
37. Celin, S., & Vasanth, K. (2018). ECG Signal Classification using various machine learning techniques. *Journal of Medical Systems, 42*, 241
38. Dimitriadis, S. I., & Liparas, D. (2018). How random is the random forest? Random forest algorithm on the service of structural imaging biomarkers for Alzheimer's disease: From Alzheimer's disease neuroimaging initiative (ADNI) database. *Neural Regeneration Research, 13*, 962–970.
39. Au, T. C. (2019). Random forests, decision trees, and categorical predictors: The "absent levels" problem. *Journal of Machine Learning Research, 19*, 1–30.
40. Sweilam, N. H., Tharwat, A. A., et al. (2010). Support vector machine for diagnosis cancer disease: A comparative study. *Egyptian Informatics Journal, 11*(2), 81–92.
41. Dietterich, T. G. (2000). Ensemble methods in machine learning. In *Multiple classifier systems, lecture notes in computer science* (Vol. 1857). Berlin: Springer.
42. Afolabi, L. T., Saeed, F., et al. (2018). Ensemble learning method for the prediction of new bioactive molecules. *PLoS One*, 208–220.
43. Menahem, E., Shabtai, A., et al. (2009). Improving malware detection by applying multi-inducer ensemble. *Computational Statistics and Data Analysis, 53*, 1483–1494.
44. Zhou, Y., Cheng, G., et al. (2020). Building an efficient intrusion detection system based on feature selection and ensemble classifier. *Journal of Computer Networks.*
45. Saini, R., & Ghosh, S. K. (2017). Ensemble classifiers in remote sensing: A review. In *2017 International Conference on Computing, Communication and Automation (ICCCA)* (pp. 1148–1152).
46. Adriano, B., Xia, J., et al. (2019). Multi-source data fusion based on ensemble learning for rapid building damage mapping during the 2018 Sulawesi earthquake and Tsunami in Palu, Indonesia. *Journal of Remote Sensors.*
47. Ju-Young, L., Lim, J.-W., et al. (2018). A study of image classification using HMC method applying CNN ensemble in the infrared image. *Journal of Electrical Engineering and Technology, 13*(3), 1377–1382.
48. Senthilnath, J., Varia, N., et al. (2020). Deep TEC: Deep transfer learning with ensemble classifier for road extraction from UAV imagery. *Remote Sensors.*
49. Hosni, M., Abnane, I., et al. (2019). Reviewing ensemble classification methods in breast cancer. *Computer Methods and Programs in Biomedicine, 177*, 89–112.
50. Sheibani, R., Nikookar, E., et al. (2019). An ensemble method for diagnosis of Parkinson's disease based on voice measurements. *Journal of Medical Signals and Sensors, 9*(4), 221–226.
51. Aayushi, V., & Shikha, M. (2017). A comparative study of ensemble learning methods for classification in bioinformatics. In *2017 7th International Conference on Cloud Computing, Data Science & Engineering* (pp. 155–158).
52. Zhou, Z.-H. (2012). *Ensemble methods foundations and algorithms.* CRC Press, Taylor and Francis Group.
53. Seni, G. (2010). *Ensemble methods in data mining improving accuracy through combining.* John Elder.

Role of Internet of Health Things (IoHTs) and Innovative Internet of 5G Medical Robotic Things (IIo-5GMRTs) in COVID-19 Global Health Risk Management and Logistics Planning

Ugochukwu O. Matthew, Jazuli S. Kazaure, Onyebuchi Amaonwu, Umar Abdu Adamu, Ibrahim Muhammad Hassan, Aminu Abdulahi Kazaure, and Chibueze N. Ubochi

1 Introduction

The prompt progressive development in Internet of 5G Medical robotics and Internet of Health Things (IoHTs) was propelled by some permutations in technological and Scientific Innovations in what could be general referred to as paradigm shift in extreme digital automation in Industry 4.0, the fourth industrial revolution that unveiled some set of technological dynamics that pushed the current society into digital realization. While focusing on the comprehensive technology implication of the ongoing digital society extreme automation and why the healthcare sector is at the verge of experiencing unimaginable robotization in the ongoing COVID-19 pandemic of the twenty century era of "global health uncertainty". The healthcare extraordinary modernism had gradually combined with numerous high-tech digital innovations, concentrating attention on the state-of-the-art blending with Artificial Intelligence (AI), Robotic technologies, Internet of Thing (IoTs), Internet of Medical Things (IoMTs), Internet of Health Things (IoHTs), 5G Network Technology and several others. COVID-19 health calamity had deliberately pushed the capacity for the current digital healthcare automation to accomplish the optimum

U. O. Matthew (✉) · O. Amaonwu · I. M. Hassan · A. A. Kazaure
Computer Science Department, Hussaini Adamu Federal Polytechnic, Kazaure, Nigeria
e-mail: matthew.ugochukwu@hafedpoly.edu.ng

J. S. Kazaure
Electrical Electronics Engineering Department, Hussaini Adamu Federal Polytechnic, Kazaure, Nigeria

U. A. Adamu
Polymer Technology Department, Hussaini Adamu Federal Polytechnic, Kazaure, Nigeria

C. N. Ubochi
Micheal Okpara University of Agriculture Umudike, Umudike, Nigeria

M. Niranjanamurthy et al. (eds.), *Intelligent Data Analysis for COVID-19 Pandemic*, Algorithms for Intelligent Systems, https://doi.org/10.1007/978-981-16-1574-0_2

public healthcare demand in its comprehensiveness. However, an executive order had emerged from the "White House Office of Science and Technology Policy" mandating encounter for the enterprise companies to assist the academic community, research community, science community and of course the scientific inventors to response proportionately to the extraordinary scientific enquiries surrounding COVID-19 pandemic escalation [10].

Also, Centres for Disease Control and Prevention (CDC) had acknowledged the capacity for technology and surveillance systems to have played significant roles in championing the public health rejoinder in the management of COVID-19 global pandemic [38]. Moreover, the Robotic innovations have motivated numerous treatment options and healthcare services automation that may perhaps generate extraordinary care for the under-protected patients' populace and accelerate intervals of the overall treatment. These paradigms are expected to couple in many more forms in excess transformation in the new digital e-society configuration [33]. Other more prospective model would fundamentally and uncompromisingly concentrate on the insufficiency of treatment opportunities in the bucolic United States of America and in the third world countries where infrastructural deficits are prevalent. The continuous implementation of the model involves embedding a treatment facility alongside the tele-robotic machine and allowing the junior ranked healthcare personnel to take charge of the operating room while in simulated networked environment with another senior technicians in a remote location. The approach was to enable the distinguished physicians that is occupationally engaged in another esteemed healthcare facility (hospital) to handle patients' care in another geographic location. The 5G wireless technology Internet of health Things will substantially perform fundamental functions in galvanizing the adaptation of e-healthcare into the mainstream on the premise that hard wired internetworking barely function within the remote locations.

More so, the prevalence and long devastating effects of COVID-19 pandemic had underscored the susceptibility tendency and ill-preparedness of the current digital society healthcare systems in responding to the pandemic from the global perspective. Such an extreme health condition that pushed the closure of the entire schools and business premises, offices, religious gathering, social connections and country's borders around the world, indicated the extend of predominance of COVID-19 pandemic which had highlighted the urgency for prompt development of man power capacity building and critical infrastructures such as healthcare facilities, vaccines, drone delivery logistics and internet of 5G Medical robots to respond to the infected patients, shift production lines speedily to manufacture medical consumables required to mitigate treatments for the infected individuals. On a serious note, the COVID-19 global pandemic had highlighted the necessity for development of smart autonomous agents that are not infectious susceptible to assist the consolidation of human efforts towards defeating the ongoing COVID-19 pandemic [47].

The most contemporary knowledge, powerfully supports the conception for having confidence in the wireless technology internet of health things development, in assisting the heart course for action (procedures). The 5G Internet of Medical robotics was used to establish connection to perfect 36 remote test coronary procedures [12]. In the experimental procedure, the medical robotic system was linked to a 5G network to operate a robotic arm in very remote location. Notwithstanding the fact that the robotic 5G network signals travelled a distance almost 3,000 miles away but no significant mechanical latency, or a delay between the instance when the transaction was committed and the time taken for the robot to return feedback. In a specific term, there are number of factors impeding the development of tele-robots for medical accomplishment, among which are: Multifaceted logistical components with respect to remote procedures, Internet consistency aspect, bandwidth quantum speed & latency, network reliability and security considerations have all converged to further preclude the extensive execution of tele-robotic surgeries up to the current moment [15]. The compounded hazards associated with the robotic procedures are expected to be resolved, taking into account what could possibly transpire peradventure the Internet linkage controlling the robotic signals were unexpectedly interrupted. Suppose the signal loss happened along the line of the surgical procedure, the effect could substantially harm the patient and that could be possible assuming the on-site surgical team do not possess the requisite mastery to perfect the procedure.

The current study was a conception aimed to survey the range of autonomous Internet of Health Things (IoHTs) technologies and Artificial Intelligence (AI) performances that could be produced in response to the ongoing COVID-19 global pandemic. From the look of things, the sudden manifestation of COVID-19, pushes the advancement of technological innovations those with Artificial Intelligence (AI) origin, together with robotics technologies to combat the overwhelming effects of coronavirus that is universally recognized as COVID-19 [44].

The current research aimed at addressing the applicability and implications of Internet of Health things and Internet of 5G Medical robotics in the identification and treatment of COVID-19 pandemic together with the enablement to manufacture and deliver medical consumables in the mist of global pandemic check-up. Contributions were made in the perspective of the ongoing COVID-19 to present solutions to the technical logistics, social-psychological and clinical procedures relevant to the healthcare industry in the ongoing COVID-19 and in the next global bubonic plague. Productive discussions were offered to push the current digital society into understanding of how Internet of Health Things, Internet of 5G Medical Robotics and Artificial Intelligence can be utilized in the early diagnosis and recognition of COVID-19 and support the framework for integrative smart systems innovation to lower tension on the healthcare possibility to delivery in the next global pandemics whenever it does occur.

1.1 Background of the Study

The prompt progressive development in Medical and Healthcare Robots was propelled by some permutations in technological and Scientific Innovations in what can be general referred to as extreme automation in Industry 4.0, the fourth industrial revolution. The twenty first century techno-innovation that cut across Automobiles, Mechatronics, Motors, Materials Science, Artificial Intelligence, Machine Learning, Internet of Things (IoTs), Wireless Sensor Technologies, 4G/5G Broadband Internet transmission, Cloud Infrastructures, Cyber Physical System, ICT, Enterprise Architectures and Frameworks, Software Engineering Development Paradigms and Control Systems Theories etc. The advancements in Medical Imaging (higher resolutions, magnetic resonance imaging, 3D ultrasound and Hitech supersonic body analysers) had offered opportunities for increase in surgeon and patient acceptance, recognition and approval of laparoscopic procedures, Medical and Healthcare Robotic assistance [17]. The newest utilization of Medical Robots are fashioned consistently as the initial stages of most technology-driven revolution [6]. When contrasted to the Industrial Robots, those that were invented 50 years ago to automate dangerous tasks, the current Medical and Healthcare Robots are planned for completely different operational environments and tasks for those that comprised straightforward interaction with human specialist in the surgical atmosphere and in the rehabilitation centres and those for family use.

The Business-related approaches and research interest in Medical and Health-care Robotics Internet of Things had witnessed significant growth in the current twenty first digital era of extreme automation. Tele robotics represent an area of Robotics Innovation with focus on the control of semi-autonomous Robots operating in a relative remoteness, predominantly utilizing Wireless Sensor Network (Wi-Fi, Bluetooth, the Deep Space Network) or tethered connections [35]. Healthcare Robotic rehabilitation systems are positively providing physical and occupational therapy, permitting a better innovation for treatment that are uninterruptedly adjustable to patient's Healthcare requirements. In a social context, Assistive Robotic (SAR) systems are currently in operation for in-clinic and in-home use in a physically, cognitive and social exercisable coaching and monitoring [28]. The recent Technological improvements in Medical and Healthcare Robotics Internet of Things have the irreversible capacity to inspire development of new treatments for a comprehensive diseases, health challenges, disorders and improve both the standard and accessibility of patients' Healthcare outcomes. The innovative achievements of Medical and Healthcare Robotics needed to improve human healthcare condition and general well-being. As the demand for Medical Healthcare services intensifies worldwide in anticipation for global relief and opportunities to overcome COVID-19 challenges, Medical automation and Healthcare Robotics design, development and manufacturing will focus on assistive healthcare, surgical, medical and other next-generation technologies for opportunities for preparedness, emergency response, healthcare risk management and recovery strategies. Healthcare Robotics Engineering paradigm will focus on design, development, technical professionalism, Healthcare system market, hardware and software services and best standard practices in respect to healthcare applications.

The current issues on the Medical and Healthcare Robotics will provide insights, analysis and experiences in the following consideration: (i) Enabling Technologies

(ii) Tools and Platforms (iii) Design and Development (iv) Management and Opportunity. It is an expectation that future investments in Medical and Healthcare Robotics Internet of Things will continue to grow and engineers, clinicians, academics and commercial requirements must collaborate to address every miscellaneous Industrial and Global demands whenever it arises just as it is presently with the COVID-19 global pandemic.

1.2 Aims and Objective of the Study

The Internet of Health Things (IoHTs) and Innovative Internet of 5G Medical Robotic Things (IIo-5GMRTs) implementation will influence the activities of the ongoing healthcare logistics expenditures and enhances the performances of the treatment outcomes, diagnosis of the COVID-19 infected patients and the twenty century digital extreme healthcare automation in Industry 4.0. For that reason, this current research was focussed on the complete applications of the well-known Internet of Things (IoTs), Internet of Health Things (IoHTs) and Innovative Internet of 5G Medical Robotics Things (IIo-5GMRTs) philosophy through expansion of the technology automation available to wrestle the ongoing COVID-19 pandemic. The noteworthy applications of IoTs were acknowledged and deliberated extensively in the context of the ongoing digital e-society reconfiguration in response to the overwhelming effects stemming from the COVID-19 global pandemic. The COVID-19 had eventually obligated the researcher's community, academicians and scientists club to propose some measures for overcoming the worrisome effects from the recent pandemic.

Apart from hospital consultations, remote monitoring of patients had assisted in reducing workload on the healthcare professionals, by stopping unnecessary hospital physical consultations and allowing medical attendant's hours absolutely redirected towards the main patient who are seriously in need of attention. Through the adoption of the Internet of Health Things (IoHTs), Internet of Things (IoTs), Innovative Internet of 5G Medical Robotic Things (IIo-5GMRTs), susceptible patients can have their electronic information assembled utilizing uninterruptedly operational wearable body sensors anywhere they may be located. The research aims and objectives were to address emergent subject matters in the broad categories but not constrained to:

i. Smart Robotics in the scientific analysis (diagnosis) of COVID-19 pandemic
ii. Smart thermometry robotics systems for automatic temperature reading
iii. Intelligent autonomous Robotics in COVID-19 sample collection and intelligence gathering to necessitate healthcare response
iv. Intelligent Robotic Innovations for Disease Prevention and Control
v. Smart Robotics technologies for the Hospital Acquired Infectious Control, Sanitisation and Decontamination of viral hot-spots in the period of COVID-19

vi. Innovative Robotic technologies and Rehabilitative robots for nursing purposes
vii. Self-driven Drones conveyance and delivery logistics for medical consumable goods in the period of COVID-19.
viii. Smart Robotic systems for precipitous society reconfiguration and adaptable manufacturing product lines and supply logistics of essential medical vaccines and healthcare product manufacturing and supply chains.

2 Literature Review

Hospital acquired infections (HAIs) constitute one of the biggest health crises, yet a disregarded occupational disturbances in the United States of America [5], and among the healthcare workers around the world. The hospital acquired infections are among the main public health concerns throughout the world, contributing to an increased morbidity, mortality and health expenditures on yearly basis. Hospitals are the foremost sources for the risk of acquiring infection during healthcare delivery. There is little evidence concerning the burden of unsafe care in developing countries, where the risk of harm to patients is likely to be greater, due to low infrastructure, technologies, and human resources. There exist quite number of researches that specifically indicated that significant number of inpatients acquire infections in the hospital premises in the ongoing COVID-19 global pandemic. However, there is limited information which specifically indicated the magnitude, barriers and factors for prevention and control practice for the hospital acquired infections in teaching hospitals [51].

Currently, the Centres for Disease Control and Prevention (CDC) made some specific announcement that healthcare's fight against HAIs had charted some mild improvement but the reality is that in the United States, nearly 100,000 people still die each year from HAIs, i.e. infections acquired in the hospital or healthcare facility that is uncommon to whatever health issues that brought the patient to the hospital in the first instance [37]. Several number of those healthcare or medical oversights are clinically avoidable. Moreover, hospital acquired infections had added in excess of $4.5 billion in superfluous health management expenditures on annual basis across the globe [21]. On this note, the American government had acted in response to the financial leakages through adjustment of healthcare performance information to ensure reasonable exploitation in containing healthcare avoidable risk [37]. The Centre for Disease Control estimated about 99,000 annual deaths arising from health acquired infections are attributable to reasonable number of people dying per day in the United States due to infections they acquired while in the premises of the healthcare facility or hospital [4]. However, as long as human beings are involved in the delivery of healthcare services, infection will always be a risk. The best approach for reducing infections in the clinical routines depend on the technologies that make each processes clean, consistent, dependable and highly automated [36].

Hospital acquired infection is part and parcel of measurement of health impact for quality of healthcare performance in the United State of America hospitals where 7 million infections take place during which patients are treated for unrelated illnesses that brought them to the hospital in 2018 [20]. All through the period of the ongoing COVID-19 global pandemic, clinicians, healthcare workers and physicians have applied preventive approaches as panacea to hospital acquired infection diligently [23]. Numerous healthcare centres (hospitals and clinics) in the United States of America have already taken measures and implemented quite a number of approaches based on their individual defensive measures in responding to the current COVID-19 pandemic even before the United States America Centres for Disease Control and Prevention (CDC) proposed measures for public safety. Notwithstanding the extra preventive procedures adopted, healthcare employees those on the front line service delivery have been inexplicably overwhelmed by COVID-19 infection, where 9282 health workers have been reported of contacting COVID-19 with consequential death of 27 health workers and 55% of the victims affirming that they were infected while on active duty according to the report available with CDC on April 9, 2020 [13]. The Intermediations to slow down the initial escalation of the COVID-19 were not sufficiently successful which developed into a death proportion in excess of 5.8% measuring in a certain populaces when contrasted with the 0.5% death rising for periodic flu in the United States of America at different times [23]. This occurrence is of interest which is why new conventions, anticipatory modus operandi and early preclusion is essentially needed to be implemented for future global bubonic plague [40].

The ongoing COVID-19 pandemic not only affected the frontline healthcare workforces on the global business of healthcare service delivery, it equally intensified the possibilities for exposure to their family members who are at risk of being infected. Corresponding to the earliest 262 cases in Beijing the capital city of China, 50.8% COVID-19 reported cases have to do with family clusters [48]. On the account of this, countless healthcare benefactors chose to quarantine themselves, where they live in isolation from their families and relatives after work, they stayed secluded in the garage or hiring a hotel apartment to evade circulating the COVID-19 virus from the hospital location.

On the other hand, the after-effects of those defensive procedures and physical distancing guidelines, naturally posed detrimental consequences on the mental health and psychological assiduity of several people. Moreover, during the last week of April 2020, report had it that two healthcare workers committed suicide, with other results traceable to mental health matters, together with apprehension, nervousness, depression and post-traumatic stress disorder intensifying progressively [50]. The global world are preparing a transition into another period of little by little reviving of the economy throughout the geographical divide. This will required total adjustment, strict compliance to the standard health safety precautions amidst COVID-19 pandemic prevalence to avoid reinfection. However, fundamental questions and careful enquiries ought to be admitted and approved:

(i) Does wearing of clinical masks meant for all the healthcare workforce and patients in all the healthcare premises be essential pending when consumable vaccine and precise diagnostic treatments are developed and made public?
(ii) Does the ongoing comprehensive and worldwide mask wearing policy transcend to the normative societal norms? All the recommended and approved procedural code of behaviour may prove advantageous taking into account of the global pandemic to put a stop to the scourge of hospital acquired infections.

The concept that had lead us into something very dramatic is the sole domain of science fiction: the Robotization of healthcare services specifically the automation of disinfection of the hospital rooms where many Health Acquired Infections occur. The Ultra Violet (UV) Robot was developed by Blue Ocean Robotics with the objective of developing new innovative solutions to lower Hospital Acquired Infections [8]. According to Chuck Dunn, the Chief Executive Officer of Memphis-based Tru-D Smart Ultraviolet C, (UVC) Robotics, he concluded that only 50% of all pathogens are effectively removed from room surfaces in a typical hospital environment by traditional human cleaning [19]. Although, it's a necessary step to be taken, but there is no way a hospital can rely solely on traditional cleaning methods to disinfect its operating environments and healthcare facilities. We definitely need something more, the Ultraviolet C disinfection Robots are needed to flood hospital spaces with a pathogen-killing ultraviolet light that is capable of killing up to 99.9% of all infectious microbes potentially lurking in the shadows of the Hospital operating rooms. Chuck Dunn was careful to point out clearly that his Tru-D product, which has undergone successful Clinical Trials at Duke University Hospital Durham, North Carolina and is now in over 300 hospitals across the country. The Tru-D product is very significant in reducing germs and pathogens in any given room, but if doctors and nurses forget to wash their hands, it's all for naught [14]. Health professionals are all human beings and not prone to replicating perfectly performed operations always, standard disinfection processes is ideal within the Healthcare facilities. Human error is a major factor in manual room disinfection, which is why Health Acquired Infections have proven to be such a major challenge to the hospital administrators [29].

The Danish company Blue Ocean Robotics is taking the fight against Hospital Infectious Disease to the next higher level. The company's UV Robot was developed in partnership with Danish State Healthcare Authorities as a solution for combating Hospital Acquired Infections. The Company Chief Executive per Juul Nielsen, described his pathogen-killing machine as "Roomba meets Rambo in the fight against hospital microbes". The "Waterborne bacterial pathogens in wastewater remains an important public health concern, not only because of the environmental damages, morbidity and mortality that they cause, but also due to the high cost of disinfecting wastewater by using physical and chemical methods in treatment plants. Bacteriophages are proposed as bacterial pathogen indicators and as an alternative biological method for wastewater treatment. Phage biocontrol in large scale treatment requires adaptive and aggressive phages that are able to overcome the environmental forces that interfere with phage–host interactions while targeting unwanted bacterial pathogens and preventing biofilms and foaming" [25]. The company's autonomous Robot is completely Mobile and equipped with a highly efficient UVC light disinfecting system.

However, all of this innovation and high-end tech is promising and potentially intriguing but the great task is for the consumers to strife and avoid exposure to hospital pathogens and reduce the chances of acquiring a healthcare-induced infection. About one in 31 people will get what is called a Hospital or Healthcare Acquired Infection (HAI), according to the U.S. Centres for Disease Control (CDC) [2]. The coronavirus reportedly can hibernate on some surfaces for up to 72 h [31]. On this account, a number of companies offer a variation on the Ultra Violet disinfection Robot model for the COVID-19 purposes. For example, a medical device company called Skytron that has been around since 1972 produced a line of UV Light Disinfection Robots that look like a bunch of light tubes vertically on a wheeled cart, refer to Fig. 1. The instrument can adjust UV dosage based on variables such as room size, layout, furnishings, and environmental characteristics. A user controls the device with a wireless handheld controller with perception of ubiquitous computing expeditions. The tech-innovation was originally developed by a company called Infection Prevention Technologies, which sold its assets and patents to the private Michigan medical company in 2017.

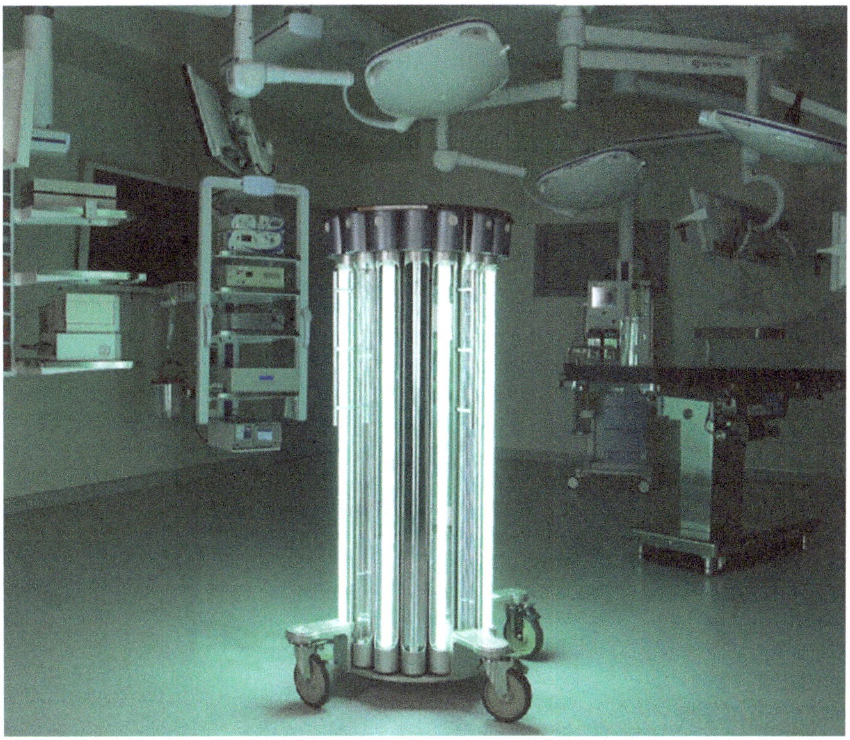

Fig. 1 Skytron UVC disinfection robot for COVID-19

Through contribution of the furthermost all-encompassing preference UVC in the consumer marketplace, Skytron had taken a lead for ideal UVC explanation in healthcare adoption that fit into the demand of any hospital in ongoing COVID-19 global pandemic, maintaining extended term durable facilities for improving diseases infectivity control techniques. In addition to the availability of four different models of UVC, Skytron satisfies all consumers' expectation in product acceptability and budget for the automation of hospital disinfection routine process. By means of applicable single cycle whole-room specific decontamination, Skytron UV dispenses extra formidability and productivity, guaranteeing comprehensive disinfection and augmented human resources workflow throughput.

3 Research Design and Implementation

Internet of Things (IoTs) generally offers substantial healthcare benefits and had turn out to become an irresistible innovative technology for the twenty first century industry 4.0 extreme digital healthcare automation and in the ongoing COVID-19 global pandemic. While the numbers of chronic diseases including COVID-19 pandemic are on the increase, IoTs had of recent found relevance and established dominance in the healthcare sector, empowering several healthcare service innovations such as Augmented Reality (AR), Virtual Reality Environment (VRE), Telemedicine, Spatial Computing, connected imaging, medication management, inpatient monitoring, connected health grid, networked healthcare workforce, digitally connected ambulance services and alongside several other healthcare innovations, refer to Fig. 2. The ongoing COVID-19 had unveiled set of computational

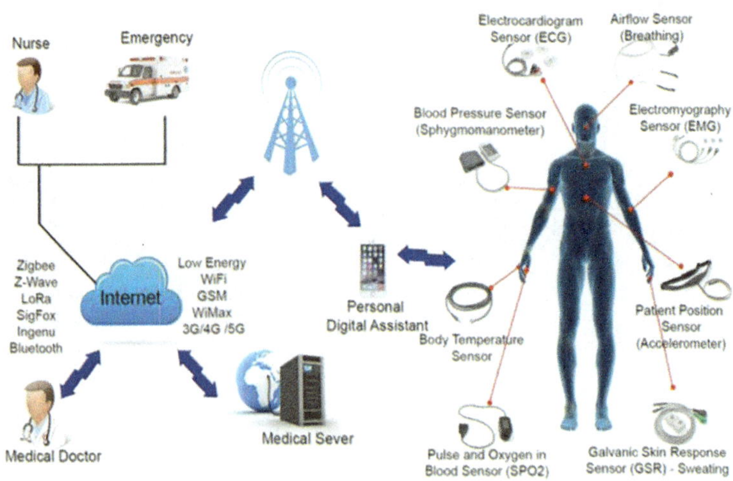

Fig. 2 5G wearable body sensors device for healthcare computing [34]

dynamics in IoTs healthcare exploration, empowering the suppliers to hurriedly perform explanations for preventing the increasing scourges and offer defence against the COVID-19 virus pandemic viral spread. The obstructive interferences of the COVID-19 pandemic have impacted adversely the whole healthcare service sectors from routine healthcare services to pharmaceutics, to COVID-19 vaccine developers, to healthcare insurance vendors and the entire hospitals management. The wide scale adoption of internet based healthcare applications such as telemedicine, augmented reality environments, remote patient monitoring, mobile medicine computing, alongside inpatient monitoring, are projected to expand considerably in the ongoing global pandemic.

Whereas COVID-19 evolution had turned into the hotspot medical research inquisitiveness, drawing attention in all aspect of medical and clinical profession with a view to finding solution to the current global scourge [11]. The emerging healthcare technology innovations will metamorphose into universal remedy for the ongoing world-wide health crisis and in the next pandemic. Internet of Things (IoTs) and more specifically the Internet of Medical Things (IoMTs) will offer a leverages to the challenges of discovery, monitoring, contact tracing and control of the ongoing COVID-19 pandemic [49]. The Internet of Medical Things (IoMTs) apply to series of internetworks of medical paraphernalia, hardware, software applications, lifeware and data peculiar to the healthcare industry. The Smartest healthcare monitoring grid is the essential aspect of the emerging IoTs application which became an applicable fit in the ongoing COVID-19 pandemic [30]. However, the Covid-19 Internet of Medical Things (CIoMTs) became a special study area of Covid-19 Internet of Things (CIoTs), meanwhile Covid-19 Internet of Things (CIoTs) was originally the extension of conventional Internet of Things (IoTs) with illustrative symbolism shown in Fig. 2. Basically, Internet of Things (IoTs) is a functionally defined technology system with set of interconnectedness and coordinated computing paradigm, having digital and electromechanical device components with natural empowerment for data transmission over a defined network carriage with no human intermediations [46]. Every Internet of Things device are naturally linked with the set of distinctive identification number to create an opportunity for self-identification within the global internetworked ecosystem. Therefore, the Internet of Things (IoTs) had become a well-established and proven technological innovation with several computational dynamics for instantaneous and ubiquitous analytics, machine learning philosophy and body sensory transmission empowerments [18].

In addition, IoTs had emerged into a functionally recognised utility grid for products or appliances serving the real-life requirements for service invention and performance upgrades which had necessitated an improved life expectancy and current industry 4.0 extreme digital automation in the healthcare management. Above all, the social aspect of human beings have also being impacted in several other ways such as; smart city configuration, IoTs wearable body sensors, security systems of the Office and home, smart switchable lighting arrangements and countless other appliances which is readily managed from side to side in our daily routines using smart speakers, body scanners, smartphones and Personal digital assistance (PDAs).

The COVID-19 pandemic will inspire IoTs technology implementation that will develop more and more in scope to optimally lower the healthcare cost and fundamentally advanced treatment options available for the infectious overwhelmed patients in the healthcare facilities. As a matter of facts, the current research is endeavoured to investigate, deliberate and underline the general applications of the intensifying IoTs philosophy in the perspective of its wide scale adoption in confronting the ongoing COVID-19 global pandemic.

Ultimately, several meaningful applications of IoTs were identified and extensively deliberated upon. The demand for IoTs innovative contributions had eventually compelled the researcher's community, academicians around the world and scientists to recommend several dynamic solutions to overwhelm the COVID-19 pandemic and return the global community to stability. In the ongoing COVID-19 pandemic circumstances, the entire countries of the world, including Nigeria, are struggling with COVID-19 while still expecting some clinically and cost-effective approaches to tackle the over stemming effects, arising from the current global pandemic. The Researchers around the world especially those from physical sciences, medical and engineering technology are mobilizing efforts to grow new theories and novel research findings to produce evidence based clinical and scientific explanations capable of paving ways for defeating COVID 19. However, the current research was intended to offer explanations on the number of innovative technologies of IoTs, IoMTs, IIo-5GMR and its substantial benefits for COVID-19 pandemic risk management.

i. **To Track Quarantine exigencies**

   Among the several decisive steps taken to control the spread of COVID-19 pandemic is the operational quarantine services for the infected or perceived to be infected persons. The adoption of IoTs and GPS empowered apps to track and when required constrict such individual passages. Numerous countries such as Poland, Hong Kong, Russia, Singapore, Germany, and South Korea are among the few countries that adopted the approach to curtail the viral spread of the COVID-19 pandemic among the general public. Country like Hong Kong kick off its quarantine operation right from the landing field of every airports within the country especially the international airports where the risk could be high. Every incoming travellers were assigned with a wrist-bands alongside a unique QR to track their way about. The travellers will download the app identified as "Stay Home Safe" into their personal Smartphones and usually scanned with the QR. While at home, the traveller had the responsibility to march all over the apartment areas to calibrate the device for virtual perimeter configuration by means of GPS, RFID, Wi-Fi, Bluetooth signal and cellular network.

ii. **The 5G Edge Body Screening and Temperature Monitoring**

   To such an extent of containing the sudden escalation of COVID-19, Beijing used 5G Patrol Robots manufactured by Guangzhou Gosuncn Robot Co., Ltd which utilized hi-tech innovative configuration to supervise face/nose mask wearing and to regulate internal body temperatures in the in the public domain, refer to Fig. 3.

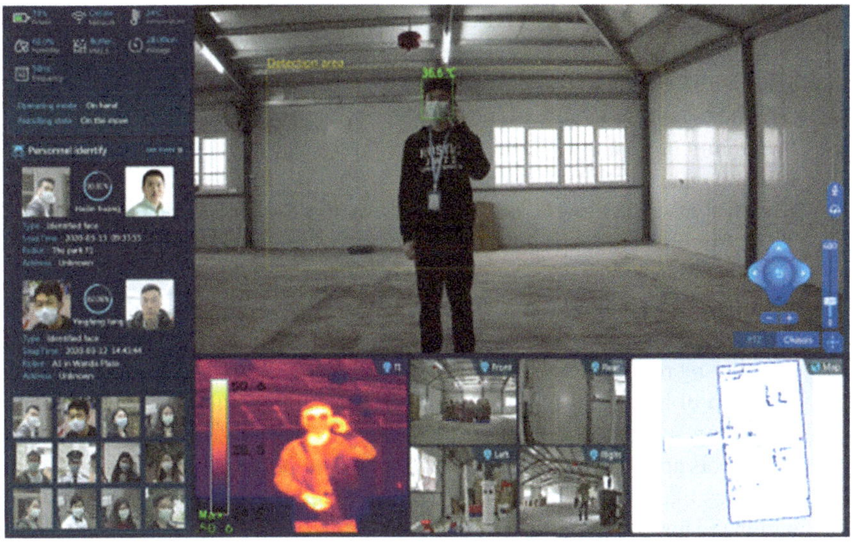

Fig. 3 5G edge smart city robot to detect COVID-19 body temperature [24]

In the wake of the outburst of COVID-19, providers of smart city Internet of Things (IoTs) manufactured goods and essential services, Guangzhou Gosuncn Robot Co modernized its 5G powered Police Patrol Robot with innovative fitness to support the frontlines law enforcement agencies on the regular duty of handling disease preclusion assessments. The direct physical reading of body temperatures will unmasks the healthcare workers to the possibility of health risks (contacting the COVID-19), but those Robots are powerfully adapted with 5G High-Resolution Cameras and Infrared Thermometers to accomplish body temperature scanning of 10 individuals instantaneously within a radius of 5 m away from each other. When the body high temperature or individual not putting on face mask is detected, the robots will deliver a signal to the appropriate agencies of the government for immediate action. Even though, those Robots are autonomous self-controllable and self-driving machines, they are equally controllable remotely, thereby saving manpower by decreasing traversing obligations and precluding the high risk and possibilities of cross infection. Not surprisingly, there are several other next-generation 5G Patrol Robots already adopted in the foremost airports and shopping malls in the urban areas of Guangzhou, Shanghai, Xi'an, and Guiyang for COVID-19 case analysis. The Chinese 5G Patrol Robots was integrated with Internet of Things, Artificial Intelligence, Cloud Computing and Big Data Technologies to conduct environmental sensing, dynamic decision-making, autonomous motion control, as well as behavioural sensing and interaction. To enable such advanced computing, 5G Patrol Robots are powered by a High-Performance Industrial Edge Computer (MIC-770) from Advantech, equipped with an 8th gen Intel Corei Processor and GPU iModule (MIC-75G20) aimed at Internet of Things Applications. The industrial-grade edge computer combined with MIC-75G20 GPU iModule provided a high-performance system for Artificial Intelligence training and inference. The device is ruggedized chassis and cast aluminium heatsink protected against vibration and shock, the passive thermal solution ensures silent operation.

iii. **Hospital Disinfection, Cleaning and Sensitization of Medical facilities**
The hospital disinfection, cleaning and sanitization are very important looking at the contagious nature of COVID-19 pandemic and the possibility of several other hospital acquired infections within the medical facilities and the isolation centres. The adoption of UVD and Xenex disinfection robotic machines, a self-driving robots that disinfect the surfaces and the medical facilities through emission of high-intensity ultraviolet light radiation, which destroys the virus by ripping separately their DNA.
The robots are 5G Wi-Fi enabled that can be manipulated through apps. Several countries like Italy, USA and China adopted and implemented the technology within the hospital facilities to combat COVID-19 pandemic and other hospital inquired infections.

iv. **Innovative Uses of Medical Unmanned Aerial Vehicles (Drones)**
Unequivocally, the adoption of Health Information Communication Technology (HICT) which implies the automation of information computation and data management processes that are facilitated by computer hardware system, software components and lifeware mechanism to handle the transactions that deal with sharing, storage, retrieval, indexing, filing and use of healthcare information, Medicare electronic records, health data and interpretation of communication procedures for an informed business decision within the healthcare management system [22]. Without doubt, the HICT had championed the contemporary digital society Healthcare extreme automation in the 4th industrial revolution regarded as industry 4.0. For the avoidance of doubt, Healthcare extraordinary mechanization or simply computerization is the combination of numerous scientific methodologies that concentrated on the inventive synchronization and interworking of Artificial Intelligence (AI), Robotic technologies, Unmanned aerial vehicles technologies, Internet of Thing (IoTs), Internet of Medical Things (IoMTs), cyber-physical systems, enterprise software engineering development paradigm and several others. The Internet of Things Drones are used to deliver Healthcare indispensable consumables being monitored from the Logistics control centres to the terminus where they are needed without interval delay. The adoption of unmanned aerial vehicle (Drones) for medical consumables delivery such as birth control items, transplantable kidney organs, blood, snake bite, vaccines, serum and other medical essentials to and from bucolic areas and having the potential to contacting patients who have need for instantaneous medical attention with in minutes which in some cases could mean the difference between life and death. The Unmanned Aerial Vehicles (Drones) use for commercial purposes has gotten much attention in the recent time due to Amazon announcing and successfully testing the use of

drones to deliver packages to customers. Such development characterized a complex and highly intriguing transformative innovation with several premeditated and unintentional development for the digital natives. The current and future utilization of drones in Healthcare delivery across nations are also highly thought provoking [42]. While the social-distancing and lock down across the countries boarders prevails, the transformations in the normal unmanned aerial vehicles (drones) have found some systematic upgrades and innovative adjustment in the ongoing COVID-19:

a. Drones were used to monitor and enforce the stay at home orders in several countries across the globe like China and Spain.
b. Drones were used in disinfecting the exceedingly infected hotspot of Wuhan province.
c. Drones were used in flying medical items and quarantine supplies in Xinchang, China in the ongoing COVID-19 during the initial lock down.
d. Drones were used in checking the temperatures of those in quarantine and isolation centres through infrared thermometers mounted on the unmanned aerial vehicle (drones) as the patients may stand at distance.

v. **Reduction in hospital acquired infection and in home infections**
The increase in awareness between people, prohibiting them from touching susceptible exteriors such as light switches, doorknobs, rail etc., was to avoid arbitrary spreading of the COVID-19 through surface contact. The IoTs technology was hurriedly adapted and configured to enable security systems, smart speakers, lights, etc. to open doors and switch on lights when it is necessary. In fact, this person recently used his smart security system to request the delivery guy to leave the package inside his house while he unlocked the door from his phone.

3.1 Research Analysis

The Research on Internet Of Things (IoTs) Drone Services for Advanced Disaster Management was implemented and tested on number of Healthcare computing assignments and situation and result proved liable and efficient especially in the countries of Africa, hence the need to communicate the findings to the academic communities, the countries policy makers, Public Healthcare Administrators, Private Healthcare Investor and all stakeholders responsible for current society healthcare extreme automation. The ongoing trend of Healthcare system automation through centralization and adaptation of the supply chain to ensure fastness, flexibility and consistent deliveries of medical consumables within healthcare facilities in the 5 regions of the selected case study. However, Logistics automation in healthcare service delivery are exceptionally impacted by the significance of demand for patient safety through maintenance of standard protocol [26]. On the merit of cost-effectiveness compared to land transportations in the urban areas, Unmanned Aerial Vehicles (UAVs) are

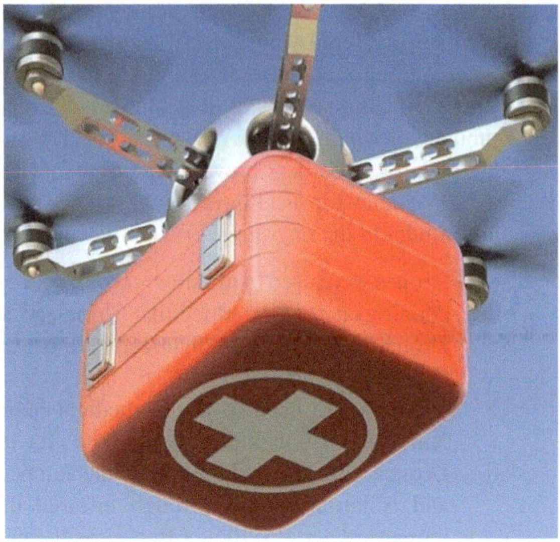

Fig. 4 The age of drones: what might it mean for health delivery of medicare items using drone [41]

more prominent means of delivery. The current research combined more appropriately findings from automated Healthcare delivery system and Logistics & Supply Chain from patient safety assessment and compared the benefits of UAVs-based delivery of medical consumables to improve current society extreme automation with respect Healthcare System Automation in Industry 4.0 era.

Zipline medical Drones innovations are at the center of the medical deliveries and logistics management in Rwanda. Zipline company operates two supply centers in Rwanda [1], and began deliveries in Muhanga in late 2016 [39], refer to Fig. 4. Rwanda has several hilly geographic formation and pitiable motorway situations compelling an Unmanned Aerial Vehicles delivery system to be more cost-effective and economize able. The expenditure of conveyance via UAVs was investigated and found comparably standard approach far better than land transportation specifically in the circumstances of disasters and emergency operations. This is on the account of pitiable public transport situations in Rwanda not minding that Rwanda is tightly inhabited with a diminutive landmass [27].

By September 2019, Zipline had completed 20,000 blood distributions and take flight beyond 1,000,000 km (620,000 mi) while in May 2019, not less than 65% of blood distributions in Rwanda separate from the capital city Kigali utilized Zipline drones to accomplish milestones [7]. Rwanda has 5 regions which include, Kigali City with total of 8 Healthcare centers (including Military Hospital and Police Hospital), Eastern region with the total of 9 healthcare centers, Western region has 12 healthcare centers, Northern region has the total of 7 healthcare centers, Southern region has the total of 12 healthcare centers, making a total of 48 healthcare centers for 12.3 million Rwandans according to record as at 2018 (Tables 1 and 2).

Zipline presently transports blood, vaccines, and test kits, medical consumables to Rwandan hospitals utilizing Unmanned Aerial Vehicles (UAVs) drones from the

Table 1 Zip line medical distribution centers in Rwanda

Location	Country	Year opened	Delivery centre
Muhanga	Rwanda	2016	Located in the center district of the country
Kayonza	Rwanda	2018	Located in the eastern district of the country

Table 2 Zipline distribution arrangement to the Rwandan 5 regional healthcare centres

Route	Distance (kilometers)	Road transport time	UAVs (drone) delivery time (min)	Time variation (min)
Zip line Muhanga District to Kigali City	53.1	3 h	6	174
Zip line Muhanga District to Southern Region	40	3 h	15	165
Zip line Muhanga District to Western Region	100.1	3 h, 30 min	25	185
Zip line Kayonza District to Eastern Region	71.4	2 h, 45 min	20	145
Zip line Kayonza District to Northern Region	163.0	4 h	40	200

company's Logistics bases in Muhanga and Kayonza districts of Rwanda. Ever since December 2016, Zipline an American conglomerated medical service distribution corporation headquartered in South San Francisco, California that invents, assembles and managed Drone aircraft operation in Africa and other part of the world had transmitted above 4000 units of blood commodities to 12 hospitals in the 5 regions of Rwanda province otherwise could have travelled several hours on transit before getting to the required hospital.

The Rwandan Government enthusiasm to collaborate with the technology professionals from the Public–private healthcare sector initiative had driven the accomplishment in incorporating extreme automation into the country healthcare system with an incredible returns on the investment. The Technology itself does not advance health equity; rather the Rwandan Government insistence on its objectiveness to put together technology and people that furthers advanced opportunities for accessing the high-tech digital automated services within the mainstream healthcare system. Such approach had driven achievement in utilizing technological modernisms to accomplish comprehensive, cost-effective and evenhanded healthcare coverage for the Rwandan citizens. Moreover, the Unmanned Aerial Vehicles (Drones) involvement into the society healthcare extreme automation, characterized a step in a positive direction for the rest of the world especially Africa. In December 11, 2019, the United

Nations (UN) Assembly adopted a resolution affirming the stoppage of the trend of catastrophic out-of-pocket health expenses through offering approaches to guarantee economic risk coverage and eradicating destitution on the account of health-related expenditures by 2030 [32].

The United Nations also beckoned on the member states to consolidate their individual country's healthcare systems, in order to support collective admittance to healthcare amenities that will support individuals that are defenseless in sponsoring their healthcare necessitates, also to formulate practically oriented training that are understandable to diverse cultures, customs, traditions and in specific to address the needs of women, children and individuals with, ill health, incapacities and disabilities. The Sendai Framework for Disaster Risk Reduction (SFDRR) 2015–2030, summarized seven unmistakable objectives and four topmost significant action to foil new and diminish prevailing catastrophic risks: (i) Comprehension of the disaster risk; (ii) Reinforcing catastrophic risk governance to manage disaster risk; (iii) Financing disaster reduction and; (iv) Improving disaster preparedness through applicable rejoinder, and to rebuild the human society in recovery, rehabilitation and modernization.

3.2 Research Discussion

The wide scale adoption of the novel 5G network technology Internet of Health Things Robots, really assisted China to expedite healthcare actions and for quick recovery in the ongoing COVID-19 global pandemic and will continue to drive innovation in Internet of Health Things (IoHTs) service delivery now and in future. The electronic Healthcare Industry will experience remarkable improvement in the recent year through sustainable investment in the novel 5G network technology. The novel 5G network technology infrastructure will enhance quick mobile connection speeds, innovative and enterprise transformation for doctor-patient relationship, recognition and adoption of essential services. The Internet of Medical Things (IoMTs) enterprise framework will enable patients to remotely transmit all useful signs to the e-Healthcare service provider for immediate choice medical action. The data workflow will enable healthcare service provider to monitor the array of patient's transmitted signs and mediate via augmented reality platform.

This will support the healthcare service provider to ubiquitously accomplish medication plans for their remote patients wherever they are. The newest treatment plans are made accessible via the fifth generation 5G wireless technology and ever progressively Internet of things framework. Moreover, the creation of the world ever novel operational 5G chips and accomplishment of the foremost clinical test of 5G connectivity implementation on the mobile device in 2017 by Qualcomm, T-Mobile, Ericsson and Sprint pushed industry transition from 4 to 5G technology. This research reviewed the existing network architecture, framework and established the basis upon the adoption of the newest 5G network technology. In accordance with provision of improved Mobile broadband (MBB) and Fixed Wireless Access (FWA),

Table 3 The varied download speed for different network generations

Network generation	Network symbol	Technology framework	Maximum download speed (A)	Typical download speed (B)
2G	G	GPRS	0.2 Mbit/s	<0.2 Mbit/s
	E	EDGE	0.4 Mbit/s	0.15 Mbit/s
3G	3G	3G (Basic)	0.5 Mbit/s	0.2 Mbit/s
	H	HSPA	7.3 Mbit/s	1.25 Mbit/s
	H+	HSPA+	21.5 Mbit/s	5 Mbit/s
	H+	DC-HSPA+	42.5 Mbit/s	9 Mbit/s
4G	4G	LTE Category 4	150.5 Mbit/s	15.1 Mbit/s
4G+	4G+	LTE-Advanced Cat6	300.8 Mbit/s	30.2 Mbit/s
	4G+	LTE-Advanced Cat9	450.1 Mbit/s	45.1 Mbit/s
	4G+	LTE-Advanced Cat12	600.1 Mbit/s	60.1 Mbit/s
	4G+	LTE-Advanced Cat16	979.2 Mbit/s	90.1 Mbit/s
5G	5G	5G	1000–10,000 Mbit/s (1–10 Gbit/s)	150–200 Mbit/s

the Standalone 5G network implementation will favour private enterprise networks and industrial internet of things (IoTs) business ecosystem most especially in the healthcare sector and robotics technologies.

Table 3 presents two discrete download speeds for different network generation ranging from 2 to 5G. The initial comparison (A), represent the theoretical maximum download speed for the different network generations. The values are based on the parameters of the technology support, supposing downloading activities are done within the network coverage area and no congestion on the service masts. Attempt was made to specify the typical download speed as the illustration of day-to-day activities. The authentic download speeds usually hinge on number of considerations which include (i) Location (indoors or outdoors) (ii) The distance from the base masts (servicing mask) (iii) The amount of congestion on the mask. In general perspective, a quicker download speed usually entail that contents from the remote location (internet server) loads more rapidly with less wait time. A quicker download speed will always favour advanced quality streaming (viewing very higher definition video in real times void of buffering effect). However, the download speeds are not necessarily the major factor affecting the responsiveness of the internet connectivity rather the latency.

From Table 4, it can be deduced that the potential of 5G network technology are not necessarily on the predominance of lowered latency and increased capacity for faster download speeds. This is on the premise that the download speeds already present

Table 4 Different network generation latency as the major factor affecting internet of health things responsiveness with respect to download speed

Network generation	Typical latency
2G	$\geqq$ 500 ms (0.5 s)
3G	$\geqq$100 ms (0.1 s)
4G	$\leqq$ 50 ms (0.05 s)
5G	$\leqq$ 1 ms (0.001 s)*

on 4G network are expeditiously sufficient for most users (15 Mbit/s is adequate for high definition video). On the other hand, regardless of faster download speeds not making any significant distinction for 5G network, the diminution in latency from 5G network technology will increase the general response time. Moreover, the reduction in latency of 5G network infrastructure will predominantly impact some of the modern interactive applications for Mobile technology [45]. The lower latency of 5G network will empower enormous technological innovations for connecting Mobile technology to be utilized within the services of Internet of Medical Things for healthcare Robotic extreme automation. Moreover, connecting people to data have potential for innovative 3D imagery, holograms, virtual reality, augmented reality and telemedicine. The 5G's low latency may perhaps advance public safety, digital activation, electronic society diffusion and security. The 5G network latency is an essential features of Wireless generation of cellular technology that considerably enhanced several applications that runs smart mobile Internet of Health Things.

4 Future Research Focus

Intensification in extreme automation, active robotisation and uncommon digitalisation presumably becomes the world agenda on the account that financial opportunities in several developing and developed countries are becoming limited. The twenty first century extreme digital automation primarily will be fanatically established in the Western industrialized nations and Southeast Asia. The industry 4.0 automation will be potentially established in those countries on the merit of technological endowments by nature and innovative service models orientation. An extra positive inclination are conspicuous for India and China, both countries are well thought-out appropriate contenders for involvement in the extreme digital revolution, owing to the fact that majority of their populations are possessing excellent knowledge of English and superlative order of IT proficiencies.

IT education or intelligence are communicated in schools as the fundamental qualification requisites in that region. Prior to the COVID-19 outbreak, majority of individuals had developed certain gradation of apprehensiveness in relation to Robots and Artificial Intelligence (AI). However, their opinions might have been originally influenced by dystopian interpretations regarding technology in science fiction, although such apprehension may have been highlighted through reasonable and unpretentious concerns. Minority of Artificial Intelligence (AI) business applications are undeniably heading to the loss of human jobs, strengthening of preconceived notions and encroachments into information privacy such as the use of military predatory drones for espionage, spying and remote combatant engagement.

Certain initially held believe have been kept aside because from the commencement of the COVID-19 pandemic, Artificial Intelligence (AI) mitigated technologies were utilized to moderate the escalation of the COVID-19 pandemic spread. The twenty first century digital e-society had witnessed an increase in rate of the adoption of robotics to perform several tasks initially meant for human beings. While human being were observing sit at home order, robots were busy working and occupying all the available workplaces originally were performed by humans. The Labour artificial intelligence swapping robots, for instance, are taking over staircase cleaning of the shopping malls, healthcare facilities killing the COVID-19 pathogen and other hospital acquired infections (HAIs), online ordering, weather forecasting, personal finance assistance, product suggestions, scheduling meetings, customer support, classifying news, search and track flights route, send money and sorting and recycle event centres [3]. Artificial Intelligence is currently promoting an enthusiastic dependence on enterprise chatbots for customer hospitality assistance at business corporations including hospital diagnostics centres and on machine guided information censoring platforms with particular reference to YouTube [16]. The Robotic telepresence podiums were currently supporting schoolchildren, undergraduates and apprentices in Japan with "in-human" university advancement experience in the ongoing COVID-19 pandemic.

With respect to data collection and analysis, artificial intelligence (AI) presently is showing capacity in immediate endeavours to supervise the infection rates and contact tracing. When finally the COVID-19 vaccines are manufactured and made public for COVID-19 treatment and the pandemic eventually retracts, it will be very hard to contemplate life beginning again as it was at the commencement of 2020. The digital society experiences and understandings in the ongoing COVID-19 will make it very comprehendible to regularize scientific automation as a component of our new society configuration that will consolidate the industry 4.0 extreme digital automation. Business establishments and companies which have already consolidated the adoption of robots at the peak of the COVID-19 crisis, may perhaps reconsider that a substantial proportion of the company workforce are not necessary to any further extent, this will lead to loss of human jobs. The current twenty first century digital society will witness some set of social adjustment, a number of individuals may possibly wish to sustain the social distancing even when COVID-19 pandemic had left the street.

However, while the digital e-society adoption of AI, Robotics and scientific automation intensifies, organizations and businesses are expected to weigh the opportunities available for preconceptions that the current society are already aware that exist in artificial intelligence (AI). Take for instance, the capacity for artificial intelligence algorithms to support the healthcare business processes and determination control are enormous in part for the reason that they are expected to be trained on the large data sets before it can be successfully accomplished. The artificial intelligence

(AI) may be ultimate solution when handling business cases where a triage evaluation are required to be expedited in an intensive care unit looking at access and who gets turn to use the ventilator for life support.

In summary, the upcoming AI application in healthcare may perhaps involve assignments that ranged from a flexible to complex operations. Predictably, the AI robots could perform the whole thing from responding to the telephone calls to medical electronic documentation and re-examination, clinical diagnosis and treatment plans, therapeutic drug and device design, citizen's health trending analytics, transcription of radiology images, and nurse caring patients. The healthcare perspective view of artificial intelligence (AI), robotics, machine learning (ML) and natural language processing (NLP) could be extremely scaring. The upcoming applications of extreme digital automation in the healthcare sector and the impressions on patient-care, clinicians routine and pharmaceutical manufacturing is superlatively intriguing on the premise that industry 4.0 extreme healthcare automation has been predicted to increase life expectancy up to 250 years from the previous 80–100 years average life cycle in the developed countries while in the less developed countries, the average life expectancy is assumed to be less than 80 years [9].

Beginning from patientcare and extended hospitality self-services to chat bots, computer aided detection (CAD) systems for clinical diagnosis and image data analysis requirement for candidate molecules identification in drug discovery, artificial intelligence (AI) is well established for extreme digital automation toward enhancing suitability, effectiveness while diminishing costs and errors susceptibility and comprehensively formulate the easy route for many patients to achieve the quantum of healthcare substantially [43]. However, the Natural Language Processing (NLP) and Machine Learning (ML) are at present being utilized in the healthcare sector to improve performances while in the future, they are expected to develop progressively toward improving life expectancy through:

i. Advancing the healthcare supply chains, clinical efficiency, throughput and excellence of patientcare.
ii. Improve patient appointment with the healthcare providers and customize patient access to medical care.
iii. Increase speed and lower the cost of evolving novel pharmaceutical drug manufacturing and medical treatments.
iv. Customize medical treatments through digital automation analytic leverages, providing approaches to substantial untapped accumulations of non-codified clinical information.

5 Recommendation

In all of these, Robots in healthcare management played significant roles in helping Medical personnel in routine tasks, persuasive obligations and assisting clinical processes to be fundamentally reliable and less detrimental to the consumers (patients). Those automated robots can equally accomplish precise surgery with minimal invasion in microscopic places and dispose hazardous substances with less human supervision. Healthcare Medical Robotic Assistants are used to monitor patients in the hospital wards and vital statistical observations are communicated to the nurses who readily evaluate the signs to determine if human attention is needed in the medical ward/rooms. This approach enables nurses to monitor several patients at once most especially during the period of COVID-19 in several healthcare units. Those Robotic assistants usually enter patient's information into the electronic health record automatically. In a similar development, robotic carts were observed traversing from beginning to end of the hospital corridors moving materials around with the capacities to observe disruptions and avoid them. The robots were helping in surgery, permitting the medical doctors to accomplish surgeries through a minimal incision as an alternative to inches-long incision previously in practice. Robots are exerting extensive influences in every areas of medicine and healthcare technology and the contributions are expected to increase amidst the current digital automation. Moreover, the Robotic innovations are performing many functions in several areas that straightforwardly improved patient care management.

Robots were utilized in disinfecting patient rooms and wards in addition to operating suites, diminishing the susceptibility for patients and clinical workforce from contacting infections in the ongoing COVID-19. Robots were seen working in clinical laboratories taking samples and moving them to the analysis department and finally storing the results. Corresponding Robotic innovation is the development of human-robotic look alike called humanoids which are used to provide tasks such a personal care, socialization and for coaching. The particular humanoid robots adopted for coaching emergency personnel to respond to distress in particular resembled a victim who screams, bleeds and even responds to treatment. Moreover, the fundamental uncertainty phenomenon for Robots in clinical, medical field and healthcare profession is whether robots might profitably takeover jobs away from humans. In that regard, possibilities exist more than a few explanations why the automated machines (Robots) will not replace their human counterparts in some classified occupations. For some reasons, most hospitals have less than 300 beds and fewer automated masterplan. They simply may not be able to afford the Robotic technology extreme automation. Some highly robotic conducted automobiles needed a supportive pathway or floor tracks and the installation of navigation devices all over the facilities. The process of such automation are exceedingly high-priced but eventually, the robotic assistant's automation may not replace indispensable human contacts and operations in the actual.

In the perspective of all the findings and ongoing development in the COVID-19 global pandemic and indispensable roles played by robots in the current digital society response to COVID-19, the following recommendations has been formulated:

i. The twenty first century digital world should continue the incremental development in the robotic research and innovation.

ii. Synergy between the academic researchers, captains of industries and government at all levels in finding more investment opportunities and policy adoption for scientific inventions.
iii. Medical, Healthcare and Clinical personnel's should accept and adapt the ongoing automation and be ready to adjust to avoid being displaced by highly automated clinical and medical robots.
iv. Unified framework and adoption strategies for robotic innovations especially in the healthcare sectors.
v. With respect to COVID-19, the current digital society should expect unavoidable in future time and therefore prepare ahead of time.

6 Conclusion

The Consequential COVID-19 global health emergency which triggered the escalation of the novel SARS-CoV-2 virus had unwittingly assembled the worldwide scientists, academicians, researchers and medical professionals to conjure several innovations such as Internet of Things (IoTs), Artificial Intelligence (AI), Machine Learning (ML), Internet of Health Things (IoHTs), Internet of Medical Things (IoMTs), Innovative Internet of 5G Medical Robotic Things (IIo-5GMRTs), 5G Network technology and Internet of Things Drone technology (IoTD) in response to the overwhelming effects of the ongoing global pandemic. Come up with advancement in few space of time, the artificial intelligence and machine learning research group are acclimatized to speedy distribution of evidence based results which had enabled appropriate adjustments in the perspective of the ongoing COVID-19 pandemic. In addition, the increasing attentiveness on AI and Machine learning models are assisting the current digital society and promoting sustainable development agenda in industry 4.0 digital extreme automation. Most important Machine Learning symposiums such as the conferences on Neural Information Processing Systems and the International Symposium on Machine Learning was held boost intensive pursuit on Artificial Intelligence for collective investment sustainability.

The health emergency caused by COVID-19 quickly got the attention of the machine learning field. Now that many of the challenges around data and model sharing, local adaptation and prioritizing work where clinical needs are greatest have been identified, more AI solutions can be expected that are inclusive and will make a global impact.

Acknowledgements The authors acknowledged the fact that the current paper does not attract any government or corporate funding and also does not have any conflict of interest.

Conflict of Interest This research does not have conflict of interest.

References

1. Ackerman, E., & Koziol, M. (2019). The blood is here: Zipline's medical delivery drones are changing the game in Rwanda. *IEEE Spectrum, 56*(5), 24–31
2. Adhikari, B., Lewis, B., Vullikanti, A., Jiménez, J. M., & Prakash, B. A. (2019). Fast and near-optimal monitoring for healthcare acquired infection outbreaks. *PLoS Computational Biology, 15*(9), e1007284
3. Albayrak, N., Özdemir, A., & Zeydan, E. (2018). *An overview of artificial intelligence based chatbots and an example chatbot application.* Paper presented at the 2018 26th Signal processing and communications applications conference (SIU).
4. Infectious Diseases Society of America. (IDSA). (2011). Combating antimicrobial resistance: policy recommendations to save lives. *Clinical Infectious Diseases, 52*(suppl_5), S397–S428.
5. Archibald, L. K., & Gaynes, R. P. (1997). Hospital-acquired infections in the United States: The importance of interhospital comparisons. *Infectious Disease Clinics of North America, 11*(2), 245–255
6. Beasley, R. A. (2012). Medical robots: current systems and research directions. *Journal of Robotics, 2012.*
7. Berkley, S. (2019). The power of vaccines and how Gavi has helped make the world healthier: 2019 Lasker-Bloomberg public service award. *JAMA, 322*(13), 1251–1252
8. Bocicor, M. I., Dascălu, M., Gaczowska, A., Hostiuc, S., Moldoveanu, A., Molina, A., Molnar, A. J., Negoi, I., & Racoviţă, V. (2017). *Technological platform for the prevention and management of healthcare associated infections and outbreaks.* Paper presented at the International Conference on Evaluation of Novel Approaches to Software Engineering.
9. Branger, J., & Pang, Z. (2015). From automated home to sustainable, healthy and manufacturing home: A new story enabled by the Internet-of-Things and Industry 4.0. *Journal of Management Analytics, 2*(4), 314–332.
10. Calisher, C., Carroll, D., Colwell, R., Corley, R. B., Daszak, P., Drosten, C., Enjuanes, L., Farrar, J., Field, H., Golding, J., & Gorbalenya, A. (2020). Statement in support of the scientists, public health professionals, and medical professionals of China combatting COVID-19. *The Lancet, 395*(10226), e42–e43.
11. Carter, J., Hoffman, C., & Wiedenheft, B. (2017). The interfaces of genetic conflict are hot spots for innovation. *Cell, 168*(1–2), 9–11
12. Chen, M., Yang, J., Hao, Y., Mao, S., & Hwang, K. (2017). A 5G cognitive system for healthcare. *Big Data and Cognitive Computing, 1*(1), 2
13. Covid, C. (2020). Characteristics of health care personnel with COVID-19—United States, February 12–April 9, 2020. https://www.cdc.gov/mmwr/volumes/69/wr/pdfs/mm6915e6-H.pdf
14. Dancer, S. J. (2011). Hospital cleaning in the 21st century. *European Journal of Clinical Microbiology & Infectious Diseases, 30*(12), 1473–1481
15. Daneshmand, M., Bilici, O., Bolotnikova, A., & Anbarjafari, G. (2017). Medical robots with potential applications in participatory and opportunistic remote sensing: A review. *Robotics and Autonomous Systems, 95*, 160–180
16. Dwivedi, Y. K., Hughes, L., Ismagilova, E., Aarts, G., Coombs, C., Crick, T., Duan, Y., Dwivedi, R., Edwards, J., Eirug, A., & Galanos, V. (2019). Artificial Intelligence (AI): Multidisciplinary perspectives on emerging challenges, opportunities, and agenda for research, practice and policy. *International Journal of Information Management*, 101994.
17. Edwards, C. C., & Bailey, R. W. (2000). Laparoscopic hernia repair: The learning curve. *Surgical Laparoscopy Endoscopy & Percutaneous Techniques, 10*(3), 149–153
18. Geng, H. (2017). *Internet of things and data analytics handbook.* Wiley.
19. Han, J. H., Sullivan, N., Leas, B. F., Pegues, D. A., Kaczmarek, J. L., & Umscheid, C. A. (2015). Cleaning hospital room surfaces to prevent health care–associated infections: A technical brief. *Annals of Internal Medicine, 163*(8), 598–607
20. Haque, M., Sartelli, M., McKimm, J., & Abu Bakar, M. (2018). Health care-associated infections—An overview. *Infection and Drug Resistance, 11*, 2321–2333

21. Hassan, M., Tuckman, H. P., Patrick, R. H., Kountz, D. S., & Kohn, J. L. (2010). Cost of hospital-acquired infection. *Hospital Topics, 88*(3), 82–89
22. Hassanalieragh, M., Page, A., Soyata, T., Sharma, G., Aktas, M., Mateos, G., Kantarci, B., & Andreescu, S. (2015). *Health monitoring and management using Internet-of-Things (IoT) sensing with cloud-based processing: Opportunities and challenges.* Paper presented at the 2015 IEEE International Conference on Services Computing.
23. Hu, L.-Q., Wang, J., Huang, A., Wang, D., & Wang, J. (2020). COVID-19 and improved prevention of hospital-acquired infection. *BJA: British Journal of Anaesthesia.*
24. Inn, T. L. (2020). Smart city technologies take on COVID-19. *World Health.*
25. Jassim, S. A., Limoges, R. G., & El-Cheikh, H. (2016). Bacteriophage biocontrol in wastewater treatment. *World Journal of Microbiology and Biotechnology, 32*(4), 70
26. Jayaraman, R., Taha, K., & Collazos, A. B. (2015). *Integrating supply chain data standards in healthcare operations and Electronic Health Records.* Paper presented at the 2015 International Conference on Industrial Engineering and Operations Management (IEOM).
27. Khanna, T. (2018). When technology gets ahead of society. *Harvard Business Review, 96*(4), 86–95
28. Kidd, C. D., & Breazeal, C. (2008). *Designing for long-term human-robot interaction and application to weight loss.* Massachusetts Institute of Technology.
29. Mehta, Y., Gupta, A., Todi, S., Myatra, S., Samaddar, D., Patil, V., Bhattacharya, P. K., & Ramasubban, S. (2014). Guidelines for prevention of hospital acquired infections. *Indian Journal of Critical Care Medicine: Peer-Reviewed, Official Publication of Indian Society of Critical Care Medicine, 18*(3), 149.
30. Nižetić, S., Šolić, P., González-de, D. L.-d.-I., & Patrono, L. (2020). Internet of Things (IoT): Opportunities, issues and challenges towards a smart and sustainable future. *Journal of Cleaner Production,* 122877.
31. Omrani, A. S., Al-Tawfiq, J. A., & Memish, Z. A. (2015). Middle East respiratory syndrome coronavirus (MERS-CoV): Animal to human interaction. *Pathogens and Global Health, 109*(8), 354–362
32. Query ID="Q3" Text="Unable to parse this reference. Kindly do manual structure" Organization, W. H. (2018). An inclusive health agenda: meeting public health challenges in South-East Asia, Selected Speeches by Dr. Poonam Khetrapal Singh, WHO Regional Director for South-East Asia, 2014–2017.
33. Ortega-Fernández, A., Martín-Rojas, R., & García-Morales, V. J. (2020). Artificial intelligence in the urban environment: Smart cities as models for developing innovation and sustainability. *Sustainability, 12*(19), 7860
34. Ostfeld, A. E., Gaikwad, A. M., Khan, Y., & Arias, A. C. (2016). High-performance flexible energy storage and harvesting system for wearable electronics. *Scientific Reports, 6,* 26122
35. Pamplin, J. C., Yeaw, R., Gilbert, G. R., Davis, K. L., Mann-Salinas, E., Salinas, J., Kral, D., & Schlachta-Fairchild, L. (2018). *Augmenting clinical performance in combat casualty care: telemedicine to automation.* Paper presented at the International Conference on Augmented Cognition.
36. Quinn, M. M., Henneberger, P. K., Braun, B., Delclos, G. L., Fagan, K., Huang, V., Knaack, J. L., Kusek, L., Lee, S. J., Le Moual, N., & Maher, K. A. (2015). Cleaning and disinfecting environmental surfaces in health care: toward an integrated framework for infection and occupational illness prevention. *American Journal of Infection Control, 43*(5), 424–434.
37. Reed, D., & Kemmerly, S. A. (2009). Infection control and prevention: A review of hospital-acquired infections and the economic implications. *Ochsner Journal, 9*(1), 27–31
38. Reeves, J. J., Hollandsworth, H. M., Torriani, F. J., Taplitz, R., Abeles, S., Tai-Seale, M., Millen, M., Clay, B. J., & Longhurst, C. A. (2020). Rapid response to COVID-19: Health informatics support for outbreak management in an academic health system. *Journal of the American Medical Informatics Association, 27*(6), 853–859.
39. Rosen, J. (2017). Zipline's ambitious medical drone delivery in Africa. *MIT Technology Review. June, 8,* 2017.

40. Roser, M., Ritchie, H., Ortiz-Ospina, E., & Hasell, J. (2020). Coronavirus (COVID-19) deaths. *Our World in Data.*
41. Sachan, D. (2016). The age of drones: What might it mean for health? *Lancet (London, England), 387*(10030), 1803–1804
42. Sandbrook, C. (2015). The social implications of using drones for biodiversity conservation. *Ambio, 44*(4), 636–647
43. Schönberger, D. (2019). Artificial intelligence in healthcare: A critical analysis of the legal and ethical implications. *International Journal of Law and Information Technology, 27*(2), 171–203
44. Shi, F., Wang, J., Shi, J., Wu, Z., Wang, Q., Tang, Z., He, K., Shi, Y., & Shen, D. (2020). Review of artificial intelligence techniques in imaging data acquisition, segmentation and diagnosis for covid-19. *IEEE Reviews in Biomedical Engineering.*
45. Simsek, M., Aijaz, A., Dohler, M., Sachs, J., & Fettweis, G. (2016). 5G-enabled tactile internet. *IEEE Journal on Selected Areas in Communications, 34*(3), 460–473
46. Singh, R. P., Javaid, M., Haleem, A., & Suman, R. (2020). Internet of things (IoT) applications to fight against COVID-19 pandemic. *Diabetes & Metabolic Syndrome: Clinical Research & Reviews.*
47. Stawicki, S. P., Jeanmonod, R., Miller, A. C., Paladino, L., Gaieski, D. F., Yaffee, A. Q., De Wulf, A., Grover, J., Papadimos, T. J., Bloem, C., & Galwankar, S. C. (2020). The 2019–2020 novel coronavirus (severe acute respiratory syndrome coronavirus 2) pandemic: A joint American college of academic international medicine-world academic council of emergency medicine multidisciplinary COVID-19 working group consensus paper. *Journal of Global Infectious Diseases, 12*(2), 47.
48. Tian, S., Hu, N., Lou, J., Chen, K., Kang, X., Xiang, Z., Chen, H., Wang, D., Liu, N., Liu, D., & Chen, G. (2020). Characteristics of COVID-19 infection in Beijing. *Journal of Infection.*
49. Vafea, M. T., Atalla, E., Georgakas, J., Shehadeh, F., Mylona, E. K., Kalligeros, M., & Mylonakis, E. (2020). Emerging technologies for use in the study, diagnosis, and treatment of patients with COVID-19. *Cellular and Molecular Bioengineering*, 1–9.
50. Watkins, A., Rothfeld, M., Rashbaum, W., & Rosenthal, B. (2020). Top ER doctor who treated virus patients dies by suicide. *New York Times, 27.*
51. Worku, W. (2017). *Hospital acquired infections and infection prevention practice in teaching hospitals in the Amhara Regional State.* Addis Ababa University.

Battling COVID-19 with Process Model of Integrated Digital Technology: An Analysis of Qualitative Data

Aastha Verma

1 Introduction

The crisis of corona has moved the financial and health status of big economies like USA, Italy, Russia, Spain, and UK. Emerging economies like India, South Africa, and China are worst hit countries. In such a scenario, authorities concerned in these economies are looking out for action plans, strategies, and policies to contain the spread of virus and limit the number of infected people's cases. WHO declared corona virus disease (COVID-19) 2020 as public health emergency at world level. This is by far the most uncontrollable disease outbreak seen in generations. A similar disease appeared in 2003 named severe acute respiratory syndrome (SARS) corona virus (SARS–CoV), 26 countries reported 8000 cases. However, COVID-19 cases worldwide are many times higher than SARS outbreak. The prime difference which exists in the two scenarios of 2003 and 2020 is of digital technology advancement as well as data production. The amount of data produced in a day then is produced within a matter of minutes today. COVID-19 pandemic is occurring when the world is much more digitized. This can be used as an advantage to enable governments, heathcare authorizes, and policy-makers to curb the spread of the disease. Digital developments have completely changed the conduct of businesses today. The need of digital transformation had been realized by marketers as soon as the technological and digital landscape revolutionized by technology upgradation. Many eminent researchers have argued that strong digital developments require quick adaptation of a digital model to deal with the situation [1]. In order to sustain and keep ahead of competition, companies are redesigning their business models and embracing digital transformation [2, 3]. Similarly, current times require such proactive measure and the use of a digital technology is to attain 4Cs (curb, control, and culminate corona). Immediately after the onslaught of corona virus, many eminent researchers presented their views on digital technology usage to fight corona, and the literature

A. Verma (✉)
South Campus, Ramlal Anand College, University of Delhi, New Delhi, India

M. Niranjanamurthy et al. (eds.), *Intelligent Data Analysis for COVID-19 Pandemic*, Algorithms for Intelligent Systems, https://doi.org/10.1007/978-981-16-1574-0_3

contribution has grown much the same way as diseases transmission. A large group of experts, scientists, and researchers from all over the globe suggested the use of technologies of industry 4.0, artificial intelligence, Internet of things (IoT), big data, mobile data, Internet data, social media, and government enforced mobile applications to tackle the pandemic [4–7]. There is a lot more generation of the literature in a short span owing to the enormity and urgency of the matter. Numerous reputed journals launched special issues covering and publishing the research on the similar theme. Wide internationally renowned magazines covered articles pertaining to the issue. Most of these studies have posited leveraging specific digital technology to tackle the situation; non-have worked towards development of an integrated model encapsulating all technologies to a single model in the form of process to combat COVID-19. In an attempt to bridge this gap, present study is designed and positioned as a qualitative study with the following aims:

- Systematic analysis of the plentiful extant literature for the development of a digital architectural background which showcases the integration of all potential digital technologies (mobile applications, artificial intelligence, big data, Internet of things (IoT), social media) which can be used to control and monitor the spread of disease.
- Exploring and augmenting technological platforms with their usage and implementation to tackle the situation of COVID-19.
- The current research proposes a "Process Model of Integrated Digital Technology" as a ready tool to adopt by authorities for detection, control and management of COVID-19.

2 Research Design and Structure

This paper adopts qualitative research methods to achieve the objectives. Study is conducted in two phases: Phase I is dedicated to systematic manual exploring, structuring, and synthesis of literature on the broad theme of "Digital Technology and COVID-19." Results are built on the research studies and articles published for the period of Jan 2020–July 2020. After a thorough search, sixty-nine articles were shortlisted for establishing, assessing, and combining all aspects of the theme—technology usage to combat disease. Author searched articles in reputed journals published by Sage Publishing, Emerald, Springer Link, Elsevier, Taylor and Francis, IGI Global. Online libraries such as EBSCO Host, Pro Quest, Jstor, and Google Scholar Mobile searched thoroughly to identify and include each article available on the theme. Articles published online from eminent publishers like Oxford University Press, Cambridge University Press, and Harvard University Press were also included. Phase I generated rich source of information related to recognize themes to get a clear vision of their interconnectedness. Phase II of this research focuses on handling the big literature with the use of computer-aided qualitative data analysis software (CAQDAS)—NVIVO and MAXQDA Analytics Pro 2020.

Qualitative research has been greatly advanced with the development of these softwares. As it allows more extensive and comprehensive review of big literature free from human bias and other limitations, this phase followed a step-wise procedure; nodes/codes/themes were created to contain common information in a structured format such as digital technology, mobile applications/data, social media, artificial intelligence, Internet of things, and big data analytics. Thereafter data was visualized through word cloud and word trees. To present a comprehensive view of interconnections between nodes, concept map was derived which leads to the development of "Process Model of Digital Integration." The use of software strengthens and confirms the underlying understanding of the relationship in data useful for creating model to combat COVID-19.

3 Digital Technology to Combat COVID-19

2020 brings significant development in digital technologies. Multiple digital tools can be used to control COVID-19 outbreak [8]. History had witnessed similar type of outbreaks like SARS 2003 controlled by extreme quarantine measures and painstaking physical contact tracing efforts. These classic prevention control public healthcare measures cannot be adapted in case of COVID-19 owing to the scale and intensity of disease. In such a case, digital technology advancement is proved to be bliss. Combination of technologies like mobile applications, artificial intelligence, IoT, big data analytics, and social media can deter the spread of disease remarkably. Most of the countries in the world have developed mobile applications dedicated to detection, treatment, prevention, and control of disease. This technology has been used widely for resisting the transmission of COVID-19 [9]. As per a report, two widely used mobile applications in China Alipay and WeChat have helped to contain the spread of the virus in a big way, and it has limited the public life as it enforces restrictions and keeps a track on the people's movement. Color codes on the screen of mobile: red, yellow, and green indicate the health status of a person [10]. Another technology gaining popularity is the combination of artificial intelligence, Internet of things (IoT), and big data analytics. It has proven its value in multiple uses starting from detection of cases, isolation of patients, and development of vaccine. Interestingly, much like the theme of the current study, Hutson [11] has reported the use of artificial intelligence (AI) by biomedical researchers and clinicians to explore COVID-19 papers/literature they need for the development of a drug. The author highlights the benefits of using AI tools to explore 28,000 articles swiftly and for extracting the specific findings from the results which is useful in the development of COVID medicine. In order to decrease the load of doctors healthcare sector is utilizing various AI-based systems. AI is also used to increase doctor to patient ratio so that no one remains deprived of medical attention when it is required the most. Additionally, mobile-based data can develop AI algorithms for detection of COVID-19. Further, artificial intelligence helps to predict the future spread of contagious disease with the help of machine learning that analyzes big data to make a pattern

[12]. Cohen et al. [13] bring to fore the use of artificial intelligence in the fight against COVID-19 by the use of biometric identification and face recognition software for diagnosis and containment.

Digital technology is capable of enhancing public health awareness with the help of social media. Government healthcare agencies can utilize the data available on these platforms (Facebook, Twitter, Instagram, and WhatsApp) and may clarify uncertainties and misinformation through the same medium [14] Singapore government has collaborated with WhatsApp to disseminate valid information to public and apprising people of all government initiatives/drives/decisions in order to eradicate COVID. Social media data can also be leveraged for prediction and thus helps in making necessary preparations in advance. Cuilian et al. [15] establish a correlation between new laboratory confirmed cases and social media search about COVID-19. According to them, Internet social media data enable monitoring of disease. The study revealed the benefits of Internet surveillance to monitor the infectious disease and claimed an accurate prediction outbreak and progress of COVID.

In order to obtain a visual understanding of literature connecting digital technology with COVID-19, a word cloud is generated with NVIVO-coded nodes created from all the sixty-two articles reviewed as shown in Fig. 1. It is observed through placement of the words that COVID-19, and digital technologies have been studied most dominantly in the literature and selected for further examination. Thereafter utilizing the same textual data word tree is generated with the software as shown in Fig. 2. Word tree produces interactive visual concordance of the word COVID-19 in its context connected with branches. A word can be navigated through its branches to assess the linkages. Software also provides a feature to locate the word in the original document through document browser enabling researcher to read and draw inferences.

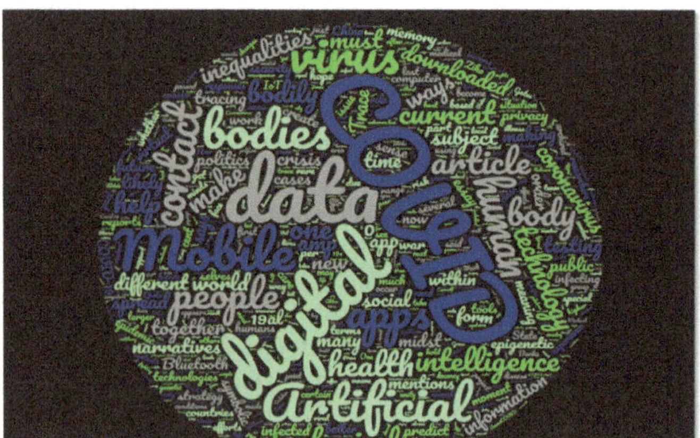

Fig. 1 Word cloud based on NVIVO analysis

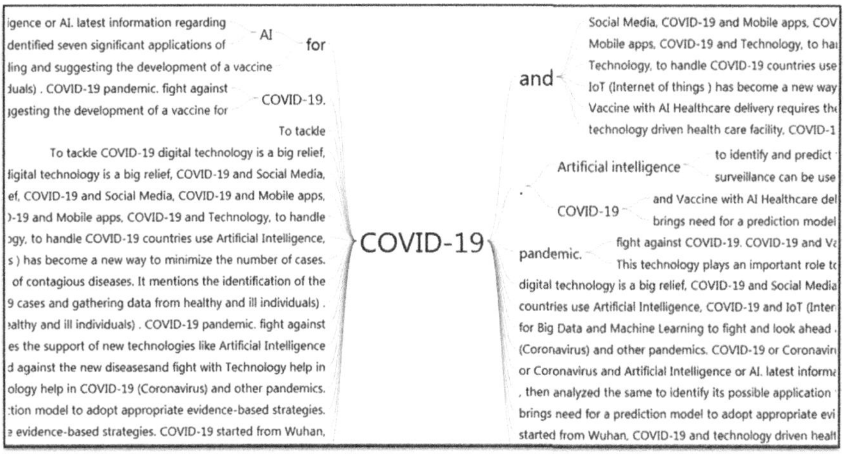

Fig. 2 Word tree indicating linkages of COVID-19 and digital technologies

3.1 *Mobile Applications and COVID-19*

Governments around the globe are testing and considering mobile applications to control COVID-19. Most European countries are developing, testing, or rolling out contact tracing applications to have a rapid COVID-19 monitoring and control system in place. Many countries have already developed these applications which are in use, for example, ArogyaSetu—India, COVID safe—Australia, COVID Shield—Canada, Alipay health code—China, Immuni—Italy, COVID watch—USA, and so on. These applications enable the governments to access important information. Mobile applications support the coordination of tests at medical institutions allowing users with a high infection risk to book a test slot directly from the application. This reduces the effort and increases the efficiency of the medical test processes. Martinez et al. [16] elaborate the usefulness of COVID symptom tracker, the mobile application built through the efforts of team of scientists called COPE consortium. Scientists with expertise in big data research and epidemiology developed this application offering data on predictive symptoms, risk factors, clinical outcomes, and geographical hotspots. This application was launched in the UK and USA in short time intervals, garnered data from more than 2.8 million users. Tibbetts [17] supports the same that smart phones and other digital devices harness latest digital technology for epidemiological and shed valuable data trails that number of nations are capturing and using as surveillance system to suppress COVID-19 outbreak. The data from phone also critically examines the travel history of the person tested positive. If any person comes in close range of the infected person's phone, then that phone owner can be spotted and screened irrespective of development of symptoms. Parker et al. [18] posited that rapid pre-symptomatic transmission of COVID-19 is raising a question on the efficiency of standard manual contract tracing procedure and also highlights the significance of mobile application enabled contact tracing. This approach adopted by China and several countries in Asia has been highly successful in reducing the number of cases. Ferretti et al. [19] conducted a study at Oxford University's big data institute to further the understanding of use of mobile application in COVID-19 control. The authors explained urgent need of mobile contact tracing application to support healthcare services as well as policy-makers to plan target interventions. Mathematical model suggests traditional public health contact tracing provide incomplete data and cannot be used in the pandemic of this scale. Authors further argued that mobile application reduces transmission at any stage peak or decline and can handle the situation until vaccines are available. The mobile applications to control the transmission of virus have been used around the globe, and their effectiveness to control can be seen through the graphs presented for countries India, China, Italy, Australia and South Korea in Fig. 3, 4, 5, 6, and 7. The graphs plot the data of active cases. The number of active cases from the month of Match till July 2020 is obtained

Fig. 3 India active cases

India Mobile App–Aarogya Setu
Launch Date – April 2020

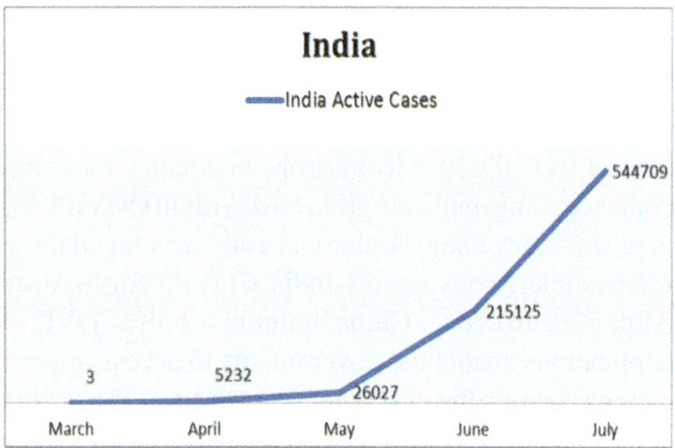

Fig. 4 China active cases

China Mobile App – Alipay Health Code Software
Launch Date – February 2020

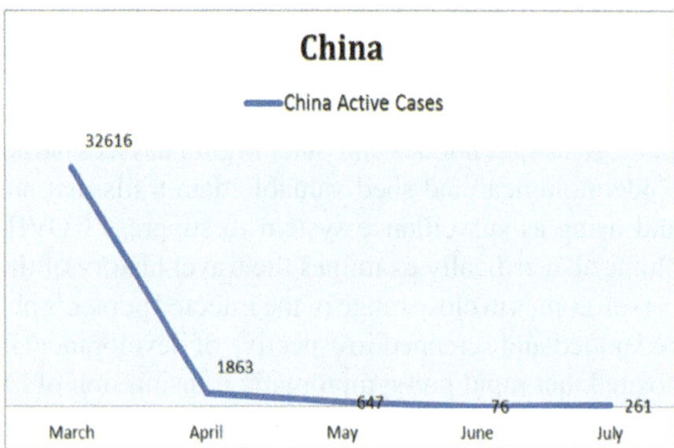

Fig. 5 Italy active cases

Italy Mobile App – Immuni
Launch Date – June, 2020

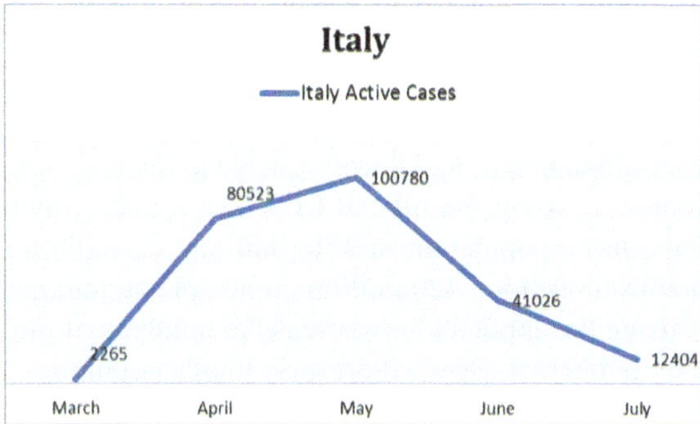

Fig. 6 Australia active cases

Australia Mobile App – Covid Safe
Launch Date – April, 2020

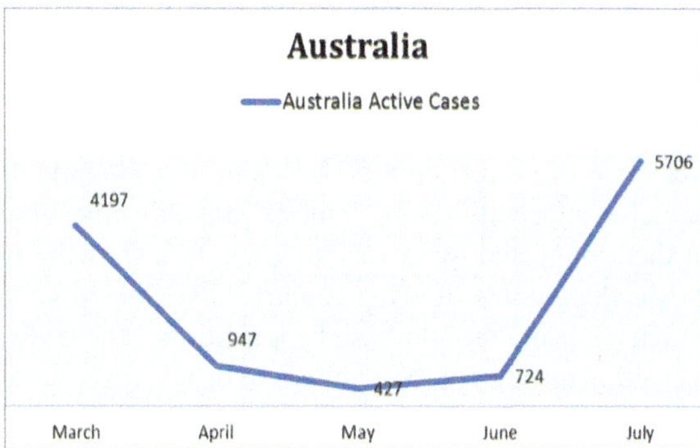

Fig. 7 South Korea active cases

South Korea Mobile App – Corona 100M
Launch Date – February, 20

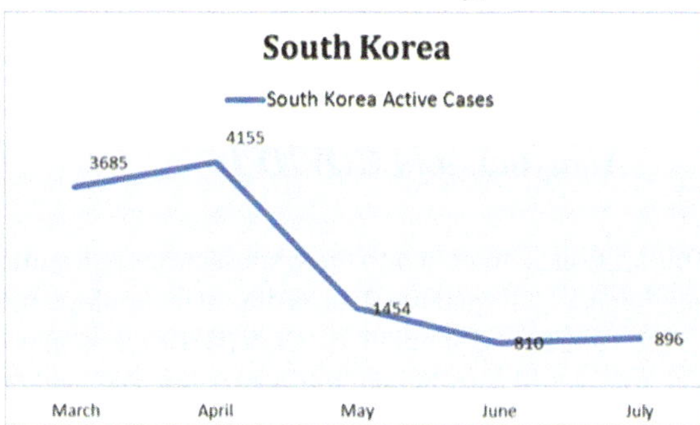

from official WHO data stream on Web site. It is observed that there is a decline in active cases soon after the introduction of mobile applications in these countries. The possibility of decline due to other control measures has not been ruled out completely though. It is seen that in all the countries there is a decline in number of cases from the month of mobile application launch except in India, where the active cases count is surging with each passing day. The reason for the same is many including population, discontinuation of lockdowns, unable to maintain social distancing, etc. However in context to using the official COVID-19 control mobile application: AarogyaSetu, India has a population of 1366 million. 75 million have downloaded the application from the total 420 million mobile phone Internet users. Only 7% of population is using the application, whereas the numbers of mobile application download and mobile Internet users with respect to other countries are more closure than these.

In an attempt to address the concern of pandemic prevention and control WHO launched two mobile applications: WHO academy application for healthcare workers and WHO info application for public use [20]. The first application provides WHO developed knowledge resources, workshops, tools, and virtual training in order to maintain a single standard worldwide for COVID control, prevention, and treatment. WHO info application provides the latest up to date news and developments. These mobile applications are free to download. Several studies all around the world have contributed different advantages of mobile applications. Figure 8 represents the word tree of mobile application using in pandemic derived from the literature. The branches attached to word "mobile" are indicative of its connection with word "apps" further connected to its various uses. It is showing how it can be used to suppress the pandemic; it is showing countries like Singapore, Germany, Australia, and China which are using mobile-based applications. There are connections implying the data collection through mobile phones to be leveraged for mathematical AI-based prediction models. Other branches on the left are showing the linkages of mobile majorly with contact tracing.

Table 1 represents the extant literature on mobile applications usage and COVID-19.

3.2 *Artificial Intelligence, Internet of Things (IoT), Big Data Analytics, and COVID 19*

This section is divided into three subsections pertaining to the discussion on artificial intelligence, IoT, and big data as digital technology instruments to battle COVID-19.

Increase in the number of COVID-19 cases and death tolls call for the use of technologies like artificial intelligence, big data, and the Internet of things as valuable tools to combat the pandemic [32]. The combinations of these digital technologies bring miraculous solutions at many fronts and strengthen the efforts in a fight with COVID-19. These technologies are often used in combination; therefore, this section discusses all three of these. The advancement of AI technology helps at many fronts

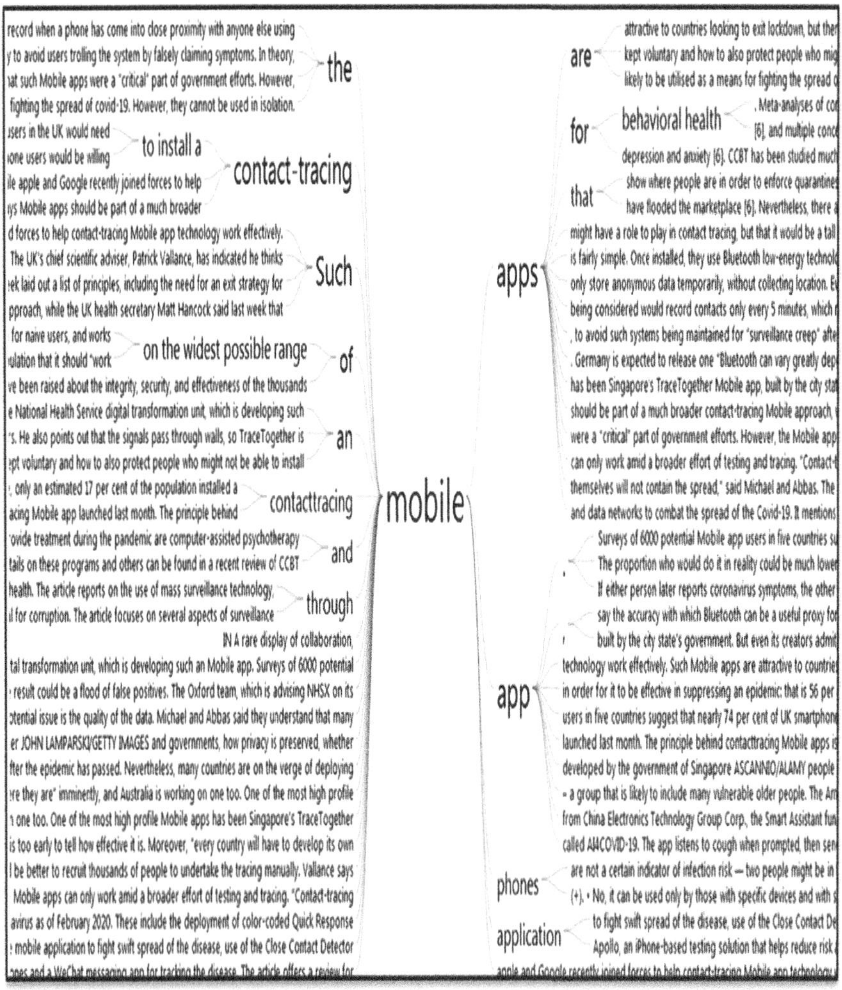

Fig. 8 Word tree of mobile application usage in COVID-19

in tackling pandemic. The use of innovative AI technology can help to fight COVID-19 pandemic. The technology is helpful in screening, tracking, and predicting the cases. It is also useful in early detection, diagnosis, proper screening, tracking, and predicting the current and future patients. The use is not only limited to this, drugs and vaccines can also be developed using artificial intelligence [24]. As per the Head, WHO Tedros Ghebreyesus—"a devastating epidemic can start at any time in any country killing millions." In order to be prepared, governments of the countries can depend upon AI. Artificial intelligence is capable of predicting the conditions and locations where spillover of a new pathogen may occur. Countries like China is using AI-based testing backed by AI-based thermal imaging cameras in crowded

Table 1 Literature on mobile applications and COVID-19

Technology: mobile applications		
Source	Country of study	Description
Whitaker [21]	UK	Author highlights the importance of applications in tracing contacts as well difficulties in implementation of NHS trace and trace app. There is an appeal to big players like Apple and Google to create a centrally held database to free from data abuse
Morley et al. [22]	South Korea, UK, Australia	Authors sought ethical justification of mobile contact tracing applications. Provided four principles of contact tracing applications; necessary, proportional, scientifically valid, and time bound
Park [23]	Singapore	The article discusses the usefulness of using smart phone applications, data analytics, and artificial intelligence in finding and treating people with infection
Martinez et al. [16]	United states and Europe	Evaluated safety and effectiveness of software-based technology implemented to safeguard public health
Vaughan [24]	Singapore	Discusses Trace together application (developed by Govt. of Singapore). Article highlights the issues of using contact tracing applications
Evans [25]	USA	Development of Apollo application with the features of testing diagnostic checks, locating closest available testing center, ease for frontline health workers to scan data through car window
Economist, April 2020	Italy, Denmark	Highlights activities of governments initiating medical testing leveraging mobile phone applications to narrow down the testing sphere

(continued)

Table 1 (continued)

Technology: mobile applications		
Source	Country of study	Description
Imran et al. [26]	USA	The authors proposed and tested an artificial intelligence (AI)-powered screening solution for COVID-19 infection that is deployable via a smartphone application. The application is called AI4COVID-19. It records the sound of cough, sends to AI engine, and produces the results in two seconds
Fava [27]	USA	The paper highlights the use of mobile applications for remote/virtual treatment success specially when in person patient treatment is
Park et al. [28]	South Korea	Authors report South Korean trace, test, and treat strategy enabled by data collected through mobile phones
Trevisan et al. [29]	Vietnam	Government of Vietnam has made it mandatory for people to download and declare their health status through a mobile app—NCOVI. The application has successful in detecting high-risk cases
Ferretti et al. [19]	USA	Contributed the mathematical model to support the contact tracing mobile applications as a great help to reduce the number of cases
Garg et al. [30]	India	Authors discuss the scope and advantages of Participatory disease surveillance application (PDA), AarogyaSetu in India's digitally isolated population and scarce healthcare resources
Coyne and Jennings [31]	Australia	Australian Government finds it imperative to develop an application as the passport for Australians, also to resume businesses application is required for safety

places such as trains and airports to identify people with high temperature. For more precision and accuracy, there are CT scan recognition technologies which can accurately distinguish between patients with COVID-19 and ill due to other problems. Further, Martinez et al. [16] report that several funded projects exploring and advancing AI transformative potential for society are underway in USA, they are working on creating proteins to deter SARA—CoV-2, search of best materials to be used in designing of face masks, privacy first approach in contact tracing mobile applications, overcoming manufacturing and supply hurdles to ensure global access of COVID-19 vaccine, finding better ways to treat COVID-19 patients on ventilators. Researchers like [33] have conducted a study in which they proposed that data collected from individuals basic travel history is much valuable for machine learning algorithms to predict the infection risk of people. This further helps in identifying cases which require to be quarantined. Authors suggested that the use of AI and data sharing helps in better management of public health during COVID-19 pandemic. Multiple benefits can be obtained through this technology in case AI is integrated with cameras installed in cities for rapid detection of outbreak. Figure 9 presents the word tree of artificial intelligence and COVID-19. Table 2 outlines recent research endeavors for the use of AI to fight virus.

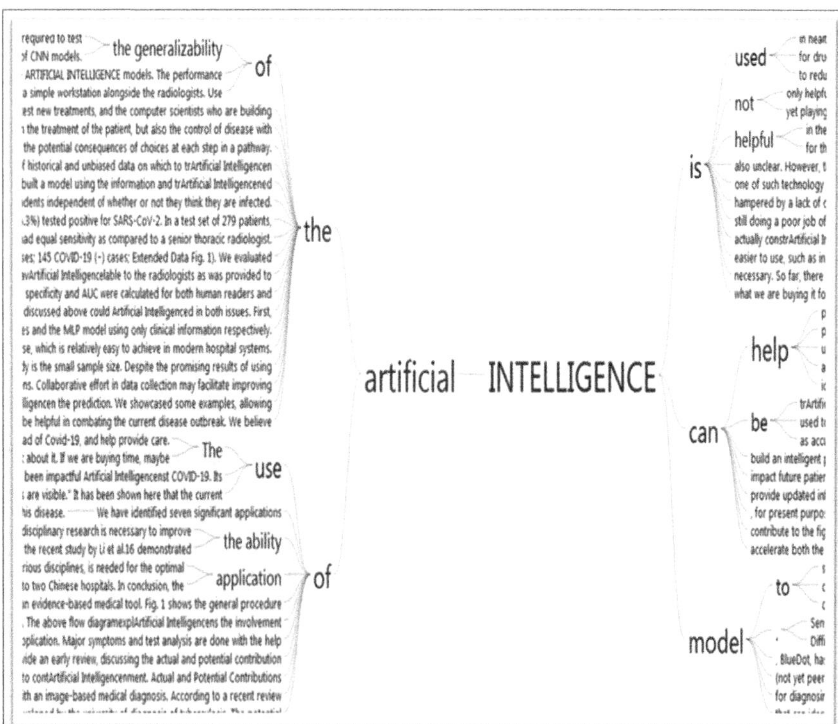

Fig. 9 Word tree of artificial intelligence application in COVID-19

Table 2 Literature review on artificial intelligence and COVID-19

Technology: artificial intelligence		
Source	Country of study	Description
Niazkar and Niazkar [34]	Iran	Authors explain multi-gene genetic programming (MGGP) as one of the artificial intelligence models to predict COVID-19 outbreak. The study suggests the development of a country-based prediction model
Pressman [12]	USA	The article reports on the use of artificial intelligence to identify and predict the spread of contagious diseases. It mentions the identification of the corona virus outbreak with the use of computer algorithms
Cohen [13]	Illinois, USA	The Article reports an artificial intelligence enabled nurse triage hotline to direct people to the medical facilities.
Shachar et al. [35]	New York, USA	Ethical implementation of artificial intelligence surveillance by physicians, public health officials, and technology companies
Vaishya et al. [36]	India	There are multiple uses of artificial intelligence. The authors have identified seven significant applications of AI for COVID-19 pandemic
Drozdiak et al. (2020)	USA	Article reports the use of biometric identification and face recognition software for diagnosis and containment
Srinivasa and Vazquez [37]	Georgia, USA	Authors propose a use of machine learning algorithm to reduce the cases of infection. They report artificial intelligence framework using mobile survey
Salman [38]	Palestine	Authors developed a model for early detection, diagnosis, and treatment of COVID-19 cases. Also helping frontline radiologists in hospitals by relieving their pressure
Nguyen [39]	USA	Author suggests ways to combat COVID-19 through artificial intelligence

IoT-enabled technologies have good results and have great potential to identify the cases, reduce the spread and eliminate the pandemic. As posited by Mishra [40] IoT devices can be used in healthcare sector by healthcare professionals ensuring their own safety by reducing direct contact with infected. Citing Wuhan Wuchang Smart Field Hospital, author explains the combination of AI and IoT used by this hospital, robots and IoT devices are being used in providing assistance like monitoring temperature, disinfecting surfaces, providing food, and medicines to isolated patients. Further, as per McKinley [41] IoT-enabled monitoring systems produces real-time patient tracking data to ensure faster decision making which is crucial for containing a virus outbreak of such scale and gravity. Such smart systems assist healthcare providers, and they can do away with the need of carrying out tests and tracing the cases in densely populated urban settlements. Srinivasa and Vazquez [37] suggested the combination of IoT and AI framework that can assess individuals and categorize them into no risk, minimal risk, moderate risk, and high risk groups. The high-risk cases found can then be isolated earlier, thus decreasing the chance of spreading the virus. A much detailed view of IoT applications during COVID-19 to healthcare sector has been contributed by Singh [6], the authors have earmarked some of the important applications of IoT, like hospitals connectivity with Internet allows integration of networks that enable a quick response of staff to patients, automated response to treatment, patients consultation through telecom, automated process of treatment, application installation in smart phones to identify COVID-19 patients, rapid screening, IoT connectivity of all medical tools and devices to deliver real-time information during treatment, accurate virus forecast. A most successfully used application of IoT with evidence of favorable results is reported by Tropea and Rango [42] in Italy, in the troubling current pandemic situation as in the month of March the number of infected people increased exponentially, which raised the need for organized IoT-enabled facility in the country. IoT being an innovative technology to fight COVID-19 pandemic can fulfill significant challenges when the whole country is in lock down state. Technology helped in capturing real-time data and other necessary information of infected patients. IoT captured health data from various locations of the infected patients and utilized virtual management system to manage. This technology helps control the data and follow up on the report attained. Furthermore, IoT had also been used to serve the purposes in public health-care system's domains like Internet of healthcare things (IoHT) or Internet of medical things (IoMT). After following up the procedures and guidelines of the facilities equipped with IoHT/IoMT, the number of resolved cases can be alleviated. Another study [43] is a step ahead in this context, authors posited turning IoT-enabled virtual assistant into emergency response system. The technology is useful for population who are not internet and techno users, therefore attaching virtual assistant (VA) to IoT brings together smart Internet-enabled objects to remind and alert people. Clubbing together of household items with VA can help grown-up people with shopping, they can find out the shortage of supplies beforehand and may organize deliveries with local stock, reducing the need for overstocking and undersupply. These could be altered at times of emergency to reflect social needs. If virtual assistant can be installed all through like homes, residential complexes, hospitals, educational institutes, shopping malls, etc., then in the situation of COVID-19 and other emergency situations, this combination of VA and IoT is capable of providing rich information. The technology of IoT serves various useful purposes in COVID times, its usage effectiveness is proved in public health departments, general public and patients. The combinations of technologies like artificial intelligence and IoT have the potential to bring revolutionary changes at the time when world is battling a non-curable and hard to prevent disease. Various applications of this technology are already being implemented and used at most parts of the world with new developments and advancements opening the doors for more opportunities. IoT technology helps to prevent and limit the spread of the virus by its efficiency in getting the work done with zero physical touch and contact. It can be thus concluded that IoT in COVID is not a luxury rather a necessity. Figure 10 presents software generated word tree of IoT and its applications (Table 3 and 4).

The infection rate is rapidly rising in most part of the world. India still has upward trend with respect to per day infection rate. The cases and their data have created a vital source of information, and this big data can be used for prediction and understanding the nature of virus. The data can be reused for developing future preventive methods. The big data regarding the number of people infected, recovered and expired provides massive amount of information to the scientists, health workers, epidemiologists so as to enable them to make informed decision to fight with the COVID-19 virus [54]. The data can be used effectively to track the virus globally as well as it continuously

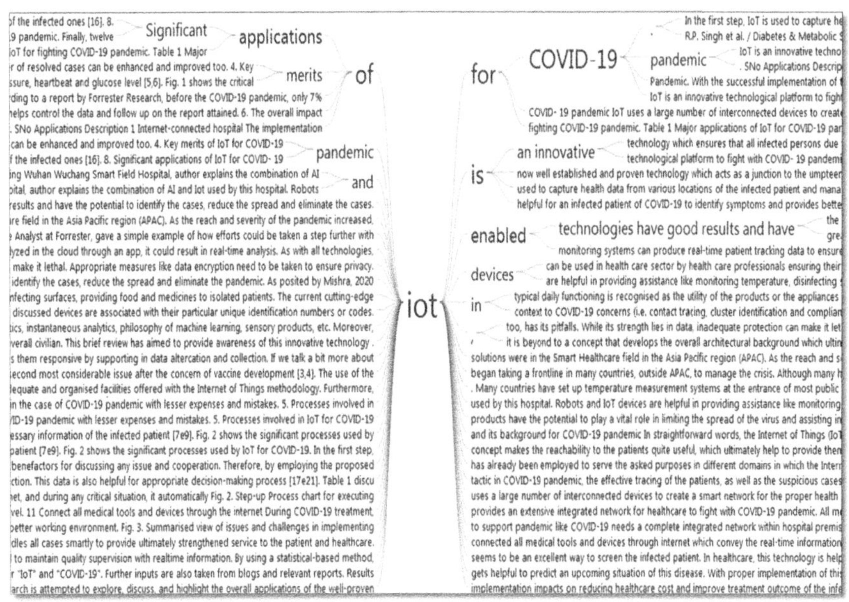

Fig. 10 Word tree of Internet of things (IoT) applications in COVID-19

Table 3 Literature review on IoT and COVID-19

Technology: Internet of Things (IoT) advantage		
Source	Country of study	Description
Srinivasa [37]	India	Suggested the categorization of individuals in low risk, moderate risk, and high risk zones through a device enabled by AI and IoT technologies
Allam and Jones [33]	USA	Authors contributed the usefulness of online collection of data from people so as to develop an AI algorithm for early detection and COVID cases
Singh [6]	India	The authors have outlines some very important applications of IoT for handling the pandemic
Yang [44]	China	The study has combined IoT with medical diagnostic. Elaborating the role of IoT in healthcare to manage patients
Mishra [40]	India	Explains the usage of IoT devices in healthcare sector for the safety of healthcare service providers during COVID-19
Wang et al. [45]	China	Authors propose the use of social Internet of things (SIoT) to suppress the infected cases
Chamola et al. [46]	India	Authors presented a comprehensive review of the COVID-19 pandemic and the role of IoT, drones, AI, block chain and 5G in managing its impact
Otoom et al. [47]	Jordan, Canada	Development of an IoT- enabled framework for COVID-19 control consisting of data collection, isolation, data analysis, and interface to health physician
Siripongdee et al. [48]	Thailand	This qualitative research analyzes and synthesizes model of blended learning (BL) with IoT technology. Authors used analysis and create tables with content analysis model
Swayamsiddha and Mohanty [49]	India	Authors generated CIoMT cognitive Internet of Medical Things. It is a disruptive technology providing real-time medical data of infected people. It also helps in contact tracing, clustering and screening, surveillance, thereby reducing workload of medical industry

Table 4 Literature review on big data and COVID-19

Technology: big data analytics		
Source	Country of Study	Description
Pham et al. [50]	South Korea	Paper provides researchers and communities with new insights into the ways AI and big data improves the COVID-19 situation, and drives further studies in stopping the COVID-19 outbreak
Wu et al. [51]	China	Article reports the use of big data technology in contain, prevent and control Corona virus.
Haleem et al. [52]	India	Big data can be used to the advantage of medical science which can track the cases at global level and innovation to medical field
Wang et al. [53]	Taiwan	Authors have highlighted the usage of big data analytics in Taiwan to combat COVID-19. The insurance data has been leveraged in Taiwan to identify cases

creates innovation in the medical field [52]. A report by Berman [2] explains the central role of big data application as Taiwan's strategy to contain the spread of virus. As corona virus-infected huge population of China, Taiwan as a neighboring country sensed the danger because each day there were many flights connected main island to China. A considerably large population of Taiwanese people is employed in China. Taiwan used technology and a robust pandemic action plan to combat COVID-19 and for minimizing virus impact in its land. Their strategy integrated national health insurance database with data from its immigration and customs database. The centralized use of data enabled the prediction of infected. They could manage to get real-time alerts related to infection possibility of an individual based upon symptoms and travel history. Additionally, the classification of traveler's infection risk was predicted by scanning and online reporting of travel and health symptoms which helped in classification of infection risk. Toll-free hotlines were also placed for citizens to report suspicious symptoms. Quick Taiwan's response with utilization of big data technology can be attributed to lower rate of infection than others despite their closeness to China. In Fig. 11, the word tree depicts the uses and various applications of data for reducing the infection of virus. The advantages of big data have also been pointed out at the University of Oxford's Big Data Institute. A study from the institute suggests advantages of mobile application that could provide valuable data for an integrated corona virus control strategy.

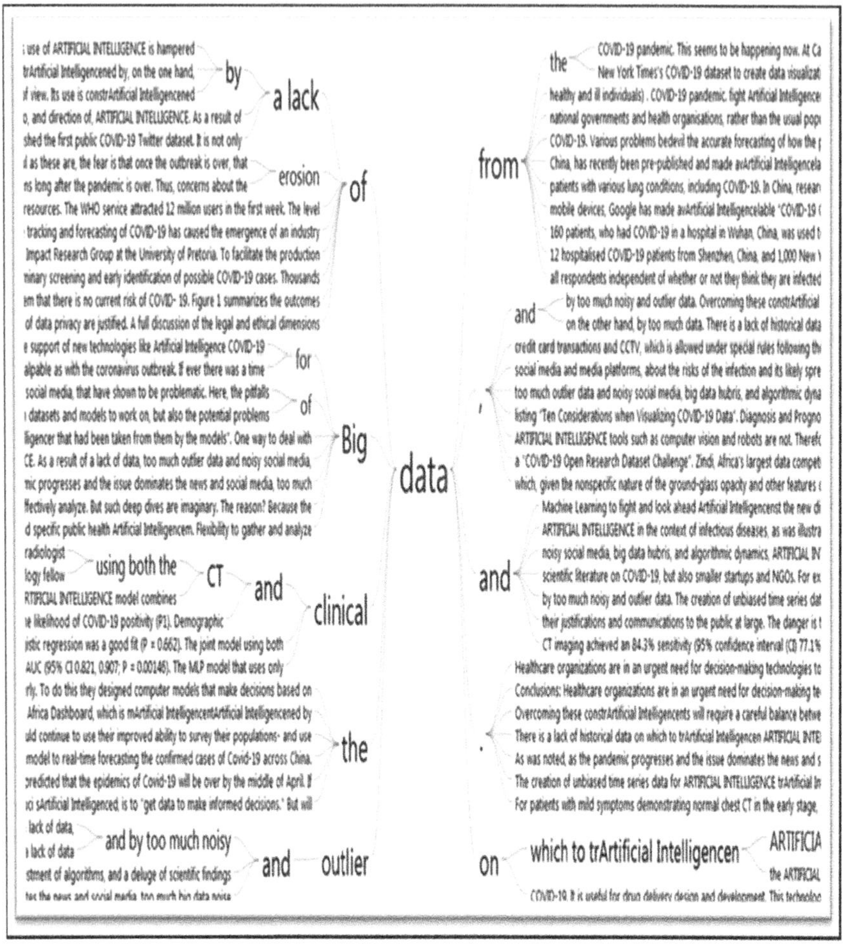

Fig. 11 Word tree of data usage in COVID-19

3.3 *Social Media and COVID*

As per a statement of Director General of WHO—Tedros Adhanom, "the battle of COVID-19 is also a battle against—trolls and conspiracy theories." A lot of misinformation is present on the social media platforms about corona virus which creates confusion and spread fear and anxiety. The misinformation is more contagious than the virus [55]. Therefore, it is required to disseminate correct information so as to have an environment free from fear. At the same time such a situation of pandemic, digital platform of social media is capable of dealing with all misconceptions. In this endeavor big corporate, Google and Facebook after understanding the severity of matter have tried to completely rule out misinformation by changing the algorithms. They have placed lie detectors in an effort to only promote placement of legitimate information on digital platform. Social media also serves as a medium to provide timely communication to public in crisis situation. To this end, Sheehan [56] added providing correct information through digital platform is one major role of social media plays in the crisis. Digital world provides an introduction to crisis communication theories and management. Authorities can use various social media platforms (e.g., Facebook and Twitter) for providing real-time updates and clarification of doubts. In Singapore, the government has partnered with WhatsApp to allow public to receive accurate information about COVID-19 and government initiatives. There is big responsibility of social media in the current pandemic situation; it has the potential to provide rapid and effective dissemination routes for key information. Researchers have also suggested correcting misconceptions about health through social media involving timely expert advice, public health awareness programs, and correction programs. There should be regular communication among general people. The word tree in Fig. 12 presents the uses of social media in COVID-19.

Table 5 summarizes the uses and concerns regarding social media in pandemic as expressed in extant literature.

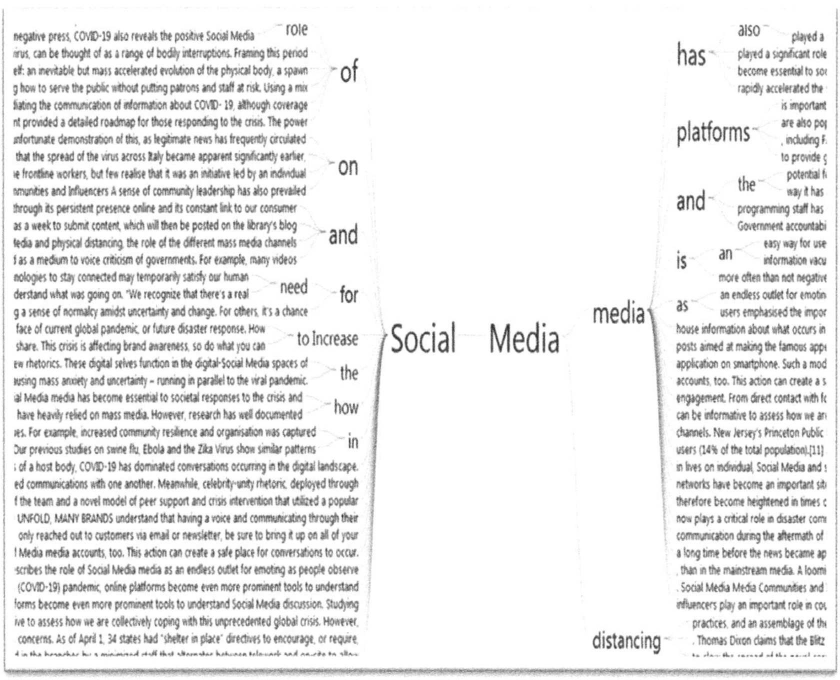

Fig. 12 Word tree of social media usage in COVID-19

Table 5 Literature on social media and COVID-19

Technology: social media		
Source	Country of Study	Description
Pennycook et al. [57]	USA	Authors tried to figure out the tendency of people for sharing misinformation about COVID-19 on social media
Gao et al. [58]	China	Authors assess the prevalence of metal health problems and examine their association with social media exposure. It is suggested in findings that government needs to pay more attention on mental health problems like anxiety and depression
Depoux et al. [59]		Authors raise the need for development of a real-time information sharing system. Utilizing multiple social media platforms in multiple languages across the globe to enhance the ability of public health bodies
Alington et al. [60]	UK	Authors posited that when unregulated social media messages may pose a health risk that is partly but not completely reducible to health related conspiracy beliefs
Zhao et al. [61]	China	Authors asserted that social media platform can immensely help government and public health departments to communicate on health-related issues and translate health needs into practice to create targeted measure for prevention and control of COVID-19
Qin et al. [62]	China	Authors collected social media search Index (SMSI) for dry cough, fever, chest distress for a period of three months. The lagged series of SMSI predicted new suspected COVID-19 case numbers during this period
Llewellyn [63]	Britain	The article gives a word to caution about following rumors and stories on social media in the pandemic situation. It highlights the ripple effect being produced related to one news on social media and its consequences
Ahmad [64]	Iraq	Majority of youth in Iraq are facing psychological anxiety. Authors found a significant positive statistical correlation between self-reported social media use and the spread of panic related to COVID-19
Machado et al. [65]	Brazil	Authors have highlighted the usefulness of social media/ telemedicine services during pandemic when physical contact is prohibited

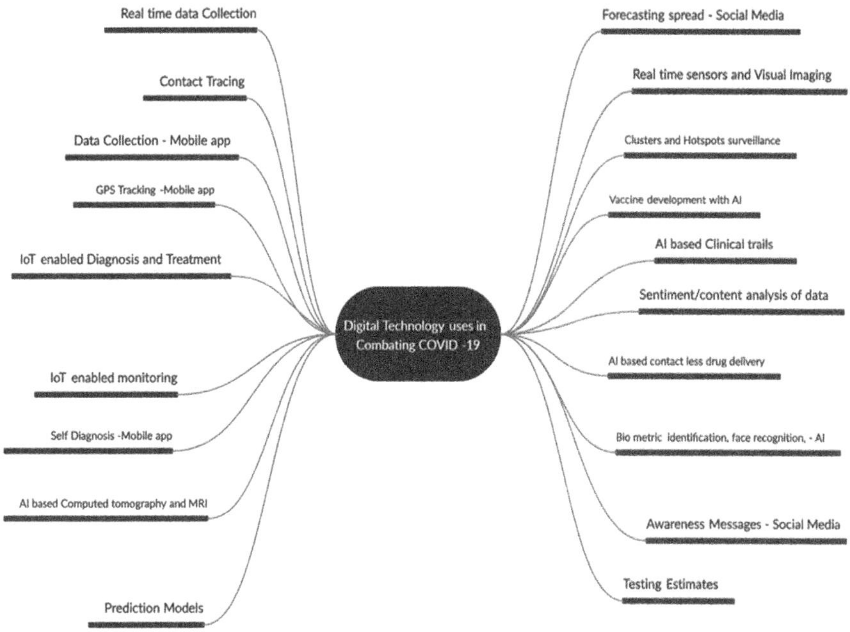

Fig. 13 Digital technologies application and COVID-19

4 Summarization of Digital Technology Applications and COVID-19

This section summarizes and derives the most significant applications of afore mentioned various digital technologies. It is obtained by careful analysis of all above software generated word trees in various sections of this study. Presented in Fig. 13 as.

5 Process Model of Integrated Digital Technology

A detailed analysis of the current literature and with the results obtained from qualitative data software, the study presents a process model of integrated digital technology as shown in Fig. 14; this explains usage of all technologies in a form of a process. Its usage is intended to be adapted by policy-makers in cities planning to develop a robust technology wall against the spread of fatal COVID-19.

The step-wise process is as explained below:

1. Technology for Control—This step identifies all digital technologies which can be instrumental in the control of COVID-19. As discussed in the sections above of the study, it is evident from the literature reviewed as well as output obtained

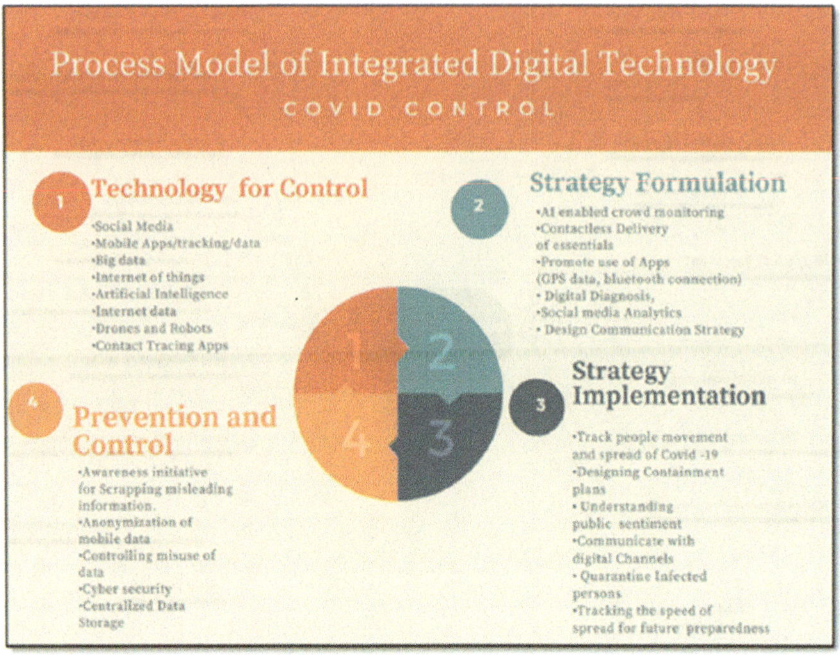

Fig. 14 Process model of integrated digital technology. *Source* Compiled by Author

from (computer-aided qualitative data analysis software (CAQDAS) that the technologies, viz. social media, mobile applications, big data analytics (data generated through mobile app/any other source), Internet of things (IoT), artificial intelligence, contact tracing applications, drones, and robots have great potential in deterring the spread of virus. The use of technology can be planned as per the requirement. For instance, installation of contact tracing application by majority of city/state/country population is to know the need for quarantine, treatment, or diagnosis. The usage of IoT and artificial intelligence is to find out the cases of infection among a larger crowd. Big data is capable of predicting the speed and volume of virus spread. Social media—In a stressful virus stricken environment, the condition gets further aggravated with a lot of threatening, baseless misinformation. Social media can be used as a medium to by authorities, public health departments, government officials to notify general public the facts about virus, simultaneously bursting the myths and rumors. There should be regular public health awareness and corrections programs through these mediums.

2. Strategy Formulation—This phase consists of planning the specific strategy with the use of a particular technology as per the case and need. Most of the countries around the globe have started unlocking, public places are allowed to be visited by general public, crowd has started gathering at transportation facilities like airports. Individual manual detection of cases seems a gigantic task. In such

a scenario, planning of installing AI enabled fever detecting cameras has the potential of mass screening to locate individuals with high infection risk. Due to pandemic, delivery of essentials in high risk areas can be envisaged through AI- and IoT-powered drones to enable contact less delivery. Social media analytics is yet another powerful tool in COVID-19 to identify the source of misinformation, velocity in which the piece of content is shared and its impact. The knowledge of same is helpful in planning of implementation measures to eradicate the misinformation.

3. Strategy Implementation—In this stage, all the designed strategies regarding decreasing the spread of virus, treatment, publishing liable, valid news/messages in public domain are executed. This entails tracking people's movement through drones and cameras, designing containment plans, understanding public sentiments, thereby communicating reliable information through digital channels, quarantine infected person—as per the information received from data, mobile applications, infrared cameras in public places, tracking the speed, and spread for future preparedness. Effective implementation of all such strategies requires the scale of coordination and management of digital data. Integration of digital technology in public and health care should be adopted.
4. Prevention and Control—All the discussed digital technologies in this study can be attached to COVID-19 control and prevention to help in preparation of future pandemics. However, there are concerns raised about collection of large public data and its privacy; recently, many countries have developed mobile applications which collect location data by global positioning system or cellular networks. Through Bluetooth proximity data is being collected. Decentralized data storage threats the security and may lead to its misuse; therefore, centralized storage of data is the measure adopted by many countries. *Anonymization* of data is another measure which can be adopted to maintain data privacy.

6 Conclusion

COVID-19 has impacted the lives of millions of people all over the globe. All the countries in the world are affected because of 2020 pandemic. With little knowledge of this newly formed pathogen, medical field has failed to provide any immediate solution to alleviate the infection rate. However, the advancement of digital technology and development of multiple digital tools can be leveraged to combat COVID-19 outbreak. Latest digital technologies are being used to sustain people's health as a response to rapidly growing virus infection worldwide. As discussed in the sections above, it includes population surveillance, infected person identification/contact tracing, utilization of large data generated through mobile phones/applications, etc., thereby evaluating suitable interventions before finalizing implementation. This study develops an integrated model with the help of CAQDAS and rich extant literature. Qualitative research provides a robust methodology to draw meaningful inferences and connections in existing theories and concepts. In the last two decades, qualitative research is used more frequently in social sciences and becoming widely accepted across a range of other disciplines. With the development and advancement of CAQDAS, qualitative research will grow exponentially in years to come. There is a consistent rise in the reporting of qualitative research studies. It is a vigorous, instinctual, and creative method of inductive research helpful in reasoning, thinking, and theorizing. The process of analyzing qualitative data in this research mostly involved coding or categorizing the data, followed by identification of patterns and subsequently building a model. Following the same, the model created in the current study is with the aim to help in formulating a strategy to fight COVID-19 with the use of digital technology. This can be seen as one of the main advantages that we have today for fighting corona virus that wasn't there in earlier times when the world was in similar situation (SARS outbreak). The technologies were there but not as advanced and sophisticated as they are today. As the virus spreads through the world, strategies used for its containment are all types of digital tools—big data, machine learning, artificial intelligence and IoT. Many counties today have engaged technology usage as their main stream strategy to control virus. China is leading the world with exploring these technologies first. The understanding gained, lessons learnt, and technology breakthroughs will continue to spread across the world. Countries are developing real-time forecasts to equip healthcare sector for developing the insights to predict the impact of virus. There is now a wide range of digital technologies that can be used as full blown strategies for improvement and enhancement in public health. The acceptance of digital tools by government and public to tackle this major global public health challenge of 2020 has increased manifold. Therefore, the model proposed in present research finds its place as a step-wise procedure for implementation. The model suggested is a framework for the application of digital technologies in current time as well as in the future for pandemic management, planning, surveillance, testing, prevention, and control. As the saying goes "crisis provides an opportunity," this great crisis of 2020 provides a great opportunity for digital technologies.

References

1. Verhoef, P. C., & Bijmolt, T. H. A. (2020). Marketing perspectives on digital business models: A framework and overview of the special issue. *International Journal of Research in Marketing, 36*(3), 341–349.
2. Berman, B. (2016). Planning and implementing effective marketing programs. *Business Horizons, 59*(4), 431–439. https://doi.org/10.1016/j.bushor.2016.03.006
3. De Haan, E., Wiesel, T., & Pauwels, K. (2016). The effectiveness of different forms of online advertising for purchase conversion in a multiple-channel attribution framework. *International Journal of Research in Marketing, 33*(3), 491–507. https://doi.org/10.1016/j.ijresmar.2015.12.001
4. Goldschmidt, K. (2020). The COVID-19 pandemic: Technology use to support the wellbeing of children, Elsevier public health emergency collection, Published online April 2020, 16. https://doi.org/10.1016/j.pedn.2020.04.013

5. Gordon, J. (2007). The mobile phone and the public sphere mobile phone usage in three critical situations. *The International Journal of Research into New Media Technologies, 13*(3), 307–319.
6. Singh, R. P., Javid, M., Haleem, A., & Suman, R. (2020). Internet of things (IoT) applications to fight against COVID-19 pandemic. *Diabetes & Metabolic Syndrome: Clinical Research & Reviews, 14*(4), 521–524.
7. Torous, J., Myrick, K., Rauseo- Ricupero, N., & Firth, J. (2020). Digital mental health and COVID-19: Using technology today to accelerate the curve on access and quality tomorrow. *JMIR Mental Health, 7*(3), e18848. https://doi.org/10.2196/18848
8. Ting, D. S. W., Carin, L., Dzau, V., et al. (2020). Digital technology and COVID-19. *Nature Medicine, 26*, 459–461
9. Pan, X. (2020). Application of personal-oriented digital technology in preventing transmission of COVID-19. China. *Irish Journal of Medical Science.*
10. Kupferschmidt, K., & Cohen, J. (2020). Can China's COVID-19 strategy work elsewhere? *Science, 367*(6482), 1061–1062
11. Hutson, M. (2020, June). *Artificial Intelligence tools aim to tame the corona virus literature.* Technology feature. https://www.nature.com/articles/d41586-020-01733-7
12. Pressman, A. (2020). Bringing A.I. to the coronavirus fight. *Fortune, 181*(4), 23–24.
13. Cohen, J. P., Morrison, P., Lan, D., Roth, K., Duong, T. Q., & Ghassemi, M. (2020). *COVID-image data collection: Prospective predictions are the future.* https://arxiv.org/abs/2006.11988, eprint= 2006.11988.
14. Chan, A., Nickson, C. P., Rudolph, J. W., Lee, A., & Joynt, G. M. (2020). Social media for rapid knowledge dissemination: Early experience from the COVID-19 pandemic. *Anaesthesia.* https://doi.org/10.1111/anae.15057
15. Cuilian, L., Jia, C. L., Xueyu, C., Mingzhi, Z., Pui, P. C., & Haoyu, C. (2020). Retrospective analysis of the possibility of predicting the COVID-19 outbreak from Internet searches and social media data, China, 2020. *Eurosurveillance, 25*(10).
16. Martinez, M. N., Wieten, S., Magnus, D., & Cho, M. K. (2020). Digital contact tracing, privacy, and public health. *Hastings Center Report, 50*(3), 43–46
17. Tibbetts, J. H. (2020). Researchers continue quest to contain spread of COVID-19: Digital technologies aim to accelerate contact tracing. *Bio Science, XX*, 1–7.
18. Parker, M. J., Fraser, C., Abeler-Dörner, L., & Bonsall, D. (2020). Ethics of instantaneous contact tracing using mobile phone apps in the control of the COVID-19 pandemic. *Journal of Medical Ethics, 46*, 427–431
19. Ferretti, L., Wymant, C., Kendall, M., Zhao, L., Nurtay, A., Abeler-dörner, L., Parker, M., Bonsall, D., & Fraser, C. (2020). Quantifying SARS-CoV-2 transmission suggests epidemic control with digital contact tracing. *Science, 368*(6491).
20. WHO. (2020, May 13). *Launch of the WHO Academy and the WHO Info mobile applications.* https://www.who.int/news-room/detail/13-05-2020-launch-of-the-who-academy-and-the-who-info-mobile-applications
21. Whitaker, P. (2020). The NHS app has been abandoned but no app is necessary to trace government ineptitude. *New Statesman, 149*(5526), 9
22. Morley, J., Cowls, J., Taddeo, M., & Floridi, L. (2020). *Ethical guidelines for COVID-19 tracing apps* (p. 582). Springer Nature Limited.
23. Park, A. (2020). Preventing the next pandemic. *TIME Magazine, 195*(11), 40–43.
24. Vaughan, A. (2020). The problems with contact-tracing apps. *New Scientist, 246*(3279), 9.
25. Evans, J. (2020). Apple design Award winner launches iPhone app to improve COVID-19 testing. *Computerworld.*
26. Imran, A., Posokhova, I., Qureshi, H. N., Masood, U., Riaz, S, Ali, K., John, C. N., Hussain, I., & Nabeel, M. A. (2020). COVID-19: AI enabled preliminary diagnosis for COVID-19 from cough samples via an app, Informatics in Medicine Unlocked.
27. Fava, G. A. (2020). The decline of pluralism in medicine: Dissent is welcome. *Psychotherapy and Psychosomatics, 89*(1), 1–5. https://doi.org/10.1159/000505085

28. Park, S., Choi, G. J., & Ko, H. (2020). Information technology-based tracing strategy in response to COVID-19 in South Korea—Privacy controversies. *JAMA, 323*(21), 2129–2130
29. Trevisan, M., Cu Le, L., & Vu Le, A. (2020). The COVID-19 pandemic: A view from Vietnam. *American Journal of Public Health, 110*(8), 1152–1153.
30. Garg, S., Bhatnagar, N., & Gangadharan, N. (2020). A case for participatory disease surveillance of the COVID-19 pandemic in India. *JMIR Public Health and Surveillance, 6*(2), e18795.
31. Coyne, J., & Jennings, P. (Eds.). (2020). After Covid-19: Australia and the world rebuild. *Australian Strategic Policy Institute, 1*, 3–59. https://doi.org/10.2307/resrep25138.5
32. Rahman, A., & Sathi, N. J. (2020). Knowledge, attitude and preventive practices towards COVID-19 among Bangladeshi Internet users. *Electronic Journal of General Medicine, 17*(5), 1–6.
33. Allam, Z., & Jones, D. S. (2020, March). On the corona virus (COVID-19) outbreak and the smart city network: Universal data sharing standards coupled with Artificial intelligence (AI) to benefit urban health monitoring and management. *Healthcare, 8*(1), 46.
34. Niazkar, M., & Niazkar, H. R. (2020). COVID-19 Outbreak: Application of Multi-gene Genetic Programming to Country-based Prediction Models. Electronic Journal of General Medicine, 17(5), em247. https://doi.org/10.29333/ejgm/8232
35. Shachar, C. Gerke, S. Adashi, E.Y (2020) AI Surveillance during Pandemics: Ethical Implementation Imperatives. The Hastings centre report. 50 (2) : 18 - 21
36. Vaishya, R., Javaid, M., Ibrahim, H. M., & Haleem, A. (2020). Artificial Intelligence (AI) applications for COVID-19 pandemic. *Diabetes & Metabolic Syndrome. Clinical Research & Reviews, 14*(4), 337–339.
37. Srinivasa, A. S. R., & Vazquez, J. A. (2020). Identification of COVID-19 can be quicker through artificial intelligence framework using a mobile phone–based survey when cities and towns are under quarantine. *Infection Control & Hospital Epidemiology, 41*, 826–830. https://doi.org/10.1017/ice.2020.61
38. Salman, F. M., Abu-Naser, S. S., Alajrami, E., Abu-Nasser, B. S., & Ashqar, B. A. M. (2020). COVID-19 detection using artificial intelligence. *International Journal of Academic Engineering Research, 4*(3), 18–25.
39. Nguyen, T. (2020). Artificial intelligence in the battle against corona virus (COVID-19): A survey and future research directions. https://doi.org/10.13140/RG.2.2.36491.23846/1
40. Mishra, S. (2020, June). *The growing role of IoT in COVID-19 response.* https://www.iotforall.com/the-growing-role-of-iot-in-covid-19-response.
41. Mckinley, J. (2020). IoT & mobile apps: How it can help in preventing Covid-19. *The IoT Magazine*, May 11.
42. Tropea, M., & Rango, F. D. (2020). COVID-19 in Italy: Current state, impact and ICT-based solutions. *IET Smart Cities, 2*(2), 74–81. https://doi.org/10.1049/iet-smc.2020.0052
43. Sheerman, L., Marston, H. R., Mussel, W. C., & Morgan, D. (2020). COVID-19 and the secret virtual assistants: The social weapons for a state of emergency. *Emerald Open Research, 2*(19). https://doi.org/10.35241/emeraldopenres.13571.1
44. Yang, T., Gentile, M., Shen, C. F., & Cheng, C. M. (2020). Combining point-of-care diagnostics and internet of medical things (IoMT) to combat the COVID-19 pandemic. *Diagnostics*. https://doi.org/10.3390/diagnostics10040224
45. Wang, B., Sun, Y., Duong, T. Q., Nguyen, L. D., & Hanzo, L. (2020). Risk-aware identification of highly suspected COVID-19 cases in social IoT, a joint graph theory and reinforcement learning approach. *IEEE Access, 8*, 115655–115661. https://doi.org/10.1109/ACCESS.2020.3003750
46. Chamola, V., Hassija, V., Gupta, M., & Guizani, M. (2020). A comprehensive review of the COVID-19 pandemic and the role of IoT, drones, AI, block chain, and 5G in managing its impact. *IEEE Access, 8*, 90225–90265. https://doi.org/10.1109/ACCESS.2020.2992341
47. Otoom, M., Otoum, N., Alzubaidi, M. A., Etoom, Y., & Banihani, R. A. (2020). *IoT-based framework for early identification and monitoring of COVID-19 cases, biomedical signal processing and control.* Elsevier. https://doi.org/10.1016/j.bspc.2020.102149

48. Siripongdee, K., Pimdee, P., & Tuntiwongwanich, S. (2020). A blended learning model with IoT-based technology: Effectively used when the COVID-19 pandemic. *Journal for the Education of Gifted Young Scientists,* 8(2), 905–917. https://doi.org/10.17478/jegys.698869
49. Swayamsiddha, S., & Mohanty, C. (2020). Application of cognitive Internet of Medical Things for COVID-19 pandemic. *Diabetes & Metabolic Syndrome: Clinical Research & Reviews, 14*(5), 911–915.
50. Pham, Q. V., Nguyen, D. C., Huynh-Th, T., Hwang, W.-J., & Pathirana, P. (2020). Artificial Intelligence (AI) and big data for corona virus (COVID-19) pandemic. *A Survey on the State-of-the-Arts.* https://doi.org/10.13140/RG.2.2.23518.38727
51. Wu J, Wang J, Nicholas S, Maitland E, Fan Q (2020) Application of Big Data Technology for COVID-19 Prevention and Control in China: Lessons and Recommendations J Med Internet Res 2020;22(10):e21980 URL: https://www.jmir.org/2020/10/e21980 DOI: 10.2196/21980
52. Haleem, A., Javaid, M., Khan, I. H., & Vaishya, R. (2020). Significant applications of big data in COVID-19 pandemic. *Indian Journal of Orthopaedics, 54*(4), 1–3. https://doi.org/10.1007/s43465-020-00129-z.
53. Wang, C. J., Ng, C. Y., & Brook, R. H. (2020). Response to COVID-19 in Taiwan: Big data analytics, new technology, and proactive testing. *JAMA, 323*(14), 1341–1342. https://doi.org/10.1001/jama.2020.3151
54. Barnard, M. (2020, April). *The vital role of big data in the fight against COVID-19.* https://www.linkedin.com/pulse/vital-role-big-data-fight-against-covid-19-coronavirus-bernard-marr.
55. Sahni, H., & Sharma, H. (2020). Role of social media during the COVID-19 pandemic. Beneficial, destructive, or reconstructive? *International Journal of Academic Medicine, 6*, 70–5.
56. Sheehan, M., & Quinn-Allan, D. (2015). *Crisis communication in a digital world.* Cambridge University Press.
57. Pennycook, G., Mc Phetres, J., Zhang, Y., Lu, J. G., & Rand, D. G. (2020). Fighting COVID-19 misinformation on social media: Experimental evidence for a scalable accuracy-nudge intervention. *Psychological Science, 31*(7), 770–780.
58. Gao, J., Zheng, P., Jia, Y., Chen, H., & Mao, Y. (2020). Mental health problems and social media exposure during COVID-19 outbreak. *Plos One, 15*(4), e0231924.
59. Depoux, A., Martin, S., Karafillakis, E., Preet, R., Annelies, S., & Larson, H. (2020). The pandemic of social media panic travels faster than the COVID-19 outbreak. *Journal of Travel Medicine,* 27(3), 1–2.
60. Alington, D., Duffy, B., Wessely, S., Dhavan, N., & Rubin, J. (2020). Health-protective behaviour, social media usage and conspiracy belief during the COVID-19 public health emergency. *Psychological Medicine,* 1–7.
61. Zhao, Y., Cheng, S., Yu, X., & Xu, H. (2020). Chinese public's attention to the COVID-19 epidemic on social media. *Observational Descriptive Study JMIR Publications, 22*(5), e18825.
62. Qin, L., Sun, Q., Wang, Y., Wu, K. F., Chen, M., Shia, B. C., & Wu, S. Y. (2020). Prediction of number of cases of 2019 novel coronavirus (COVID-19) using social media search index. *International Journal of Environmental Research and Public Health, 17*, 2365
63. Llewellyn, S. (2020). Covid-19: How to be careful with trust and expertise on social media. *BMJ, 368*, 1160.
64. Ahmad, A. R., & Murad, H. R. (2020). The impact of social media on panic during the COVID-19 pandemic in Iraqi Kurdistan: Online questionnaire study. *Journal of Medical Internet Research, 22*(5), e19556.
65. Machado, R. A., de Souza, N. L., Oliveira, R. M., Martelli Júnior, H., & Bonan, P. (2020). Social media and telemedicine for oral diagnosis and counseling in the COVID-19 era. *Oral Oncology, 105*, 104685.

High-Fidelity Intelligence Ventilator to Help Infect with COVID-19 Based on Artificial Intelligence

Jamal Mabrouki, Mourade Azrour, Driss Dhiba, and Souad El Hajjaji

1 Introduction

COVID-19 refers to "coronavirus vector 2019", a virus of the Coronaviridae class, SARS-CoV-2. This contagious disease is a debated zoonosis that appeared in December 2019 in the city of Wu-han, Hubei Province, China. It spread rapidly, first throughout China and then abroad, causing a global epidemic. COVID-19 is a potentially fatal pulmonary disease in patients debilitated by age or other chronic disease. It is transmitted through close contact with infected individuals. The disease could also be passed on by asymptomatic patients, but there is no scientific evidence to demonstrate this with absolute confidence.

Respiratory infections and respiratory failure caused by injury are major public health problems in both developed and underdeveloped countries. Asthma, chronic obstructive lung disease (COPD) and other chronic respiratory diseases are very common. Air pollution, smoking and fuel biomass combustion have exacerbated these diseases, all of which are on the rise in developing countries [1].

J. Mabrouki (✉) · S. E. Hajjaji
Laboratory of Spectroscopy, Molecular Modeling, Materials, Nanomaterial, Water and Environment, CERN2D, Faculty of Science, Mohammed V University in Rabat, Avenue Ibn Batouta, BP1014 Agdal, Rabat, Morocco

S. E. Hajjaji
e-mail: souad.elhajjaji@um5.ac.ma

M. Azrour
Moulay Ismail University, Department of Computer Science, Faculty of Sciences and Techniques, IDMS Team, Errachidia, Morocco

D. Dhiba
International Water Research Institute IWRI, University Mohammed VI Polytechnic (UM6P), Benguerir, Morocco
e-mail: Driss.DHIBA@um6p.ma

M. Niranjanamurthy et al. (eds.), *Intelligent Data Analysis for COVID-19 Pandemic*, Algorithms for Intelligent Systems, https://doi.org/10.1007/978-981-16-1574-0_4

Patients with underlying lung disease will develop respiratory failure in a variety of situations and may benefit from mechanical ventilation. Such machines mechanically assist the patient to breathe in and out, allowing the exchange of oxygen and carbon dioxide in the lungs, a process known as artificial respiration [2]. This process is called artificial respiration [2]. Although the ventilators used in modern American hospitals are very advanced in terms of function and technology, their purchase costs are very high (up to US$30,000) [3]. The high cost of these machines and equipment makes them too technically complex, making them prohibitively expensive for resource-poor countries. In addition, they are generally fragile and easily damaged in continuous use, requiring expensive service contracts with manufacturers. In developing countries, this has led to practices such as sharing fans between hospitals and purchasing less reliable products in refurbished units. Because these countries' medical resources are concentrated in the centers of large cities, in some cases, mechanical ventilators cannot be used at all in rural and outlying areas [4].

Therefore, the most important issue is the need for low-cost transport fans. In developed countries with large medical centers, the nature of the problem is different. Although there are sufficient ventilators for normal use, preparations for large-scale casualties (such as influenza pandemics, natural disasters and large-scale releases of toxic chemicals) are inadequate. In developed countries, the cost of storing and deploying advanced mechanical ventilators for high casualty environments is prohibitive.

According to the National Pandemic Preparedness Plan released by President Bush in November 2005, the USA will require 742,500 fans in the worst-case pandemic scenario. Compared to the 100,000 currently in use, it is clear that the system is failing [5]. One example is the shortage that occurred during Hurricane Katrina, when the number of fans was less than 5 and staff was forced to rely on manual ventilation of MVB6. Since then, steps have been taken to increase preparedness, including the Centers for Disease Control and Prevention (CDC) recently purchased 4,500 portable emergency ventilators for the national stockpile [6]. However, due to the low number of ventilators in stock and limited availability, there is a need for an inexpensive portable ventilator that can be upgraded as needed.

2 Operating and Revision Modes

Patient treatment during COVID-19 faces serious problems of lung injury, and ventilators must be able to cope with rapid changes in lung compliance and the risk of collapse and fusion. The ventilator power is a key factor in patient prognosis [7]. Particularly, when using low tidal volume, drive pressure is a significant predictor of risk of death in hospital [8].

Due to the high importance of pressure monitoring, the HEV ventilator has a target pressure control mode. This includes PRVC control (pressure regulating), SIMV-PC mode (synchronized mandatory intermittent intermittent pressure release). There is also a basic mode of function: continuous positive airway pressure (CPAP). The design of HEVs also provides for end-of-life CPAP (CPAP), which is not a means of ventilation per se, but is designed to maintain a constant low positive airway pressure in the lungs. CPAP is the standard for commercial ventilation, used to regulate tidal volume at the low airway pressure. If the tidal volume is not obtained at a particular pressure setting due to changes in the patient's airway resistance or pulmonary compliance, the tidal volume can be adjusted incrementally. The SIMV-PC mode permits patients to take and assist breathing when they breathe spontaneously. This mode uses an auxiliary sensor to detect the negative pressure caused by the patient's breathing. If the respiratory rate of the patient does not reach the target value, use equipment to ventilate the patient [9].

Our ventilator will also have a basic non-invasive mode of operation that can provide a fixed pressure for the patient. Although the national definitions are not the same, they are consistent with the definition of CPAP in the literature [10, 11] from drug and health product regulatory agencies. PEP can be used in all modes of operating, which is important for patient management to avoid alveolar collapse. The design of the ventilator described here is not intended to replace the necessary high-end ventilator with the most intensive phase of treatment, but for mild symptoms or in-hospital care and rehabilitation, the ventilator should be appropriate and useful long.

3 Design and Condition of the Instrument

The system design makes patient safety a priority, so that any failure puts patient security at the forefront. In particularly, if the pressure maintenance stop mode is selected, the respiratory ventilator will automatically switch to ventilation mode, as shown in Fig. 1. The device uses as input standard pressurized air or mixed air

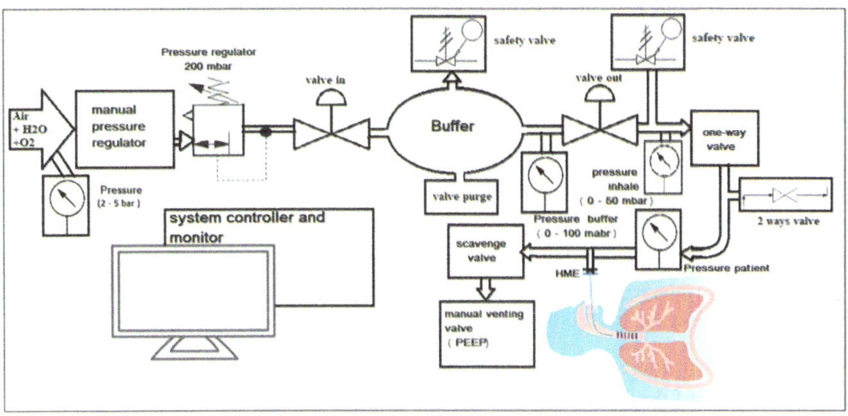

Fig. 1 Conceptual design ventilator

available in the input device. The supply pressure is generally expected to be between 2 and 5 bar. The connection to external I/O provided by the equipment will meet the standards of the hospital. The supply air pressure is reduced to approximately 200 mbar by a pressure regulator. The concept of the system is based on a buffer volume of about 2 L. The filling of the buffer is controlled by the water inlet valve (water inlet valve). By controlling the opening time, the desired target pressure in the buffer can be reached, and then, the valve (inlet valve) can be closed. This filling of the buffer occurs during the exhalation part of the breathing cycle. If the buffer is within the tolerance of the required pressure, the outlet valve is opened, thus initiating the breathing cycle. The breathing rhythm, inhalation time (corresponding to the breathing rhythm of the buffer) and breathing time (corresponding to the breathing rhythm of the buffer) are displayed as the valve opening time, and the pause time can be controlled. If the PEEP pressure is the lung pressure if defined, the lung pressure will be at least the PEEP pressure. We define P1 as the pressure in the buffer before the start of the aspiration cycle and P2 as the pressure in the buffer at the end of the aspiration cycle when the valve is closed. Then, the amount of air (tidal volume) inhaled by the patient can be calculated by knowing P1, P2 and the fixed amount of buffer and tubing.

During operation, all parameters are monitored. If the minute volume is below the programmed value, you can increase the pressure P1 in units of 1 to 2 mbar until the target minute volume is reached or the maximum permissible pressure is reached.

For the CPAP operating method, all valves are kept open and the manual setting of the regulator is set to a fixed low pressure. The safety valve can directly protect the patient from overpressure. The safety valve can open 80 cm of water column. In addition, the pressure sensor in the buffer memory (P buffer) also checks the overpressure. If the pressure in the buffer is too high, open the solenoid valve (valve outlet) to discharge the contents and refill it to the appropriate level. If the surge valve (valve closed) or the power supply fails, the two-way on/off valve will connect the patient to the atmosphere so that the patient can breathe without assistance. During the exhalation cycle, the purifier valve will open, allowing air in the lungs to flow to the purification system. The mechanical design will be based on this concept and will reach a unit size of approximately 500 × 500 × 350 mm. The size and location of the device are shown in Fig. 2.

Figure 3 shows the control concept based on the integrated controller, which receives signals from the captors and valves, and the touch screen interface with the clinician. The user interface includes an intuitive panel that displays the necessary information and executes commands dynamically and continuously. The commands and alarms described here are very preliminary and only give an idea of how the system works. They will appear during the prototyping phase. The display will include the following elements:

- Adjustment of the volume of the minutes of inspiration.
- Adjustment of the number of breaths per minute.
- Display of the tidal volume, based on the two previous parameters.
- Adjustment of the inspiration time.

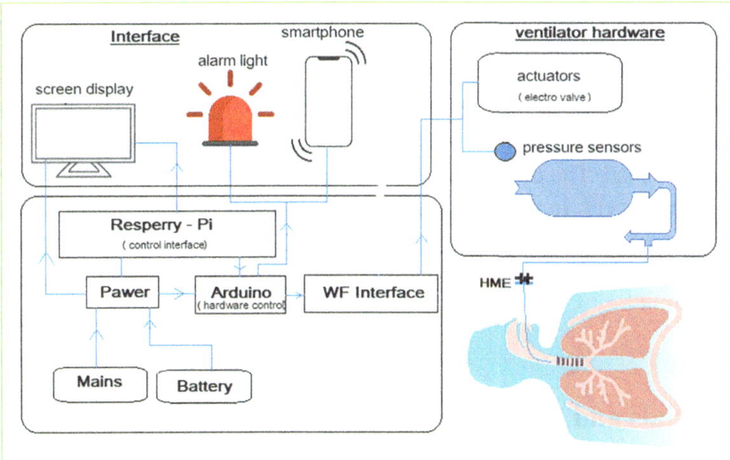

Fig. 2 Conceptual layout of the controls and interface

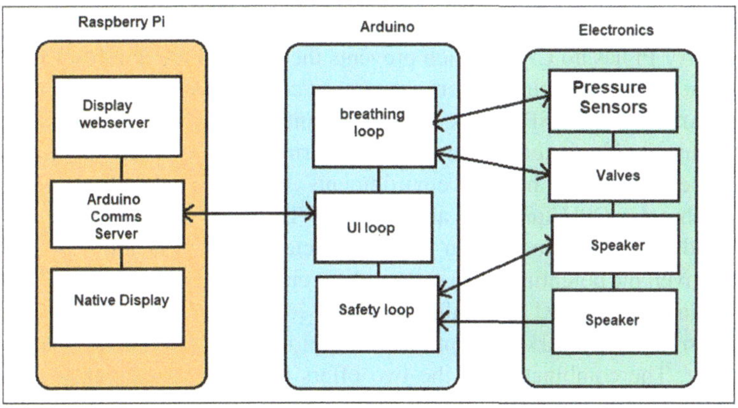

Fig. 3 Core software components and their interconnections

- Adjustment of the pause time.
- Display of expiration time based on the two previous parameters.
- Volume of elapsed minutes.
- Display of airway pressure based on P2 reading.
- PEEP setting.
- Trigger sensitivity to patient-triggered breathing.
- The following will be plotted as a continuous graphical display.
- Volume versus time.
- Pressure versus time.
- Flux versus temps.

HEV will pay particular attention to the MV Leak Alert, which is a standard alert in hospitals, but is essential for highly infectious diseases such as COVID-19, which can protect staff and patients. It will be very sensitive to trigger any leak in the circuit, which may be caused by a leaking balloon in the patient's airway, a disconnection or loose tubing. In the current version, the O_2 concentration is not measured, but is actively researched. The display format will be similar to a typical display seen in a hospital environment. In pressure maintenance mode, if the patient stops breathing, the ventilator will sound an alarm and enter forced ventilation. For all modes, if the respiratory rate or volume of breaths per minute is below an acceptable level, an alarm will sound.

4 Materials and Technology

A variety of solutions for onboard controllers are currently being studied, including Arduino, Framboise Pi and ESP32. Each has its advantages and limitations. Raspberry Pi offers a superior human–machine interface and graphics capabilities, as well as HDMI support for larger displays.

Raspberry Pi has no CAN, which prevents the use of some devices. On the plus side, the need for operating systems increases complexity, which reduces overall stability. Arduino and ESP32 have several variants of ADC and Wi-Fi features, but most graphical add-ons tend to have smaller form factors (5 inches or less), which may not be suitable for hospital environments. ESP32 is an Arduino-compatible device with extra CPU functions and memory. The supply of spare parts is under review, and availability may be an important determinant of technology choice. In addition, given the potential use in several different geographical locations, different variants can be developed to suit that location.

The current benchmark concept uses Arduino for control and Raspberry Pi for monitoring. The combination of the two offers the most functionality, and many developers already own one or two of these devices when working at home. If the platform needs to be changed, the code will be written on the handheld device.

4.1 Typical Parts Needed

For the mechanical structure, the objective is to use as many standardized parts as possible. A list of standard parts is included as follows:

- Solenoid valve with an internal diameter greater than 22 mm. This is the supposed patient supply hose diameter.
- Fast-acting electrovalve for air inlet to the buffer volume.
- Solenoid valve for ventilation. This can be a small volume which, in the event of overpressure, releases only a very small quantity of air.

- Buffer volume of 2 L.
- Pressure control from 2–5 bar to 200 mbar.
- Five pressure detectors.

4.2 Arduino Nano Compatible V3.0 ATmega328

The Arduino Nano is a small, a user-friendly and extensive table using the ATmega328. It has more or less the same characteristics as the Arduino Duemilanove, but in a different packaging. All that is missing is a DC power plug, and it works with a USB Mini-B cable instead of a standard cable [12] (Fig. 4).

The Arduino Nano is a low-cost and portable electronic prototyping platform for electronic design [12]. It uses the ATmega328 microcontroller from Atmel. The main characteristics of the Arduino used in this work are described as follows:

- Atmel ATmega328 microcontroller.
- I/S: 14 digital pins and eight analog pins.
- USB 2.0 port.
- FLASH memory of 32 KB.
- Low cost.
- Portable design.

4.3 Electronic Motor Speed Controller

It controls the frequency speed of a DC motor by adapting the pulse rate modulating (PWM). It is perfectly suitable for use on areas such as car windshield wiper engine

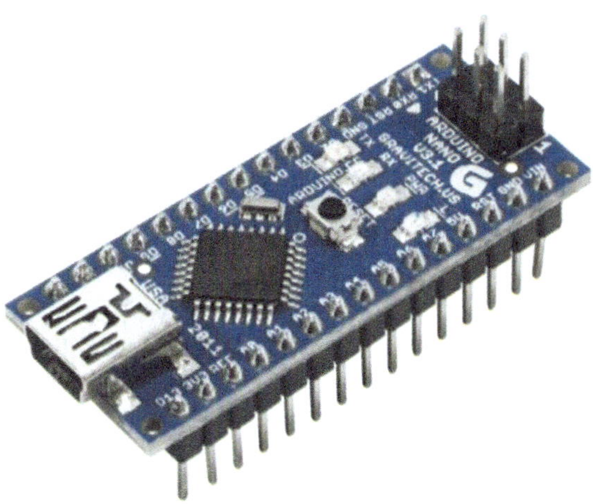

Fig. 4 Arduino cards nano

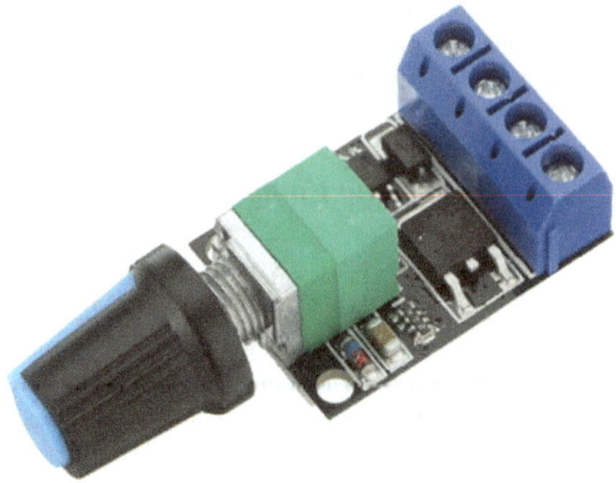

Fig. 5 Electronic motor speed controller

and muffler blower by ensuring good control of the motor frequency speed. These features are as follows:

- Material: Electronic components
- Working voltage: DC 4.5–28 V
- Output current: 0–5 A
- Output power: 90 W (maximum)
- Standby current: 7u A (standby state)
- PWM duty cycle: 1–100%.
- Frequency PWM: 20 khz (Fig. 5)

4.4 Wi-Fi Module

In this case, we used the ESP8266 Wi-Fi protocol module, which has a TCP/IP proxy stack embedded on the chip. Therefore, it can allow any other microcontroller to connect to the Wi-Fi network. The ESP8266 is a preset SOC, and any firmware microcontroller must communicate with it via the UART interface. Its operating voltage is 3.3 V. The module is parameterized with AT commands, and the microcontroller must be programmed to send AT commands in the order required to configure the module in client mode. The module can be used in both client and server mode [13].

After you have connected it to the Wi-Fi network, get an IP address that can be accessed on its local network. The module will also have two GPIO pins next to the UART pins. The module also has one GPIO pin next to the UART pins. It also integrates the SPI protocol by using two UART pins as data lines and configuring the two GPIO pins as control lines and clock signals. It also has an embedded 1 MB flash memory and a power management unit with all controllers and PLLs inside. The processor-on-chip is a 32-bit processor [14] (Fig. 6).

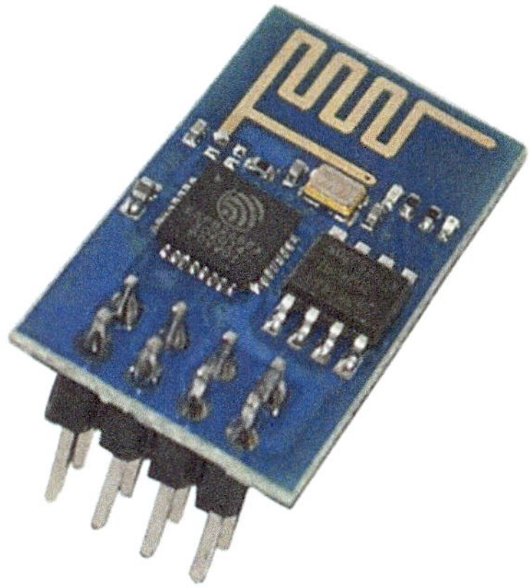

Fig. 6 ESP8266 pin details

5 Results and Discussion

It is a comprehensive system including mask, test tube, pump, 12 V battery and power switch. However, I would highly recommend using it with a DC power supply as the battery can only be used for about 3–4 h. The use of a facepiece when the battery is discharged may cause a dangerous buildup of carbon dioxide. This special battery can be charged and powered at the same time as a serial backup battery for wall power.

This is a close-up of the extracted blower. It is just a BLDC motor, used to drive the blower. A small ESC and an Arduino are connected to it. It is equipped with a conical tube adapter that is printed in 3D to fit the pipeline. You can use the Arduino IDE to program the microcontroller software. The software will go through a short initialization process to configure the ESC. Then, start with the lowest CPAP setting. You can use the switch to switch from one pressure level to another and then press twice to switch from one operating mode to another.

The first step in prototyping is to prove that the alternating filling and emptying of the pad works correctly and that the fan can operate within the required pressure and time range. Please note that the demonstrator is composed of ready-to-use parts, so the mechanical aspects of the unit visible in these pictures are completely different from the final design. Based on the experience gained during the operation of the demonstrator, the ideal physical characteristics of the pressure regulator, valve and pressure sensor can be improved, and the system is currently in the prototype development stage.

The open respirator in the human respiratory tract is not good. If possible, filtration is preferable. These components were initially used in electrical air purification equipment (PAPR). However, the addition of a filter will certainly affect the output pressure. The ability of the motor to handle the extra load will depend on the fan you are using. Depending on the drop height of the fans I tested, these PAPR fans may be capable of handling the filter while reaching the target pressure. However, I did not use a solid filter for long-term high-pressure thermal testing. These adapter plates can be glued with a lot of hot glue and then wrapped with vinyl tape to obtain a reasonable seal. My fan housing is not airtight, so it is very difficult to guarantee that 100% of the air only passes through the filter. By setting the fan to a lower PAP pressure and keeping the mask port open, it can be used reasonably as a PAPR.

6 Conclusion

By saving the installed gadgets in nature for checking, self-insurance of the earth is empowered. This is accomplished by conveying sensors in nature for information assortment and investigation. By sending sensors in nature, we can bring the earth into reality; for example, it can associate with different items through the system. The data collected and the results of the exams will then be made available to the end customer via Wi-Fi. The smart method to screen nature and an effective and economical implanted framework are given various models in this report. In the proposed engineering, the elements of various modules have been analyzed. The framework for the control of agitation and air pollution with the idea of the IoT has been provisionally tested for the observation of two boundaries. It also sends the limits of the sensors in the cloud. This information will be valuable for future examinations and can be communicated effortlessly to opposing end customers. This model can be used to monitor urban communities and modern regions, a work in progress for contamination control. To protect the general welfare against contamination, this model offers an efficient and inexpensive answer for persistent ecological observation.

References

1. Cano, N. J., Pichard, C., Roth, H., Court-Fortuné, I., Cynober, L., Gérard-Boncompain, M., Cuvelier, A., Laaban, J. P., Melchior, J. C., Raphaël, J. C. & Pison, C. M. (2004). C-reactive protein and body mass index predict outcome in end-stage respiratory failure. *Chest, 126*(2), 540–546.
2. Fernández-Pérez, E. R., Yilmaz, M., Jenad, H., Daniels, C. E., Ryu, J. H., Hubmayr, R. D., & Gajic, O. (2008). Ventilator settings and outcome of respiratory failure in chronic interstitial lung disease. *Chest, 133*(5), 1113–1119
3. Borges, J. B., Hedenstierna, G., Larsson, A., & Suarez-Sipmann, F. (2015). Altering the mechanical scenario to decrease the driving pressure. *Critical Care, 19*, 342
4. Arnal, J. M., Saoli, M., Garnero, A. (2019). Airway and transpulmonary driving pressures and mechanical powers selected by INTELLiVENT-ASV in passive, mechanically ventilated ICU patients. *Heart Lung*. November 14, 2019 pii: S0147-9563(19)30533-3. https://doi.org/10.1016/j.hrtlng.2019.11.001.
5. Chunsuttiwat, S. (2008). Response to avian influenza and preparedness for pandemic influenza: Thailand's experience. *Respirology, 13*, S36–S40
6. Powelson, S. K. (2010). Design and prototyping of a low-cost portable mechanical ventilator (Doctoral dissertation, Massachusetts Institute of Technology).

7. Amato, M. B., Meade, M. O., Slutsky, A. S., Brochard, L., Costa, E. L., Schoenfeld, D. A., et al. (2015). Driving pressure and survival in the acute respiratory distress syndrome. *The New England Journal of Medicine, 372*(8), 747–755
8. Bellani, G., Laffey, J. G., Pham, T., Fan, E., Brochard, L., Esteban, A., et al. (2016). Epidemiology, patterns of care, and mortality for patients with acute respiratory distress syndrome in intensive care units in 50 countries. *JAMA, 315*(8), 788–800
9. Laffey, J. G., Bellani, G., Pham, T., Fan, E., Madotto, F., Bajwa, E. K., et al. (2016). Potentially modifiable factors contributing to outcome from acute respiratory distress syndrome: the LUNG SAFE study. *Intensive Care Medicine, 42*(12), 1865–1876
10. Medicines and Healthcare products Regulatory Agency (MHRA), Rapidly Manufactured Ventilator System, April 2020
11. Grieco, D. L., Chen, L., Dres, M., & Brochard, L. (2017). Should we use driving pressure to set tidal volume? *Current Opinion in Critical Care, 23*(1), 38–44
12. ArduinoNano Board. (2020). Available online: https://www.arduino.cc/en/Main/ArduinoBoardNano. (Accessed on April 30, 2020).
13. Thaker, T. (2016). ESP8266 based implementation of wireless sensor network with Linux based web-server. In *2016 symposium on colossal data analysis and networking (CDAN)* (pp. 1–5). IEEE.
14. Vujović, V., & Maksimović, M. (2015). Raspberry Pi as a sensor web node for home automation. *Computers & Electrical Engineering, 44*, 153–171

Boon of Artificial Intelligence in Diagnosis of COVID-19

Simran Bhatia, Yuvraj Goyal, and Girish Sharma

1 Introduction

Amidst the current global urgency, healthcare workers, scientist, and clinicians are looking for the most recent and advance technologies to terminate the COVID-19 pandemic chain. Major challenges faced by the society worldwide includes economic downfall, difficulty in managing records of patient, spread of fake news, and steady process of development of new vaccines. Need of the hour is an immediate solution to properly diagnose and curb this deadly disease. Traditional methods used for detection are time consuming and less effective. Therefore, bringing together the traditional approaches with present-day outlook may work for the betterment of society. Modern approaches such as artificial intelligence (AI) and machine learning (ML) can play a vital role in this aspect. The chapter discusses about how applications of artificial intelligence (AI) assist in rapid diagnosing COVID-19 by screening, preventing, and managing its spread. It may take days to receive results from laboratories thus AI and its models reveal their smartness and accuracy. Worldwide government of all the countries are contributing their best by dealing with all such challenges. Various countries have launched different mobile applications to track the infection and maintain records of individuals who might have been in close proximity of affected person. Contact tracing has proved to be advantageous in the early stages of infection. Benefits of AI may include early screening as well as detection, predicting outcomes beforehand by putting algorithms in use for data mining and machine learning intended for accurate predictions and processing enormous data.

S. Bhatia · Y. Goyal · G. Sharma (✉)
Center for Medical Biotechnology, Amity Institute of Biotechnology, Amity University Uttar Pradesh, Noida 201313, India
e-mail: gsharma3@amity.edu

G. Sharma
Amity Center for Cancer Epidemiology and Cancer Research, Amity University Uttar Pradesh, Noida 201313, India

M. Niranjanamurthy et al. (eds.), *Intelligent Data Analysis for COVID-19 Pandemic*, Algorithms for Intelligent Systems, https://doi.org/10.1007/978-981-16-1574-0_5

Apart from screening, this robust system is also beneficial in not only development of drugs and vaccines but also in repurposing of drugs as well. Additionally, reviewed statistics show global augment in infected cases and keeping a track facilitates in maintaining data for choosing appropriate diagnostic strategy for early detection of this fatal disease.

2 Novel Coronavirus (SARS-CoV-2)

A novel coronavirus (COVID-19) has spread from Wuhan a city of China in December 2019. This virus belongs to the family *Coronaviridae* and subfamily *Coronavirinae*. Coronaviruses are enveloped, and single-stranded RNA viruses (ranging 27–32 kb) also responsible for causing respiratory tract infections, dyspnea, fever, and dry cough. The coronavirus family has given three major highly pathogenic viruses in past two decades, and severe acute respiratory syndrome (SARS) and Middle East respiratory syndrome (MERS) caused epidemic diseases in 2002 and 2012, respectively, and currently severe acute respiratory syndrome coronavirus 2 (SARS-CoV-2) has been declared as a pandemic by the WHO. The vital structural protein of SARS-CoV-2 is Spike protein which has "crown"-like appearance, thus named corona as detailed in Fig. 1 [1]. Spherical-shaped virions have a diameter of approximately 125 nm. There are 29,727 nucleotides in the genome of SARS-CoV [2], which includes four major proteins: spike (S) glycoprotein, membrane (M) protein, small envelop (E), and nucleocapsid (N) protein. The expansion of SARS-CoV-2 has been more grievous than its two predecessors. Proliferating infected droplets through sneezing or cough are responsible for transmission of the disease from infected person to normal individuals. Once an individual is exposed to novel coronavirus, 2 to 14 days

Fig. 1 Structural proteins of SARS-CoV-2 [1]

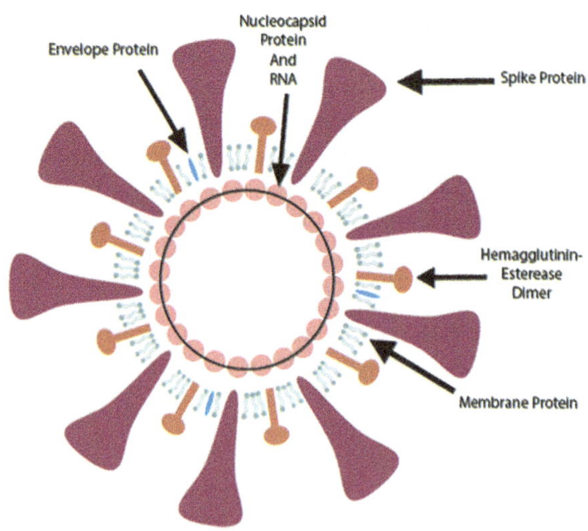

is its average incubation period [3]. Prime symptoms include high fever, cough, cold, breathlessness, and fatigue. Existing illness affects patients, distinctively suffering from respiratory diseases, and in addition cardiovascular diseases, hypertension, and diabetes can make the condition more critical.

The coronavirus pandemic has affected over 14 million people worldwide. The number of covid cases has always shown an increased growth since December 2019, and a complete set of infected cases from December 2019 to July 31, 2020 has been gathered in Fig. 2 [4]. To cope up with such circumstances, it is very important to recognize the disease as early as possible not only for an individual suffering but to avert the threat from spreading further.

To detect COVID-19 infection in early stages, a diagnostic method known as reverse transcription polymerase chain reaction (RT-PCR) is considered as gold standard. In this technique, the basic steps involves the specimen collection from upper and lower respiratory tract essentially oropharyngeal swabs (OP), bronchoalveolar lavage, nasopharyngeal (NP) and sputum followed by producing a complementary strand of DNA (cDNA) out of SARS-CoV-2 RNA via reverse transcription and subsequently its amplification. The cDNA is labeled with specific probes; after loading of samples, results are observed. Positive results indicate the higher frequency or it crosses the threshold frequency, on the other hand, negative results do not. This method is time consuming and may take a few days to deliver final results which can be inaccurate sometimes due to survival rate of pathogens (pathogens may not survive for many hours). Other limitations, such as contamination and degradation, can also alter the outcomes. Due to consequent constrains, use of artificial intelligence (AI) has gained its significance as an alternative approach for better outcomes and even more reliable diagnostic technique. Although chest CT is unable

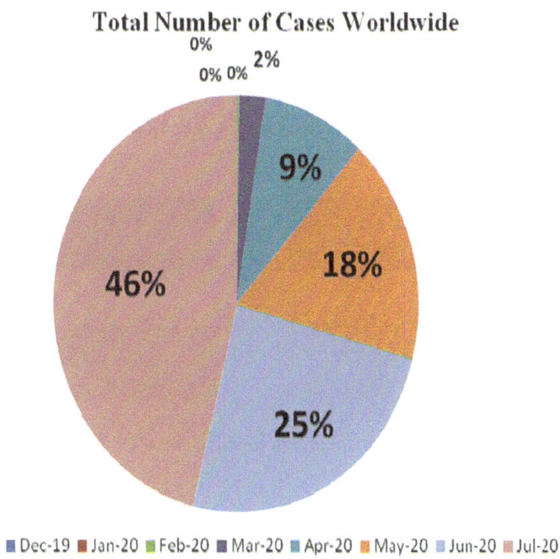

Fig. 2 Total number of active cases worldwide till July 31, 2020 [4]

to distinguish between viruses, yet it is considered the most conventional method to balance the management of disease [5]. CT alone can have bounded predictive value. AI has massive potential for analyzing and responding to loads of data quickly. Combing computed tomography (CT) and artificial intelligence (AI) can augment the procedure of diagnosis.

3 Evolution of Artificial Intelligence

Artificial intelligence is a technique that permits a machine to revive human actions. It is a field of computer science that makes a system mimic human intelligence. It is basically bringing together different technologies on indistinguishable platform that help machines to act similar to the intelligence of humans. AI works with algorithms which do not require preprogramming rather they work with their own intelligence. Figure 3 shows the evolution of artificial intelligence which originated in USA in 1956. John McCarthy coined the term AI in his first conference which was entirely dedicated to artificial intelligence. Later in 1972, Medical Biology welcomed AI in its world. A competition named *ImageNet* is held annually wherein AI proclaimed victory and ultimately in 2020 standing against this pandemic. Since the origin of AI, it has gone through many up and downs, it failed initially but has shown tremendous growth with time.

Potentially AI can be classified as:

3.1 Strong AI

It is not specific and applicable to wide range of activities. It works without the human intervention when exposed to difficult task and incorporates complex algorithms. Basically existence of this kind is rare but in near future it will achieve great heights.

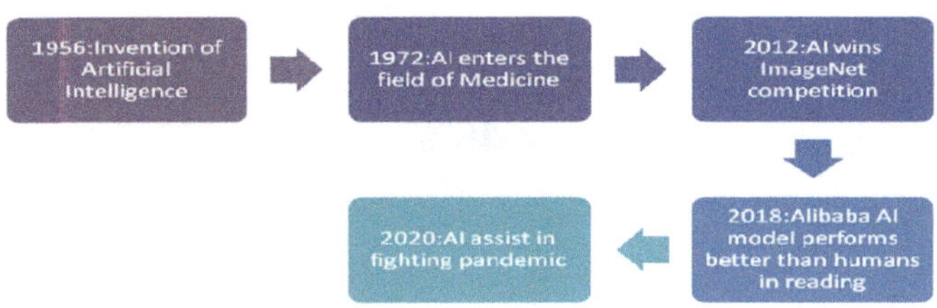

Fig. 3 Evolution of artificial intelligence since 1956–2020

3.2 *Weak AI*

It is simple and requires preprogramming by humans. It is very specific in nature and is applicable to narrow range of activities, e.g., personal assistants such as Apple's Siri and Amazon's Alexa.

AI offers compelling opportunities in realm of diagnosis. Huge amount of data can be investigated, mixed, and produced together with precision and accuracy. In the struggle against COVID-19, field of biotechnology has taken lead by adapting strategies such as artificial intelligence, machine learning, and big data to provide better facilities [6]. AI merged with big data works with algorithms to locate patterns in big data. It is basically virtual library, and enormous amount of data is stored and analyzed under this application [7]. AI and big data go hand in hand and have certain maneuver which includes:

(a) **Spotting peculiarity**: AI can inspect big data to identify any deviation in dataset.
(b) **Probability of upcoming results**: Any event that can influence ensuing conditions or has probability of doing so can already be detected by calculating present scenario.
(c) **Precise recognition**: AI can detect big data to search for patterns that a human supervision may undetect sometimes.

Machine learning is a portion of AI that works on the principle of learning from past experiences or data. It allows the machine to make predictions and take decisions using authentic data. During current pandemic, machine learning can be beneficial in predicting likelihood of patients infected with COVID-19 besides threat of mortality. It also shows excellence in developing drugs at a faster speed and can make clinical trials more efficient and better predictions.

4 Applications of Computational Techniques

4.1 *Speed Up Diagnosis*

AI assists in early detection of disease and helps doctors to take prompt decision. Use of algorithms replaces traditional diagnosis which is time consuming and designs new techniques. Machine learning, a subset of AI, accelerates medical imaging techniques such as computed tomography (CT), magnetic resonance imaging (MRI), and chest X-ray.

4.2 Computerized Tracking

AI sets platform which predicts the extent of infection and automatic treatment. A specialized network called *neural network* can be build which helps in detection of visual features of disease and this would give benefit in true monitoring and treatment of infected individuals.

4.3 Tracking of Infected Individual

AI helps in determining the infection level by identifying the hotspots. It also helps in identifying travel history of the infected person and tells the future course of the disease.

4.4 Prediction of Incidence Rate and Mortality Rate

From the available data on various social media platform and other Web sites, it can predict the nature of virus as well as can tell about the risk and spread of infection. Moreover, artificial intelligence helps in analyzing the incidence and mortality rate of a particular region. This technique also enables us to recognize the most affected regions and people.

4.5 Designing and Development of New Drugs and Vaccines

AI helps in development of drugs and vaccines from the available data related to COVID-19 [8]. In comparison to the traditional techniques which require a lot of time for the same, AI speeds up the process of drug discovery. It also helps in carrying out different phases of clinical trials quicker than the actual time taken for vaccine development.

4.6 Lowering the Work Load

Due to the spread of COVID-19, healthcare workers have very high workload owing to the increase in the number of infected individuals. With the help of AI, this workload can be reduced as this helps in early diagnosis and automatic treatment.

4.7 Prevention of Infectious Disease

For healthcare workers, AI helps in providing the information with help of real-time data analysis, which in turn is helpful not only in prevention of the disease but also to analyze the infected sites during pandemic. In future, this will be an important and useful technique to fight against various epidemics and pandemics.

5 Traditional Diagnostic Methodology

Various procedures are currently active in diagnosis of COVID-19. One such method is **molecular testing**, which involves collection of samples, such as swabs and sputum, and subsequently examining it if an individual is infected with the viral strain or not [9]. Based on molecular methodology, RT-PCR is one such technique that involves analyzing of molecules, for instance, protein, DNA, and RNA in a tissue of the infected individual for the detection of disease [10]. In this technique, the cDNA is labeled with specific probes, after loading of samples, results are observed. The steps to perform RT-PCR are depicted in Fig 4 [11]. Although it is not well grounded since it is unable to govern the detection of an individual who has just recovered from disease and also cannot determine the presence of virus if in very low amount in the body.

(a) Swab sample is collected.
(b) Extraction of RNA from samples.
(c) Generating DNA using RNA template by reverse transcription.
(d) RT-PCR amplification.
(e) Results obtained, if it crosses the threshold frequency, the test is positive.

Serological testing is another approach opted to investigate the existing infection; it includes blood-based testing for the diagnosis of viral infections. Serum, a component of blood which does not play a role in clotting, is analyzed, and this in turn informs about the presence of antibodies against the disease causing microorganism (pathogen). Enzyme-linked immunosorbent assay (ELISA) and lateral flow immunosorbent assay are the techniques considered under serological testing. One such type of serological test is **rapid antibody testing** for the detection of antibodies in the immune system against the COVID-19. This tells about the past infection of the viral disease. The sample used for the analysis is serum which is collected by pricking the finger, and it takes about 15–30 min to obtain the results. **Enzyme-linked immunosorbent assay (ELISA),** another serological test, provides the information about the antigen–antibody interaction as depicted in Fig 5 [12]. In order to detect the active antibodies, antibodies are sandwiched in the viral protein of interest and reporter antibodies. The sample used can be blood, plasma, or serum and sample is collected by venipuncture, and it takes usually 2–5 h for results.

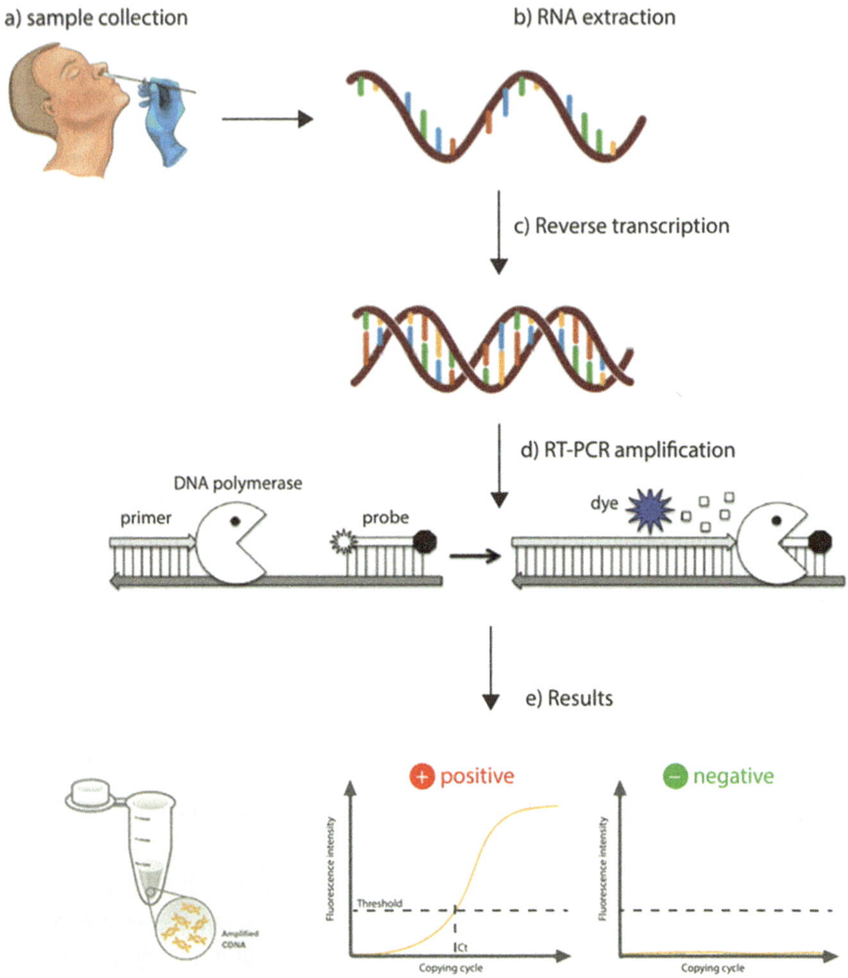

Fig. 4 Steps involved in RT-PCR [11]

1. Antibody binds to ELISA plates.
2. Antigen in sample binds to antibody.
3. Wash microplate.
4. Add detection antibody.
5. Wash microplate.
6. Substrate.
7. Read the plate.
8. Results.

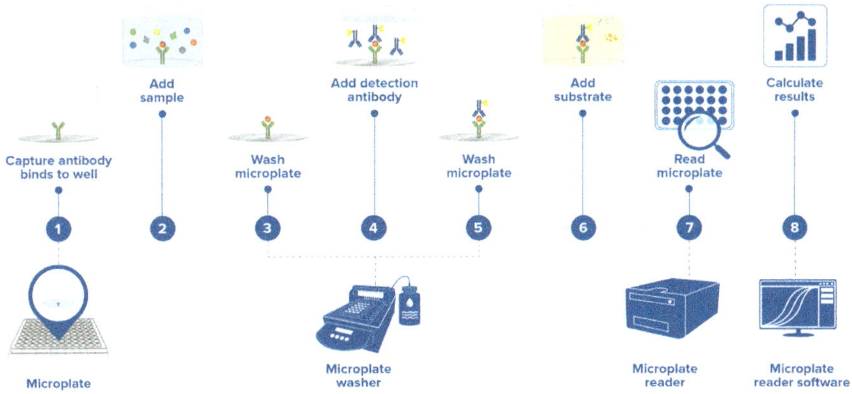

Fig. 5 Steps involved in ELISA [12]

5.1 *Lateral Flow Immunoassay (LFIA)*

It is a calorimetric assay for qualitative analysis of the antibody present. The blood sample runs over the membrane which contains target antigens. If the sample contains the antibodies specific to the antigens, which are present on the surface, they form the complex and colored band is visible, similar to the pregnancy test kits. This test is also known as *rapid diagnostic test*. Sample used for analysis is blood or serum collected by venipuncture, and result is obtained within 10–30 min. Figure 6 depicts the LFA kit [13].

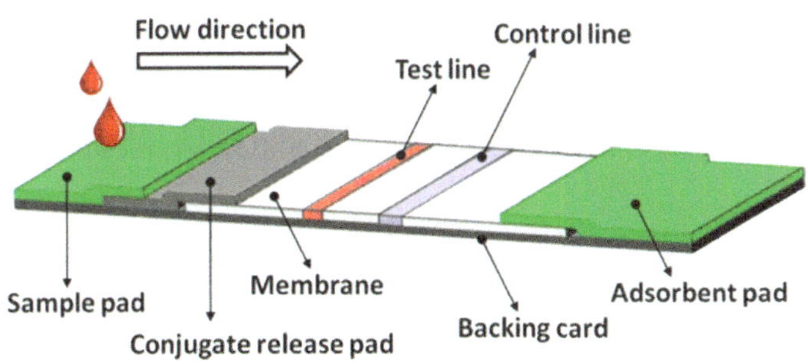

Fig. 6 Lateral flow immunoassay kit and its elements [13]

5.2 *Chemiluminescent Immunoassay (CLIA)*

It is basically a fluorescent assay that identifies the presence of antibodies to disease causing microorganisms with the help of fluorescent dyes. Since it is a type of serological test, sample used for testing is blood or serum, taken with help of venipuncture and time taken is 1–2 h for analyses.

5.3 *Neutralization Assay*

It is another type of serological test used to inspect the presence of active antibodies by analyzing the viral growth inhibited with the help of antibodies of infected individual in the laboratory as detailed in Fig. 7 [14]. Blood is used for testing and is collected from the vein. It takes minimum 3 days and maximum 5 days to obtain results. All of these approaches come with certain limitations because it is difficult to detect antibodies in patients with mild or asymptomatic version. Table 1 differentiates the types of testing as well as time consumed for testing [15].

In order to fulfill the expectations of patients, healthcare department anticipates what is to be confronted. Meeting the expectations of a patient helps fulfilling satisfactory results and better treatment. For some medical imaging and biochemical test, there are innumerable procedures carried out for detection. An individual surely keeps high assumptions of accuracy, less painful methods opted, and should be cost effective (Fig. 8).

Looking at present situation and keeping high expectations, few techniques do not carry out satisfactory results with number of limitations and providing reasons for picking several other methods over conventional ones. One of the best solutions for ongoing devastation is speedy diagnosis using artificial intelligence and its subsets—machine learning and big data. With availability of several expert system, identification of disease has been a lot more easier. Besides, it can also contribute

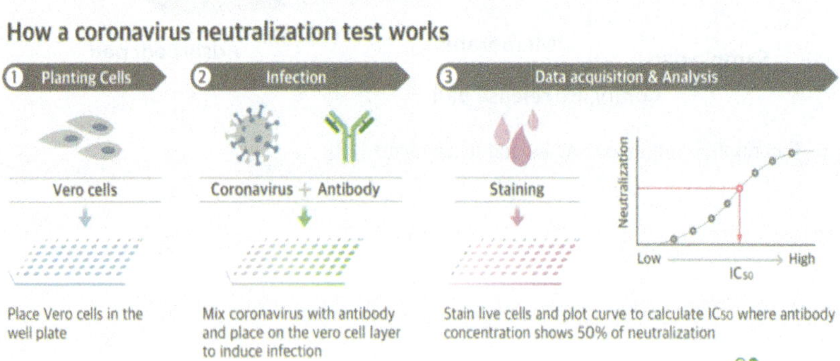

Fig. 7 Steps involved in neutralization test [14]

Table 1 Molecular and serological-based test for detection of COVID-19 [15]

Method of diagnosis	Type of test	Indicates	Sample	Utilizes	Time taken
Real time—PCR	Molecular	Current infection	Mucus and saliva	Swab technique	4–6 h
Rapid antibody test	Serological	Past infection	Blood or serum	Prick on finger	15–30 min
ELISA	Serological	Antigen–antibody interaction	Blood, serum, or plasma	Venipuncture	2–5 h
Lateral flow immunoassay	Serological	Antibody presence (Colorimetric)	Blood, serum, or plasma	Venipuncture	10–30 min
Chemiluminescent immunoassay	Serological	Antibody presence (fluorescent)	Blood, serum, or plasma	Venipuncture	1–2 h
Neutralization assay	Serological	Active neutralizing antibodies	Blood, serum, or plasma	Venipuncture	3–5 days

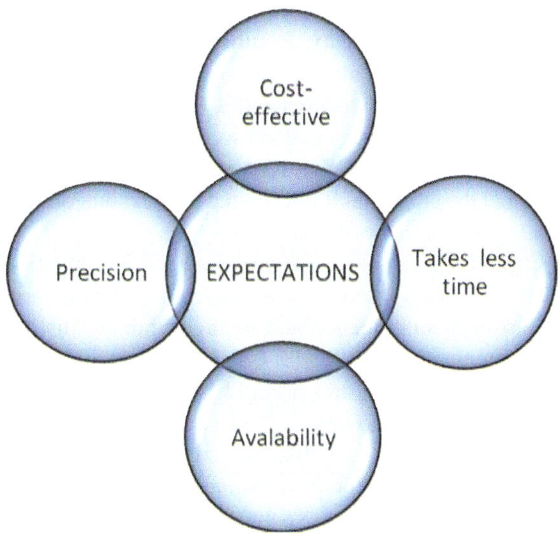

Fig. 8 Parameters defining expectations from a good diagnosis

in manufacturing and repurposing of drugs. Taking example of the gold standard, RT-PCR diagnostic technique posses certain limitations. It is important to interpret the complete history of the disease, evaluate past infection, and track the virus as it can develop asymptomatically. Also, the virus is present in the body for a limited period of time, the method only detects the **ongoing infection.** RT-PCR machines are required to carry out the testing although the procedure takes less time but transporting, taking samples, labeling, and collecting may take time. Additionally, it calls for trained staff for **handling advanced instruments** unlike antibody testing, which only needs a kit for testing. While handling samples and operating reagents and dye, utmost attention is demanded since it may result in contamination, thus emerging issues of **false positive** and **false negative results.** Therefore, to deal with similar constraints, a new AI approach has been adapted over conventional methods. Various study shows that CT findings can predict prolong infected period of an individual [16] along with recovery of patients. It also provides a better visualization about genome of the virus which in turn can help in targeting it better. There are a number of applications in context of differentiating patients on the basis of infected and non-infected, availability of ICU and better healthcare system as well as in detecting and opting treatment methods accordingly.

6 Machine Learning

Machine learning accelerates the decision making following a better diagnosis and treatment. The target detection and categorization are two main chores where deep learning put an entreaty. Resulting in accurate predictions through already existed data is the main venture. A group of researchers conducted a study to evaluate the efficiency of ML by detection of COVID-19 images on chest radiographs. They took more than 1500 images which were suspected to possess COVID-19 infection [17]. Chest radiography (CXR) is an efficient formula applied along with AI algorithms to combat the situation. It interpreted the best outcomes and resulted in faster diagnosis and treatment as well.

Another team of researchers avail the manipulation of imaging techniques which are particularly used for early screening. Computed tomography (CT) makes use of artificial intelligence and its algorithms to distinguish between images of viral pneumonia and COVID-19. CT images may imbricate with several other inflammatory lung diseases, and it could be a laborious task to differentiate them. Convolutional neural network (CNN) is one such algorithm [18] used in deep learning system which has expertise in recognizing images and able to identify differences. By the assistance of preprogrammed data filled in, it fortunately captures the temporal dependencies as well as spatial organization. They originated certain features using neural networks in the first part and using the same outcomes to differentiate between pneumonia-infected patients.

Data mining (DM) is a subset of machine learning and provides valid and hidden information from a large dataset. It connects and relates among datasets in a uniform pattern [19]. DM not only helps in recognition but also develops a future prediction about development and spread of disease to an extent. It has already set its prints in previous outbreaks like MERS and SARS-CoV. A huge amount of data mining and analyzing is performed worldwide everyday to produce better patterns and resolve the current pandemic. In medical management, DM provides an insight of recovery pattern, health outcomes, predicting, and planning as well as stability [20]. It uses different algorithms to correlate and work.

6.1 *Algorithms*

Algorithm acts as "problem solver," and it can process massive data in one go. Algorithms are crucial part of artificial intelligence and machine learning, and they help in calculations, processing, analyzing, and predictions. They work on principle of taking commands and execute the same. While using machine learning and artificial intelligence, there is a set amount of work to be done by computer [21] that is the responsibility of algorithm to get the work done using commands and already processed data. It makes life easier and smarter. Decision trees, K-nearest neighbor, support vector machine (SVM), Naive Bayes, and random forest are some of the most common used algorithms in 2020 [22]. Some of the algorithms with their latest publications are summarized in Table 2.

6.2 *Random Forest*

It is a supervised learning algorithm that is mainly used for regression (prediction) and classification. Multiple inputs are composed together without any correlation [23]. It allows an individual to examine association between multiple variables and provide an average outcome. Use of random forest algorithm divides data into smaller branches [24] and further into leaves as a result creating a similar decision tree. It has already set its imprints in the field of bioinformatics; therefore, because of its admirable identification, now elucidating disputes in ongoing required time. It has proved to give better outcomes in differentiating blood samples and discriminate patients possessing symptoms of COVID-19 with 0.9795% accuracy for cross-validation set prediction. A study carried out which showed cohort data haphazardly split into prediction model and a training set 30% and 70%, respectively, for availability of ICU hospital within 24 h [25]. For the same purpose, RF model was upskilled which resulted in providing accurate results.

Table 2 Summary of some recent algorithms used for COVID-19

S. no.	Approach adopted	Title	Publication date	References
1	Support vector machine	Classification of coronavirus images using Shrunken features	Apr-20	[28]
2	Support vector machine	COVID-19 detection using deep learning models to exploit social mimic optimization and structured chest X-ray images using fuzzy color and stacking approaches	Jun-20	[29]
3	Support vector machine	Automated systems for detection of COVID-19 using chest X-ray images and lightweight convolutional neural networks	Apr-20	[30]
4	Random forest	COVID-19 patient health prediction using boosted random forest algorithm	Jul-20	[24]
5	Random forest	Detection of COVID-19 infection from routine blood exams with machine learning: A feasibility study	Jul-20	[31]
6	K-nearest neighbor (KNN)	Using K-nearest neighbor classification to diagnose abnormal lung sounds	Jun-15	[32]

6.2.1 Support Vector Machine (SVM)

A study carried out using SVM algorithm which depicts the detection of patients infected with coronavirus [26] using X-ray images. The methodology opted was to classify patients into healthy, pneumonia, and COVID-19 infected patients which makes the diagnosis effortless. SVM classifier uses deep features produced from fully connected layer of convolutional neural network (CNN). Previously in MERS-CoV dataset, SVM acquires highest accuracy. This technique has favorable results in development of computer-aided systems and decision making in clinical field.

6.2.2 K-Nearest Neighbor (KNN)

A subset of data mining classifier, as the name suggests it determines the closest datasets to produce accurate outputs. KNN is proved to be highly capable of solving complex problems rapidly. During current outbreak, it saves the precious time of the healthcare workers. A study was conducted in which KNN was used as a problem solver [27] where it was given CT images to locate and relate. By analyzing images, it extracts features thus filtering the patients infected from COVID-19 and helps in decision making more accurate and brisk.

7 Contact Tracing

To control the spread of novel coronavirus, various countries did their part by launching different mobile applications in order to track the infected individuals and people coming in contact. This helps in better prevention [33] and awareness; WHO suggests the basic spread of virus through droplets, contact transmission, and saliva. Contact tracing is efficient way of managing this disease. It provides information such as number of infected individuals in a particular area, predicts future spread, keeps an eye on active cases, and even monitors bed's availability. The latest digital contact tracing can serve nation with use of artificial intelligence. Some of the countries with their mobile applications launched amidst the pandemic are detailed in Table 3.

8 Detection Through Smell

A variety of molecular and serological diagnostic methods is being performed today to get rid of this pandemic. Currently, research is going on across the globe to detect the virus as early as possible in order to avoid infection in community. A study by Leachien proved that anosmia (loss of smell) is prompt indication of presence of viral strains [44]. They analyzed the data of African population and European population. Leachein and his coworkers carried out the study of 417 infected individuals of 19 years to 77 years of age group with 263 females and 154 males. The outcome of the study resulted in 284 patients which were anosmic and the symptoms appeared early in 11.8% of the sample size. Another group of scientists, Gane and his team, postulated that occurrence of a fourth common syndrome of COVID-19 infection which is isolated sudden onset anosmia (ISOA). They conducted a study on UK-based population [45]. Research workers of Weizman Institute in collaboration with scientists of Edith Wolfson Medical Center [46] developed online platform as smell tracker which help in the self examination of one's sense of smell.

Table 3 Applications launched by different countries for better management of COVID-19

S. no.	Country	Application name	Launch date	Objective	References
1	India	Aarogya Setu	April 2, 2020	This app helps in contact tracing syndromic mapping and self-assessment	[34]
2	Italy	Immuni	June 1, 2020	The app aims to notify users at risk of carrying the virus as early as possible—even when they are asymptomatic	[35]
3	Australia	COVIDSafe	April 14, 2020	This is helpful in identifying people exposed to coronavirus and helps in protecting you, your family, and your loved ones	[36]
4	Iran	AC19	April, 10, 2020	Objective of AC19 is promising detection of symptoms of COVID-19	[37]
5	New Zealand	NZ COVID Tracer	May 20, 2020	It is advantageous in contact tracing	[38]
6	Malaysia	MySejahtera	April 6, 2020	This allows user to perform self-assessment of themselves and family members and helps to detect COVID-19 cases in 1 km radius	[39]
7	Singapore	TraceTogether	March 20, 2020	This facilitates the contact tracing process and tells about who are in close contact of COVID-19 cases more quickly	[40]

(continued)

Table 3 (continued)

S. no.	Country	Application name	Launch date	Objective	References
8	UAE	TraceCovid	March 20, 2020	Motive is to slow the spread of coronavirus by helping tracing people who have come into close proximity with an infected individual	[41]
9	Colombia	CoronApp	April 12, 2020	This will advice on prevention and timely information about the virus	[42]
10	Norway	Smittestopp	April 16, 2020	This is designed to help health authorities to limit the spread of deadly coronavirus	[43]

9 Conclusion

Since the outbreak of SARS-CoV-2, people across the globe have been fighting against this disease. Worldwide scientists have been engaged in exploring for all possible techniques to cure and alternative strategies to screen, detect, and prevent it. With the same approach, artificial intelligence is signified to excel and identified to be useful as a tool in early detection and monitoring of the infection and its spread. AI/ML-based models use algorithms to process large amount of data swiftly and accurately. It improves the identification of transmission and monitoring, besides enabling rapid diagnosis of COVID-19. Medical imaging is a technique opted for analysis of body images of an infected individual. Artificial intelligence has capability of upgrading the system, and it has proved to analyze and work on large amount of data itself. Computed tomography (CT), an image-based technique, has been combined with AI for societal benefit. With the help of AI, drones are being used for transportation of medicines and food during the lockdown, thereby maintaining social distancing. Thinking of reducing stress on healthcare workers and clinicians, machine learning and deep learning enhance the procedure of detection by refining false positive and false negative results, which is one of the major drawbacks of conventional approaches. Contributing enormously for the benefit of society, AI and its subsets have left remarkable impression in our life. Thus, utilization of AI-based techniques has made life easier and self-sufficient (Atmanirbhar) fulfilling the demands and making world a better place.

References

1. Holmes, K. (2003). SARS-associated coronavirus. *New England Journal of Medicine, 348*(20), 1948–1951.
2. Wu, X. (2004). The spike protein of severe acute respiratory syndrome (SARS) is cleaved in virus infected Vero-E6 cells. *Cell Research, 14*(5), 400–406.
3. Singhal, T. (2020). A review of coronavirus disease-2019 (COVID-19). *Indian Journal of Pediatrics, 87*(4), 281–286.
4. Coronavirus Cases. (2020). https://www.worldometers.info/coronavirus/?utm_campaign=homeADemocracynow%282020%29+dvegas1%3F. Last accessed September 03, 2020.
5. Li, Y. (2020). Coronavirus disease 2019 (COVID-19): role of chest CT in diagnosis and management. *American Journal of Roentgenology, 214*(6), 1280–1286.
6. www.ETHealthworld.com. https://health.economictimes.indiatimes.com/news/diagnostics/to-combat-covid-19-india-adopted-intelligent-testing-strategy/75996797, Last accessed May 26, 2020.
7. Shrestha, P. (2020). https://explorebiotech.com/applications-of-big-data-in-biotechnology/. Last accessed July 22, 2020.
8. Vaishya, R. (2020) A. Artificial Intelligence (AI) applications for COVID-19 pandemic. *Diabetes & Metabolic Syndrome: Clinical Research & Reviews, 14*(4), 337–339.
9. Kubina, R. (2020). A. Molecular and serological tests for COVID-19 a comparative review of SARS-CoV-2 coronavirus laboratory and point-of-care diagnostics. *Diagnostics (Basel), 10*(6), 434.
10. Carter, L. J. (2020). Assay techniques and test development for COVID-19 diagnosis. *ACS Central Science, 6*(5), 591–605.
11. IDTechEx. (2020). The worldwide test for Covid-19. https://www.globalbiotechinsights.com/articles/20247/the-worldwide-test-for-covid-19. Last accessed August 01, 2020.
12. Enzyme-Linked Immunosorbent Assay (ELISA). (2020). https://www.moleculardevices.com/applications/enzyme-linked-immunosorbent-assay-elisa. Last accessed August 09, 2020.
13. Koczula, K. (2016). Lateral flow assays. *Essays in Biochemistry, 60*(1), 111–120.
14. HospiMedica International. (2020). Celltrion developing 'super antibody' targeting potential SARS-CoV-2 mutations. https://www.hospimedica.com/covid-19/articles/294781720/celltrion-developing-super-antibody-targeting-potential-sars-cov-2-mutations.html. Last accessed November 07, 2020.
15. Administrator, J. (2020). Global progress on COVID-19 serology-based testing. https://www.centerforhealthsecurity.org/resources/COVID-19/serology/Serology-based-tests-for-COVID-19.html. Last accessed August 03, 2020.
16. Health IT Analytics. (2020). Artificial intelligence could speed COVID-19 detection, treatment. https://healthitanalytics.com/news/artificial-intelligence-could-speed-covid-19-detection-treatment. August 03, 2020.
17. Murphy, K. (2020). COVID-19 on the chest radiograph: A multi-reader evaluation of an AI system. *Radiology, 296*(3), 166–172.
18. Wang, S. (2020). A deep learning algorithm using CT images to screen for Corona Virus Disease (COVID-19). https://www.medrxiv.org/content/. https://doi.org/10.1101/2020.02.14.20023028v5. Last accessed November 07, 2020.
19. Muhammad, L. J. (2020). Predictive data mining models for novel coronavirus (COVID-19) infected patients recovery. *SN Computer Science, 1*(4).
20. Jeffs, A. (2020). Using data mining as a weapon in the fight against Covid-19. https://www.processexcellencenetwork.com/big-data-analytics/articles/using-data-mining-as-a-weapon-in-the-fight-against-covid-19. Last accessed August 01, 2020.
21. Stephen, F. (2020). Artificial intelligence: How algorithms make systems smart. https://www.wired.com/insights/2014/09/artificial-intelligence-algorithms-2/. Last accessed August 09, 2020.

22. Top 20 AI and machine learning algorithms, methods and techniques. https://www.ubuntupit.com/machine-learning-algorithms-for-both-newbies-and-professionals/. Last accessed August 09, 2020.
23. Chakure, A. (2020). Random forest and its implementation. https://towardsdatascience.com/random-forest-and-its-implementation. Last accessed August 09, 2020.
24. Iwendi, C. (2020). COVID-19 patient health prediction using boosted random forest algorithm. *Frontiers in Public Health, 8*(357), 1–9.
25. Cheng, F. Y. (2020). Using machine learning to predict ICU transfer in hospitalized COVID-19 patients. *Journal of Clinical Medicine, 9*(6), 1668.
26. Sethy, P. K. (2020). Detection of coronavirus disease (COVID-19) based on deep features and support vector machine. *International Journal of Mathematical Engineering and Management Sciences, 5*(4), 643–651.
27. Shaban, W. M. (2020). A new COVID-19 patients detection strategy (CPDS) based on hybrid feature selection and enhanced KNN classifier. *Knowledge-Based System, 205*, 106270.
28. Ozturk, S. (2020). Classification of coronavirus Images using Shrunken features.
29. Toğaçar, M. (2020). COVID-19 detection using deep learning models to exploit social mimic optimization and structured chest X-ray images using fuzzy color and stacking approaches. *Computers in Biology and Medicine, 121*, 103805.
30. Alqudah, A. M. (2020). Automated systems for detection of COVID-19 using chest X-ray images and lightweight convolutional neural networks. https://www.researchsquare.com/article/rs-24305/v1. Last accessed November 07, 2020.
31. Brinati, D. (2020). Detection of COVID-19 Infection from routine blood exams with machine learning: A feasibility study. *Journal of Medical Systems, 44*(8), 135.
32. Chen, C. (2020). Using K-nearest neighbor classification to diagnose abnormal lung sounds. *Sensors (Basel), 15*(6), 13132–13158.
33. Lalmuanawma, S. (2020). Applications of machine learning and artificial intelligence for Covid-19 (SARS-CoV-2) pandemic: A review. *Choas, Solitons & Fractals, 139.*
34. Jhunjhunwala, A. (2020). Role of telecom network to manage COVID-19 in India: Aarogya Setu. *Transactions of the Indian National Academy of Engineering, 5*(2), 157–161.
35. Italy launches COVID-19 contact-tracing app amid privacy concerns. https://in.reuters.com/article/us-health-coronavirus-italy-app/italy-launches-covid-19-contact-tracing-app-amid-privacy-concerns-idINKBN2383EW. Last accessed August 01, 2020.
36. Australian Government Department of Health. (2020). COVIDSafe app. https://www.health.gov.au/resources/apps-and-tools/covidsafe-app. Last accessed August 01, 2020.
37. Desk, W. (2020). Iran's coronavirus 'detection' app could have spied on users: Researcher. https://www.theweek.in/news/world/2020/03/10/irans-coronavirus-detection-app-could-have-spied-on-users-researcher.html. Last accessed August 01, 2020.
38. Mahmoud Elkhodr Lecturer in Information and Communication Technologies. New Zealand's COVID-19 Tracer app won't help open a 'travel bubble' with Australia anytime soon. https://theconversation.com/new-zealands-covid-19-tracer-app-wont-help-open-a-travel-bubble-with-australia-anytime-soon-139026. Last accessed August 01, 2020.
39. Tariq, Q. (2020). Govt launches pilot project to monitor spread of Covid-19 pandemic via app. https://www.thestar.com.my/tech/tech-news/2020/04/06/govt-launches-app-to-monitor-spread-of-covid-19-pandemic. Last accessed August 01, 2020.
40. Singapore government launches new app for contact tracing to combat spread of COVID-19. https://www.mobihealthnews.com/news/asia-pacific/singapore-government-launches-new-app-contact-tracing-combat-spread-covid-19. Last accessed August 01, 2020.
41. Al Arabiya English. (2020). UAE's coronavirus tracing app—Is it compulsory and other questions answered. https://english.alarabiya.net/en/coronavirus/2020/04/20/UAE-s-coronavirus-tracing-app-Is-it-compulsory-and-other-questions-answered. Last accessed August 01, 2020.
42. Colombian president launches app to track COVID-19. https://www.aa.com.tr/en/americas/colombian-president-launches-app-to-track-covid-19/1759011. Last accessed August 01, 2020.
43. Nikel, P. (2020). Smittestopp: How Norway's new coronavirus app works. https://www.lifeinnorway.net/smittestopp-coronavirus-app/, Last accessed August 01, 2020.

44. Lechien, J. R. (2020). Olfactory and gustatory dysfunctions as a clinical presentation of mild-to-moderate forms of the coronavirus disease (COVID-19): A multicenter European study. *European Archives of Oto-Rhino-Laryngology, 277*(8), 2251–2261.
45. Gane, S. (2020). Isolated sudden onset anosmia in COVID-19 Infection. A Novel Syndrome? *Rhinology Journal, 58*(3), 299–301.
46. www.ETHealthworld.com. Self-monitoring your sense of smell may help detect Coronavirus-ET Health World. https://health.economictimes.indiatimes.com/news/industry/self-monitoring-your-sense-of-smell-may-help-detect-coronavirus/75048602. Last accessed August 30, 2020.

Artificial Intelligence and Big Data Solutions for COVID-19

Rehab A. Rayan, Imran Zafar, and Christos Tsagkaris

1 Introduction

COVID-19, resulting from the novel coronavirus, has affected considerably healthcare economy, education, transportation, politics, and among other sectors worldwide. COVID-19 cases usually suffer chest conditions and could be managed with supportive therapy. However, COVID-19 has turned highly transmissible among humans. So far, the virus has spread rapidly in 216 countries, causing 24,854,140 and 838,924 confirmed cases and deaths, respectively, where the USA on the top of all countries in both confirmed cases and deaths [1]. Yet, there is neither a preventive vaccine nor effective therapeutics for such a viral infection. Both the Centers for Disease Control and Prevention (CDC) and the World Health Organization (WHO) have been releasing public recommendations and technical guidelines regarding the novel coronavirus [2, 3]. The collaborative efforts of national states and large companies might considerably minimize the risks of the COVID-19 pandemic. For instance, Google released a portal for the COVID-19 that includes useful information like the virus spot maps, updated statistics, and the commonly asked questions (www.google.com/covid19). Google, Amazon, IBM, and Microsoft collaborated with the White House in designing a coronavirus research supercomputer [4]. Besides, several publishers enabled freely accessible papers, operational standards, and further reports about coronaviruses, while Web

R. A. Rayan (✉)
Department of Epidemiology, High Institute of Public Health,
Alexandria University, Alexandria 21539, Egypt
e-mail: rayanr@alexu.edu.eg

I. Zafar
Department of Bioinformatics and Computational Biology,
Virtual University of Pakistan, Lahore 57000, Pakistan

C. Tsagkaris
Faculty of Medicine, University of Crete, 18233 Heraklion, Greece

M. Niranjanamurthy et al. (eds.), *Intelligent Data Analysis for COVID-19 Pandemic*,
Algorithms for Intelligent Systems, https://doi.org/10.1007/978-981-16-1574-0_6

archiving services such as medRxi, arXiv, and bioRxiv continue to gather preprints about COVID-19 [5]. Artificial intelligence (AI) and big data are applied in many disciplines such as computer science, banking, agriculture, and health; hence, such techniques might play key roles in addressing the coronavirus pandemic worldwide.

Lately, many research articles, addressing the COVID-19 pandemic, have been published. This paper reviews how the techniques for AI and big data are effective solutions against the COVID-19 pandemic, along with the special focus on some applied AI and big data techniques. Besides, it highlights the limitations of the available AI and big data techniques that lead to suggesting recommendations for future research, states, and communities.

This chapter starts with background information on COVID-19, AI, big data, and the reason for choosing AI and big data. Then, it reviews applying AI and big data in managing the coronavirus pandemic, such as detecting cases, monitoring the outbreak, investigating new drugs, and enhancing therapeutic regimens. Afterward, it describes some AI and big data-centered models for fighting the COVID-19, a phone-built model for detecting and surveillance of COVID-19, and a data-centered technique applying AI to identify antibody sequences. Ultimately, it highlights recommendations and limitations to be addressed for the future.

2 The COVID-19 Pandemic

The pharmaceutical industry is looking for innovative developments in this public health situation to track and regulate the spread of the COVID-19 (coronavirus) pandemic. AI is a tool to investigate the transmission of this virus, detect high-profile patients, and help to constantly search for this contamination. By breaking down previous patient records, researchers can also estimate mortality. Simulated intelligence helps us fight this epidemic by controlling the population, revealing, and guiding disease control guidelines [6, 7]. Such development may increase the organization, care, and outcomes of COVID-19 patients, as it is a validated treatment. Artificial information is an important and long-awaited method for detecting early coronavirus diseases and also helps to track the circumstances of infected patients. By making useful algorithms, experts can improve the precision and dynamics of the treatment. However, artificial intelligence is more than useful for their ethical monitoring in the treatment of patients suffering from COVID-19. We can monitor the COVID-19 emergency situation on different scales, for example, clinical, subatomic, and epidemiological applications. It is also beneficial to promote studies on this infection by dissecting available knowledge. The development of proper healthcare regimens, preventive programmers, drug, and antibody advances helps with simulated intelligence [8].

It is exceptional to establish new COVID-19 cases. An important source of data and knowledge about cases and health events is this accelerated manipulation. Many data on different storage strategies from these conditions need to be easily processed. This expertise is used to address and respond to and break with infectious diseases, pandemics, and behavior. Big data is a fantastic invention that allows patients to store knowledge accurately as an artificial system, pattern and association, and similarity analysis tools. Knowledge can also be sought regarding the diffusion and administration of this virus. A fine headlight can be added to reduce the risk of spreading this infection [7, 9]. Good info big data will now be included. Several data on these people infected with this COVID-19 contaminant can be stored by supercomputers. It helps to recognize the infection. Knowledge can be retrained to build potential plans to mitigate. This invention is used to store details from a good deal of COVID-19 affected cases (contaminated, retrieved, and finished). These statistics will be used to identify situations and to assist in the allocation of assets for improved general welfare insurance [10, 11]. Various advanced information strategies can be digitized and used to generate down-to-earth information both in the population and in the segment, including tolerant fields, the city, extensive travel, morbidity, physiological understanding, and current indications.

Big data provides academics, social security practitioners, and healthcare providers with a variety of data and helps them make wise decisions to combat COVID-19. This expertise can be used to continuously monitor infection and development in the clinical sector through AI. It seeks to predict and lead to groundbreaking research in all regions and the entire COVID-19 population on new clinical practices. Big data will also provide channels and tools to planned individuals, making it easier to manage upheavals. In short, innovation from AI offers knowledge about science and management processes for health, growth, and disease propagation [12]. Details are also given about the invention of AI.

In some places, big data provides data to distinguish similar incidents. It helps to provide a viable method of preventing pathogens and concentrating other important information. Big data will then enable the public, analysts, other researchers, and commentators to identify the infection and analyze the COVID-19 tool. Big data helped to investigate how this crisis could possibly be alleviated or cleared, and helped to upgrade assets, and helped solve correct and expensive choices. The latest IA is used to create a constructive and effective COVID-19 test method for experts and researchers.

3 AI and Big Data Techniques for COVID-19

AI could be used to detect, diagnose, monitor COVID-19 outbreak, info-veillance, info-demics, and developing therapeutics. The AI-based models are very efficient in mitigating COVID-19 pandemic effects, for the availability of enormous quantities of data on COVID-19 via different technologies and efforts. Yet, AI frameworks are neither tested clinically nor adopted widely, they are useful for the rapid responses and the beneficial data provided to healthcare providers and decision-makers. There are several limitations in developing AI algorithms since both the volume and the quality of COVID-19 datasets need more enhancements with further research efforts

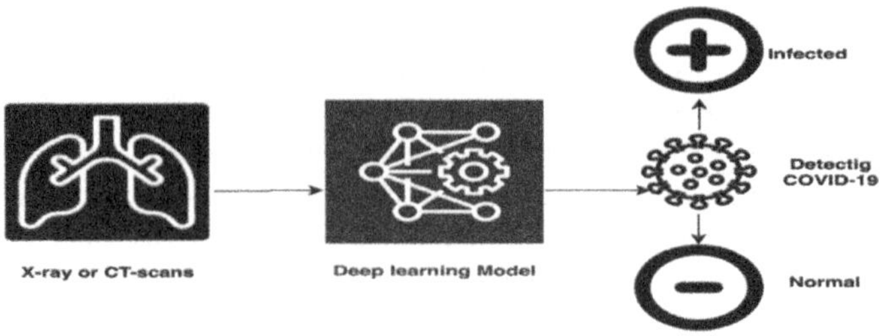

Fig. 1 AI-derived DL-model to detect COVID-19

to provide reliable and high-quality data. Figure 1 explains AI-derived applications, DL-based model, in detecting COVID-19.

Big data holds a key role in fighting the COVID-19 pandemic via many potential solutions, involving forecasting the outbreak, monitoring transmission, diagnosing and treating the infection, and developing drugs and vaccines as shown in Fig. 2. Big data could forecast the outbreak through data analytics on large datasets gathered from both international and local health organizations worldwide [13]. Big data could monitor COVID-19 transmission via integrating smart machine learning (ML) and deep learning (DL) techniques [14] to design frameworks for forecasting; enabling states to track a likely COVID-19 outbreak. Big data could enable healthcare professionals early diagnosing, analyzing, treating, and predicting therapeutic responses of coronavirus infection [15]. Ultimately, big data could discover promising targets for effective drugs or vaccines against COVID-19 [16, 17].

4 AI and Big Data Applications for COVID-19

4.1 Early Detecting and Finding COVID-19 Cases

Computer-based intelligence can quickly detect unexpected side effects and other "warnings" [18]. It makes cost-effective and complex decisions easier. AI help is developing a method to evaluate and monitor COVID-19 events using useful calculations. AI also helps to classify affected cases, such as CT, MRI, to analyze individual regions of the corpora that are compromised or not, using clinical imaging techniques.

4.2 Early Detecting and Finding COVID-19 Cases

The programmed inspections and predictions of this infection are focused on a brilliant level of mentally dependent units. It is also possible to suppress the sensory

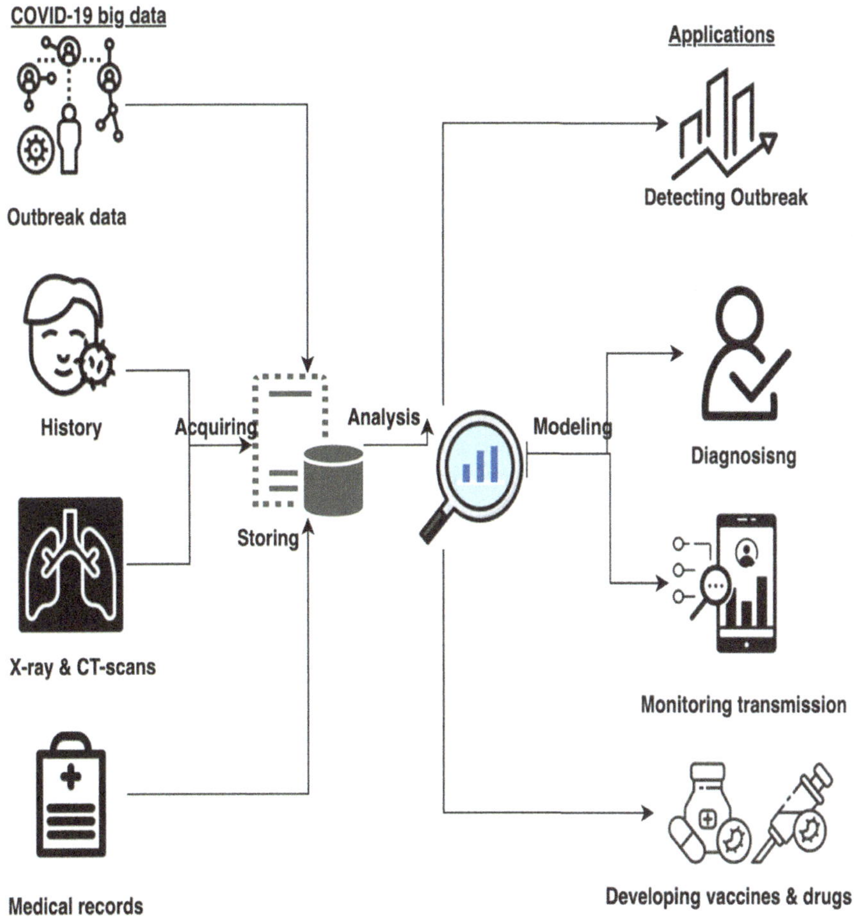

Fig. 2 Big data for addressing the coronavirus pandemic

properties of this disorder and to adequately monitor and manage patients with the nervous system [6]. It warns patients regularly and responds to COVID-19 pandemic.

4.3 Following Up Contacts

Artificial information can continue to analyze the disease issue for this infection by identifying between congregations and "problem areas" and contacting and screening individuals. You can expect this infection to improve and possibly replicate in future.

4.4 Projection of Cases and Moralities

This innovation makes it possible, through open information, interpersonal structures and the media, to control the risks of disease and its transmission and expectations of infection. In any place, the number of positive cases and deaths can also be predicted. AI helps to recognize and track the most vulnerable areas, populations, and nations to solve problems.

4.5 Reducing the Workload on Healthcare Workers

With the number of COVID-19 patients growing significantly and enormously, specialists in social security still have a lot of work to do. Here, AI is used to reduce the unresolved burdens on healthcare professionals [15]. The purpose of the research is to early define and control the current epidemic with the help of computerized techniques and the science chosen. Machine-driven system intelligence can impact potential therapies for patients and address potential challenges that minimize the remaining roles of specialists.

4.6 Prevention of the Infections

AI would provide updated results, useful in countering this crisis, using further data analysis. It can be used very easily to predict potential emission destinations, floods, bed needs, and social security experts during this crisis. Artificial knowledge is useful for detecting future illnesses with previous knowledge, coached at different times in common details. It identifies characteristics, sources, and factors for the spread of emissions. Eventually, this will be a significant step forward in dealing with the countless future pandemics. It is a preventative measure that can address several diseases. In order to provide specific and preventive health services in future, AI would play an important role.

5 A Proposed Model of AI and Big Data for COVID-19: Smartphone for Surveillance

With the late progress in developing hardware, growth in 5G wireless connectivity, and the rising cloud computing; mobile phones are promising during this outbreak, for instance, in determining the outbreak, detecting, diagnosing, and managing infected cases, and preventing disease. A proposed smartphone-based model was introduced for the coronavirus surveillance [19], as presented in Fig. 3. Globally, wireless

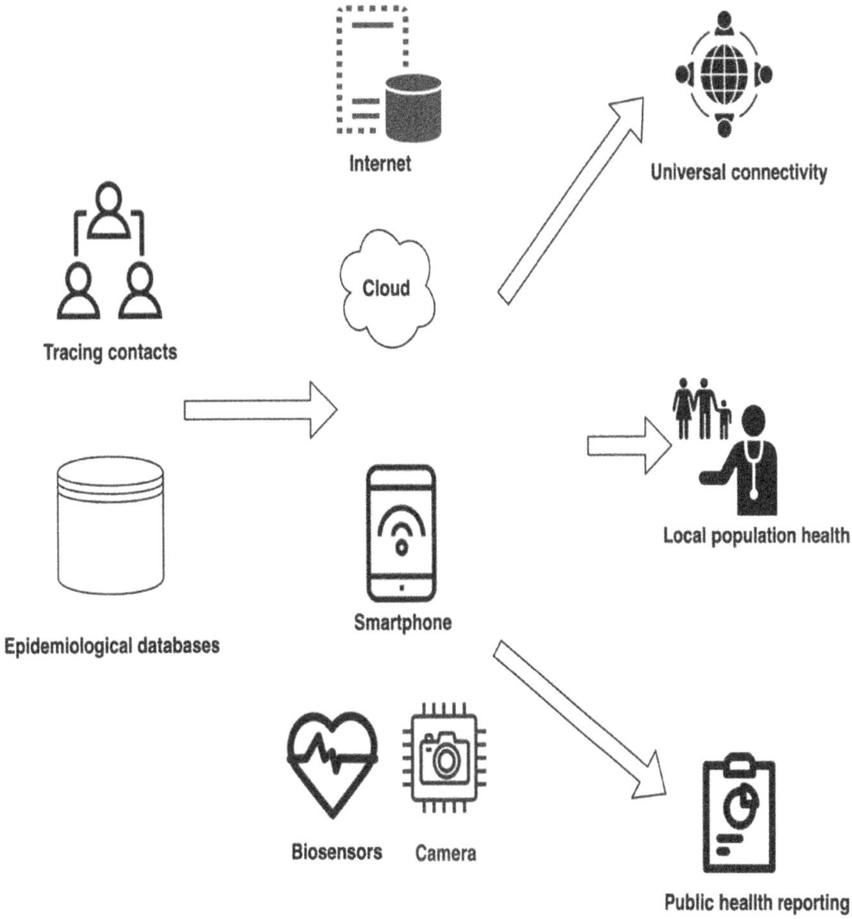

Fig. 3 AI-based model applying smartphone for COVID-19 diagnosis and surveillance

communications, such as Wi-Fi, 4G, or 5G, have been broadly adopted, enabling smartphone owners connected to the Internet performing several online activities [20]. The cloud-based DL framework could be trained [21], for instance, by embedding sensors and cameras, a smartphone could capture personal data such as scans of X-ray or CT, coughing sounds, or heart rates that could be encoded and squeezed prior to pushing for the cloud [22]. The enormous amount of Internet-connected smartphones would overcome the challenge of limited data from individual smartphones. Cisco's recent annual Internet report [23] estimated that over 70% of the people would access the mobile Internet where almost 29.3 billion connected devices would be online, including 23% smartphones and 3% tablets worldwide by 2030.

However, the many potentials, many limitations need to be tackled for the success of such a model [24]. For example, the capacity and accuracy of both software and hardware used in smartphones for medical purposes which could be addressed via developing standard smartphones with special sensing and computing elements. Besides, the protocols for gathering and storing health-related data, and the mechanism of building consumers' trust, particularly, if they preferred direct face-to-face communications with their healthcare providers. For instance, based on the local policies, the gathered health-related personal data from an area should be sent and stored at local servers instead of a cloud, one that could train the DL framework for universal communication. Ultimately, assessing the cost-effectiveness of these models is challenging since the outcomes of applying phone-based models are often debatable and nonparallel to those obtained from direct examinations.

6 Discussions

COVID-19 has been a source of controversy across several disciplines. The previous months have proved that disruptive innovation is necessary to tackle the pandemic. However, the same innovation seems to undermine privacy, confidentiality, and civil rights. For instance, remote working can violate personal and family privacy, while a tracing of contacts can pose a threat to confidentiality [25]. The situation is more complicated with AI. Although Europe is considered as one of the most privacy-friendly regions, a white paper issued by the European Commission in February 2020 suggested that there is a considerable deficit in policy and legal infrastructure for AI [26, 27]. AI has already contributed in the fight against COVID-19 and can play a greater role in the proximal future.

South Korea, China, Iran, Israel, Italy, Poland, Singapore, and Taiwan have used location data from cellphones while dealing with the pandemic. Apart from states, Big Tech entities such as Google, Apple, and Facebook are working toward tracing population movements. Their interest includes but is not limited to contact-tracing applications, local alert features, and emergency response services. Developers all over the globe are also using relevant toolkits to contribute in this effort [28, 29]. Although this technology focuses on travel patterns, potential outbreak hot-spots, chains of infections or immunity strategies, in the long-term AI and ML can enact social monitoring and control strategies. Beyond the containment of COVID-19, short-term policy regulations enable not only state authorities but also private companies and skilled individuals to monitor other individuals and communities. Protecting citizens from public health emergencies, terrorist attacks, or civil criminality can be an excuse to implement privacy violations [29, 30].

Even if governments intend to withdraw these policies after the pandemic, some modalities have the potential to become a trend. Online education and conferencing have received positive feedback by institutions, researchers, and students. AI has played a part there in administration and data analysis from grading assignments to supervising experiments [31, 32]. Being cost-effective most of these modalities are sustainable to make education and research accessible to people from remote areas or socially vulnerable groups.

Besides their benefits such practices set in peril the privacy and personal space of educators, students, and researchers worldwide, and several scholars and institutions have already issued relevant warnings [33]. On top of them, introducing immature AI modalities without prior testing to smaller sets of population and enforcing them by law can work as a dangerous precedent. Pensioners have a hard time dealing with AI-based call centers and applications of banks and public administration. Patients' well-being and lives have been set at risk while dealing with AI-based screening systems. Authorizing medicines before testing them properly increases the risk for unforeseen side effects and the same goes with innovative technology. Even if there are no systemic pitfalls, digital illiteracy can make AI-based technology ineffective or even dangerous [30, 34].

Hence, is there no space for AI during and after the management of the pandemic? In fact, the pandemic represents a chance not only to implement AI but also to resolve problems related to the trust of the public and the potential harassment of civil rights and liberties. Policy and education can play a key role toward a sustainable AI transformation of modern societies. Policy can safeguard privacy through anonymization. Public health authorities need to have access to information about crowded places or regions with a high transmission rate. They also need to track individuals who tested positive in order to track their contacts. However, nobody who is not authorized can have access to such information. Data security experts have urged for anonymization protocols while decentralized modalities including blockchain can increase the level of confidentiality [34, 35].

Several countries, including Austria, Switzerland, and Italy have announced their intention to incorporate decentralized structures and networks produced by Apple and Google in their COVID-19 response, and Norway have built their data storing and management strategies focusing on central servers (centralized systems). The UK has also shown preference to the NHSX, an app of the National Health Service based on centralized data storage. This app enables healthcare workers to track and communicate with potentially infected individuals. As important as it may seem, the processes of collecting, storing, and using the data remain obscure to date. What makes things more complicated is that for Brexit, it is not clear whether the UK will keep complying to the General Data Protection Regulation (GDPR) of the EU from 2021 onwards [29, 36]. The origin of many apps, either centralized or decentralized is questionable. On top of institutional efforts, a wide variety of modalities have been developed by non-accredited professional or even amateur developers in hackathons or challenges. Such modalities are currently under development, reaching out to citizens and requesting them to volunteer their personal data in an—often—controversial privacy and security context. Stakeholders should make quality control a priority in this context [29].

Education, in terms of digital literacy and human rights, is important considering the conspiracy theories about 5G. Ignorance creates room for fear and irrational personal and public attitudes [37]. What if AI is condemned in public conscience? Or, what mechanisms are available to make sure that everybody will be knowledgeable enough to interact with AI-based technologies? Germany, in the light of ongoing public debate and repeated warnings from privacy experts, recently declined a centralized solution leaning toward a decentralized framework instead. To conduct public dialogue of such level, the public needs to be aware of the benefits and drawbacks of such technological modalities. Nowadays, this is an endeavor for both formal educational institutions (universities, schools) and informal educational entities (NGOs, youth groups, etc.) [29, 33].

7 Future Insights

Leveraging AI with big data analytics could enable determining more about the COVID-19 such as viral structure and pathological pathways. Hence, both are key drivers for states in addressing any likely coronavirus outbreak in the upcoming years. Some guidance in fighting COVID-19 include: more optimizing AI and big data algorithms for improving consistency and precision of the data analytics thus enhanced COVID-19 detection and therapy; involving AI and big data with further growing techniques enabling novel efficient intervention for fighting COVID-19, such as Oracle cloud computing data analytics in developing a novel vaccine candidate against COVID-19 pandemic [38]. Lately, China has leveraged drones in responding to COVID-19 in the form of several applications, like transporting test samples and goods, and monitoring individual activities to track the outbreak [39]; and nontechnical measures like social distancing, adopted, and controlled by the states, contributes significantly in limiting the viral transmission and managing future pandemics [40].

8 Conclusions

Techniques for AI and big data would contribute significantly in addressing the COVID-19 pandemic via various attracting solutions, ranging from monitoring the outbreak, detecting the viral infection to diagnosing and managing. AI could address the coronavirus pandemic in many methods, for instance, AI could support info-demiology and info-veillance by optimizing learning-centered technologies of DL and ML from COVID-19-based modeling, sorting, and forecasting. AI could boost developing vaccines and drugs via using the datasets of healthcare institutions, states, clinical laboratories, and patients where AI optimizes smart analytics for designing safe, effective, and affordable vaccines and drugs against COVID-19. Meanwhile, big data could address the COVID-19 pandemic though potentially several promising applications where it assists healthcare professionals in different clinical tasks from early diagnosing, analyzing disease to identifying therapeutic responses. This work discussed some interventions in addressing the coronavirus pandemic.

References

1. WHO. (2020). Coronavirus disease (COVID-19) situation report—209.
2. CDC. (2020). Coronavirus disease 2019 (COVID-19). https://www.cdc.gov/coronavirus/2019-ncov/index.html. Last accessed July 09, 2020.
3. WHO. (2020). Coronavirus disease (COVID-19)—World Health Organization. https://www.who.int/emergencies/diseases/novel-coronavirus-2019. Last accessed July 09, 2020.
4. Guess, A. R. (2020). White House announces new partnership to unleash supercomputing resources to fight COVID-19. https://www.dataversity.net/white-house-announces-new-partnership-to-unleash-supercomputing-resources-to-fight-covid-19/. Last accessed July 09, 2020.
5. arXiv: arXiv announces new COVID-19 quick search|arXiv.org blog, https://blogs.cornell.edu/arxiv/2020/03/30/new-covid-19-quick-search/. Last accessed July 09, 2020.
6. Haleem, A., Javaid, M., & Vaishya, R. (2020). Effects of COVID 19 pandemic in daily life. *Current Medicine Research and Practice*. https://doi.org/10.1016/j.cmrp.2020.03.011
7. Bai, H. X., Hsieh, B., Xiong, Z., Halsey, K., Choi, J. W., Tran, T. M. L., Pan, I., Shi, L.-B., Wang, D.-C., Mei, J., Jiang, X.-L., Zeng, Q.-H., Egglin, T. K., Hu, P.-F., Agarwal, S., Xie, F., Li, S., Healey, T., Atalay, M. K., & Liao, W.-H. (2020). Performance of radiologists in differentiating COVID-19 from viral pneumonia on chest CT. *Radiology, 200823*. https://doi.org/10.1148/radiol.2020200823
8. Hu, Z., Ge, Q., Li, S., Jin, L., & Xiong, M. (2020). Artificial intelligence forecasting of Covid-19 in China. ArXiv200207112 Q-Bio.
9. Wang, C. J., Ng, C. Y., & Brook, R. H. (2020). Response to COVID-19 in Taiwan: Big data analytics, new technology, and proactive testing. *JAMA, 323*, 1341–1342. https://doi.org/10.1001/jama.2020.3151
10. Anshari, M., Almunawar, M. N., Lim, S. A., & Al-Mudimigh, A. (2019). Customer relationship management and big data enabled: Personalization and customization of services. *Applied Computing and Informtics, 15*, 94–101. https://doi.org/10.1016/j.aci.2018.05.004
11. MacLaren, G., Fisher, D., & Brodie, D. (2020). Preparing for the most critically Ill patients with COVID-19: The potential role of extracorporeal membrane oxygenation. *JAMA, 323*, 1245–1246. https://doi.org/10.1001/jama.2020.2342
12. Amini, S., Gerostathopoulos, I., & Prehofer, C. (2017). Big data analytics architecture for real-time traffic control. In *2017 5th IEEE International Conference on Models and Technologies for Intelligent Transportation Systems (MT-ITS)* (pp. 710–715). https://doi.org/10.1109/MTITS.2017.8005605.
13. Tátrai, D., & Várallyay, Z. (2020). COVID-19 epidemic outcome predictions based on logistic fitting and estimation of its reliability. ArXiv200314160 Q-Bio.
14. Castorina, P., Iorio, A., & Lanteri, D. (2020). Data analysis on coronavirus spreading by macroscopic growth laws. ArXiv200300507 Phys. Q-Bio.
15. Li, C., Debruyne, D. N., Spencer, J., Kapoor, V., Liu, L.Y., Zhou, B., Pandey, U., Bootwalla, M., Ostrow, D., Maglinte, D. T., Ruble, D., Ryutov, A., Shen, L., Lee, L., Feigelman, R., Burdon, G., Liu, J., Oliva, A. … Liu, Z. (2020). Highly sensitive and full-genome interrogation of SARS-CoV-2 using multiplexed PCR enrichment followed by next-generation sequencing. bioRxiv. 2020.03.12.988246. https://doi.org/10.1101/2020.03.12.988246
16. Banerjee, A., Santra, D., & Maiti, S. (2020). Energetics based epitope screening in SARS CoV-2 (COVID 19) spike glycoprotein by Immuno-informatic analysis aiming to a suitable vaccine development. bioRxiv. 2020.04.02.021725. https://doi.org/10.1101/2020.04.02.021725
17. Ge, Y., Tian, T., Huang, S., Wan, F., Li, J., Li, S., Yang, H., Hong, L., Wu, N., Yuan, E., Cheng, L., Lei, Y., Shu, H., Feng, X., Jiang, Z., Chi, Y., Guo, X., Cui, L. … Zeng, J. (2020). A data-driven drug repositioning framework discovered a potential therapeutic agent targeting COVID-19. bioRxiv. 2020.03.11.986836. https://doi.org/10.1101/2020.03.11.986836
18. Ai, T., Yang, Z., Hou, H., Zhan, C., Chen, C., Lv, W., Tao, Q., Sun, Z., Xia, L. (2020). Correlation of Chest CT and RT-PCR Testing in Coronavirus Disease 2019 (COVID-19) in China: A report of 1014 Cases. *Radiology*, 200642. https://doi.org/10.1148/radiol.2020200642

19. Udugama, B., Kadhiresan, P., Kozlowski, H. N., Malekjahani, A., Osborne, M., Li, V. Y. C., Chen, H., Mubareka, S., Gubbay, J. B., & Chan, W. C. W. (2020). Diagnosing COVID-19: The disease and tools for detection. *ACS Nano, 14*, 3822–3835. https://doi.org/10.1021/acsnano.0c02624
20. Pham, Q.-V., Le, L. B., Chung, S.-H., & Hwang, W.-J. (2019). Mobile edge computing with wireless backhaul: Joint task offloading and resource allocation. *IEEE Access, 7*, 16444–16459. https://doi.org/10.1109/ACCESS.2018.2883692
21. Pham, Q.-V., Fang, F., Ha, V. N., Piran, M. J., Le, M., Le, L. B., Hwang, W.-J., & Ding, Z.: A survey of multi-access edge computing in 5G and beyond: Fundamentals, technology integration, and state-of-the-art. ArXiv190608452 Cs Math.
22. Srinivasa Rao, A. S. R., & Vazquez, J. A. (2020). Identification of COVID-19 can be quicker through artificial intelligence framework using a mobile phone-based survey when cities and towns are under quarantine. *Infect Control Hosp Epidemiol*, 1–5. https://doi.org/10.1017/ice.2020.61
23. Cisco. (2020). Cisco Annual Internet Report (2018–2023) White paper.
24. Wood, C. S., Thomas, M. R., Budd, J., Mashamba-Thompson, T. P., Herbst, K., Pillay, D., Peeling, R. W., Johnson, A. M., McKendry, R. A., & Stevens, M. M. (2019). Taking connected mobile-health diagnostics of infectious diseases to the field. *Nature, 566*, 467–474. https://doi.org/10.1038/s41586-019-0956-2
25. Kahana, E. (2020). AI and COVID-19: Securing the intensified reliance on AI prime operational qualities. https://law.stanford.edu/2020/03/25/ai-and-covid-19-securing-the-intensified-reliance-on-ai-prime-operational-qualities/. Last accessed August 29, 2020.
26. Pierce, N., Stockton, J., & Chambers, C. (2020). Beyond HIPAA: inside the use of AI to collect COVID-19 information from employees. https://www.benefitspro.com/2020/06/25/beyond-hipaa-inside-the-use-of-ai-to-collect-covid-19-related-information-from-employees-412-100012/?amp=1
27. Pagán, J., Mokhtari, M., Aloulou, H., Abdulrazak, B., & Cabrera, M. F. (Eds). (2019). How AI impacts urban living and public health. In *17th International Conference, ICOST 2019*, NY, USA, October 14–16, 2019, Proceedings. Springer International Publishing.https://doi.org/10.1007/978-3-030-32785-9
28. Dorsten, A.-M., Sifford, K. S., Bharucha, A., Mecca, L. P., & Wactlar, H. (2009). Ethical perspectives on emerging assistive technologies: insights from focus groups with stakeholders in long-term care facilities. *The Journal of Empirical Research on Human Research Ethics (JERHRE), 4*, 25–36. https://doi.org/10.1525/jer.2009.4.1.25
29. Howard, P., & Neudert, L.-M. (2020). AI can battle coronavirus, but privacy shouldn't be a casualty. https://social.techcrunch.com/2020/05/26/ai-can-battle-coronavirus-but-privacy-shouldnt-be-a-casualty/. Last accessed August 29, 2020.
30. Gopal, G., Suter-Crazzolara, C., Toldo, L., & Eberhardt, W. (2019). Digital transformation in healthcare—architectures of present and future information technologies. *Clinical Chemistry and Laboratory Medicine, 57*, 328–335. https://doi.org/10.1515/cclm-2018-0658
31. Dimitrov, D. V. (2016). Medical internet of things and big data in healthcare. *Healthcare Informatics Research, 22*, 156–163. https://doi.org/10.4258/hir.2016.22.3.156
32. Tian, S., Yang, W., Grange, J. M. L., Wang, P., Huang, W., & Ye, Z. (2019). Smart healthcare: Making medical care more intelligent. *Global Health Journal, 3*, 62–65. https://doi.org/10.1016/j.glohj.2019.07.001
33. Stanfill, M. H., & Marc, D. T. (2019). Health information management: Implications of artificial intelligence on healthcare data and information management. *Yearbook of Medical Informatics, 28*, 056–064. https://doi.org/10.1055/s-0039-1677913
34. Michalopoulou & Associates: Artificial Intelligence|Covid-19|data protection rights|privacy concerns|Greece. https://lawgroup.gr/artificial-intelligence-covid-19-data-protection-rights-privacy-concerns-greece/. Last accessed August 29, 2020.
35. Bues, M. (2020). What AI in law can and can't do. https://europe-legaltech.org/what-ai-in-law-can-and-cant-do/. Last accessed August 29, 2020.

36. COVID-19 Data Protection and Privacy Resources • UN Global Pulse. https://www.unglobalpulse.org/policy/covid-19-data-protection-and-privacy-resources/. Last accessed August 29, 2020.
37. Warren, T. (2020). British 5G towers are being set on fire because of coronavirus conspiracy theories. https://www.theverge.com/2020/4/4/21207927/5g-towers-burning-uk-coronavirus-conspiracy-theory-link. Last accessed August 29, 2020.
38. Atiqah, A. (2020). A potential COVID-19 vaccine is being developed through AI and Cloud Computing. https://www.imapac.com/en/a-potential-covid-19-vaccine-is-being-developed-through-ai-and-cloud-computing/. Last accessed July 22, 2020.
39. Chaturvedi, A. (2020). The China way: Use of technology to combat Covid-19. https://www.geospatialworld.net/article/the-sino-approach-use-of-technology-to-combat-covid-19/. Last accessed July 22, 2020.
40. Nussbaumer-Streit, B., Mayr, V., Dobrescu, A. I., Chapman, A., Persad, E., Klerings, I., Wagner, G., Siebert, U., Christof, C., Zachariah, C., & Gartlehner, G. (2020). Quarantine alone or in combination with other public health measures to control COVID-19: A rapid review. *Cochrane Database Systematic Review*. https://doi.org/10.1002/14651858.CD013574

Emerging Trends in Higher Education During Pandemic Covid-19: An Impact Study from West Bengal

K. Mourlin

1 Introduction

The arrival of the Covid-19 has posed numerous challenges to education around the globe, particularly to Higher Education. The Higher Educational Institutes (HEIs) are found to be stagnated with teaching–learning gaps. Due to pandemic impact, the traditional instructional mode in HEIs has become less effective and is found to be weakened. The pandemic has affected the educational systems, the learning of students, and the teaching patterns.

The research of Marshall and Wolanskyj-Spinner [1] has indicated that the closure of educational institutes has widened the gap in teaching–learning and having no access to study materials, library books and journals, laboratory learning with teaching inputs and the absence of evaluative methods. These realities have impacted on the educational system to discover newer alternatives to meet the demands of the students and the faculties.

The current pandemic situation has paved a way to use technology-enabled platforms to create a student-centered learning and helping them to shape their learning. In the context of present research, the academic programs and activities of many Higher Educational Institutes particularly in West Bengal were frozen and encountered a problem of instructions. HEIs are trying to grapple with pandemic posed challenges and to find innovative solutions to bridge the teaching–learning gaps. HEIs in West Bengal have observed that teaching–learning has a major shift from offline to online mode of communication. The faculties are unable to connect with students due to unfamiliarity of the online mode of interactive teaching.

The current research paper discusses the influence of Covid-19 on Faculties of Higher Educational Institutes in West Bengal. It has further posed to introspect the road ahead to engage purposefully and to meet the demands of students to help in

K. Mourlin (✉)
Xavier Business School (XBS), St. Xavier's University, Kolkata, India
e-mail: mourlin.ksj@sxuk.edu.in

M. Niranjanamurthy et al. (eds.), *Intelligent Data Analysis for COVID-19 Pandemic*, Algorithms for Intelligent Systems, https://doi.org/10.1007/978-981-16-1574-0_8

their careers. The paper attempts to answer the questions, namely how HEIs are engaging online, tracking the progress of students, conducting examinations through virtual platform. It is also to study the development of online data management system using artificial intelligence and particularly computational intelligence in the context of education in HEIs. Thus, HEIs are learning to explore newer avenues to help the students and faculties to adopt teaching–learning strategies, using artificial–computational intelligence, cloud-based applications, and new programming to meet the demands of the students online. Many HEIs are using virtual solutions to connect the students with learning. The current research aimed to explore the usage of ICT tools and techniquesand to enhance teaching–learning instructional purposes. It is further to delve into how Higher Educational Institutes (HEIs) in West Bengal are employing the digital platforms to enable both teaching faculties and students to meet the challenges of imparting quality education during the pandemic epoch, which has paralyzed the atmosphere and the environment of curriculum designing, researching and the mode of teaching.

2 Research Background Literature

The Covid-19 has brought the closure of total cessation of business, education, and other activities. It has been observed that the lives have been stranded, business handcuffed and education systems frozen. Cohen and Kupferschmidt [2] have indicated that the closure of schools is increasing and affected largely. UNESCO report 2020 indicates that there is an alarming situation across the globe regarding education. It reports that there are 1,215,881,292 affected learners, which is nearly 70% of total enrolled learners and around 162 country-wide closures of educational institutes. It has really shaken the global educational institutes and hampered teaching–learning. Burgess and Sievertsen [3] have indicated in their research that the pandemic influence has made the Educational Institutes to meet the closure of complete schooling, and other activities have been marooned. Nicola et al. [4] have indicated that many postgraduate programs and research projects have been suspended due to the influx of Covid-19. Rundle et al. [5] have indicated that Covid-19 has impacted on more health hazards among the students and causing obesity risk in them as they stay at Home.

In the context of India, Sintema [6] has observed that the pandemic Covid-19 influence has affected the performance of the students. Burgess and Sievertsen [3] have voiced that Covid-19 has affected the learning environment as well as the key assessment period of learners with promotion. Crawford et al. [7] have given a new insight that the pandemic Covid-19 has affected the university and colleges who are not using online for their learning and teaching purposes. Sahu [8] has enumerated that the outbreak of Covid-19 has impacted on all types of education, psychological well-being, and mental framework of pupils and the teaching faculties. Research studies have revealed that there is a sharp decline in teaching–learning in education sector. Ozili [9] has provided a crucial view of Covid-19 that Covid-19 is leading to structural weakness in economics, infrastructure, and services like education and access to health systems. Rundle et al. [5] have been matched with findings of Sahu [8] who indicated that the closing of educational institutes has impacted on students, academic staff, universities programs, and career opportunities. Cao et al. [10] have indicated that the sudden termination of academic institutes has delayed in final year project completions and caused psychological and mental pressures on students. Chick et al. [11] indicated that pandemic Covid-19 has led the HEIs to discover alternative models of providing educational opportunities to the student fraternity. Bansal-Parul [12] proposed an alternative route to revival of Higher Educational Institutes in the pandemic closure. He further indicated that there is a sharp rise on online teaching–learning process, enhancing students with performance and outcomes.

The research findings of Huang and Cambria [13] indicated that Higher Educational Institutes use the online technical solutions and services to instruct students with more flexibility in time and in space. Thus, the research findings have indicated that there is an acute gap between the completion of studies, pursuing higher studies or availing job opportunities, and the need for new strategies. Mame and Tarush [14] have indicated that the tiny adventure of a few individuals with Covid-19 has brought massive disruptions in Indian educational system. He further argued that the educational system in India is being nailed to closure and leading to have multiple layers of teaching–learning gaps. Lu et al. [15] have indicated that the need of computational intelligence in real-time learning, reasoning and cognition development is the sole focus in education system. It is also furthered that convergence of computational intelligence is important and urgent need of educational system. Hanne and Dornberger [16] have indicated that the role of CI is to improve the outcomes of learning and helping students to adopt the application of CI in solving problems and attempting to find solutions. The insights of Williamson [17] have revealed that the usage of CI has contributed to build knowledge-based digital laboratories to develop new insights in CI and its application in education. Yunanto et al. [18] have indicated that the application of natural language processing in the concept of non-player in English education games, which are successful in engaging students and help them to learn new outcomes of teaching–learning English. Salem and Nikitaeva [19] have argued that the influence of CI paradigms in smart tutoring system has enhanced the system of teaching and learning outcomes. Thus, in the context of educational institutes, it invites all of us to strategize new methodologies, curriculum design, and outcome-based education models using ICT tools and techniques along with AI and CI applications in online education. It calls for an alternative model to enhance education and revive educational practices among the faculties. Educational institutes are inviting faculties to be creative and innovative in curriculum transaction exercises. Thus, the above research insights have enabled the researcher to understand the pandemic situation and its influences on Higher Education, the need for technology-enabled solutions to reduce gaps in teaching–learning and promote healthy learning environment for the students online.

3 Methodology

3.1 Research Gaps

The review of literature has facilitated to identify considerable gaps in the literature, which justifies the rationale for carrying out a research work on the topic under study. Due to obvious reasons, existing literature largely focuses on different aspects of ICT tools and techniques in educational sectors. The scant research is also found in CI-based teaching–learning and their applications in the field of education in West Bengal. Furthermore, there is paucity of the literature on technology-enabled teaching–learning paradigm in Higher Educational Institutes in the generic context, and particularly, CI-based applications in HEIs of West Bengal are weak. It has been further noticed that CI-based teaching–learning and their applications are on the rise with minimum focus and less explored.

3.2 Research Objectives

The research gaps have paved a way to comprehend the technology-enabled teaching–learning of HEIs and contextualize the CI usage and applications in HEIs in West Bengal. It is also to discover the role of CI applications in the context of educational systems and how to train HEIs' faculties to create interest for learning. In light of the insights drawn from the Research background literature coupled with the considerable research gaps, the research objectives have been formulated. The aim of the objectives of the current research is to examine the road map of the research and to understand the role of ICT tools and techniques, faculty orientation toward ICT, organizational orientation toward computational intelligence.

The research objectives are: to study the overall influence and nature of relationships among identified aspects used by Higher Educational Institutes (HEIs), to examine the strategic relationship between HEI variables in control situation like different Higher Educational Institutes (HEIs) and experience of establishment, to study the usage and the application of computational intelligence in HEIs, to extract the different dimensions (Factors) of technology-enabled teaching–learning and CI application of HEIs, to form the cluster associations based on their proximity and the areas of Computational Intelligence in HEIs, to study the role of ICT components and the usage of CI application in St. Xavier's University, Kolkata, through a case study.

Table 1 Sample size of Higher Educational Institutes in West Bengal

	Frequency	Percent	Valid percent
Affiliated colleges	105	73.4	73.4
Universities	4	2.8	2.8
B-Schools	10	7.0	7.0
Technical institutions	24	16.8	16.8
Total	143	100.0	100.0

3.3 Sample Design

The current research has used the web portal of the Department of Higher Education, Government of West Bengal (www.wbhed.gov.in*) along with the list of colleges received from the College Admission Web page (*www.collegeadmission.in*). The random sampling methodis employed to screen the colleges.* Accordingly, a list of 200 HEIs has been prepared. These HEIs were divided into small sections, namely affiliated colleges, universities, business schools, and technological institutes. A well-defined questionnaire was administered and was sent to those listed HEIs. Table 1 indicates the number of sample responses received from the types of Higher Educational Institutions in West Bengal. The responses are varying from 73 to 2.8% of HEIs in West Bengal. It has been observed that affiliated colleges both private and government colleges are having higher responses nearly 73.4% of the total responses. The second highest is technical institutions having 16.8% from West Bengal who could share the information for the benefit of the current research. A few responses have been rejected as it was found to be half-filled and returned with no answers and that accounts for 3% of the responses.

3.4 Research Approach

A two-prolonged research approach was used, involving a questionnaire coupled with 61 aspects administered through an electronic medium (Email) and a qualitative approach of using interviews to collect information from the principals and the directors of select HEIs through online platforms like ZOOM application, Google Meet, and Microsoft Team. The data collected was corroborated, computed, interpreted with statistical tools along with SPSS software. The present paper also has an in-depth case study of SXUK, as an organization using ICT tools and CI-based applications for instructional and other purposes. The case study is to elaborate the nature of online platforms used by SXUK to help the students to learn effectively. Reliability Analysis.

Lee Cronbach has proposed the concept of alpha to measure the internal uniformity and cohesiveness of a scale. Santos [20] has explained that the research construct is checked through the significance of Cronbach's alpha and used as a measuring tool

Table 2 Research construct

The value of identified aspects	N of items
0.936	60

to identify the reliability of the scales of the items included in a research instrument. The values of Alpha coefficient range from 0 to 1. Nunnally [21] has pointed out that the values of Alpha coefficient 0.7 are an acceptable reliability coefficient of the items and found to be important for assessing the strength of the research construct. Table 2 indicates the reliability of different items identified. Table 2 indicates the reliability of the entire identified aspects in the current research having 0.936 with higher validity of the research variables construct.

3.5 Research Tools Usage in Current Research

In the view of the research objectives, suitable quantitative techniques have been employed in order to draw meaningful conclusions. The objective-wise quantitative techniques employed are shown in Fig. 1. Figure 1 gives an overview of quantitative techniques employed in current research.

The researcher has used a multiple statistical framework for the data analysis. Pearson's correlation analysis to analyze the relationship between the variables and establish the correlation between identified aspects of the research to validate the data received. The factor analysis helps us to converge the aspects of ICT tools and CI components into factors that enable us to understand the dimensions of the current research that is proactive in the context of HEIs.

The cluster analysis is used to form the HEIs based on closeness and proximity and to enable researcher to identify the closeness of HEIs with regard to their commonality and differences in following CI and ICT tools and techniques that are essential for online tutoring and management of students.

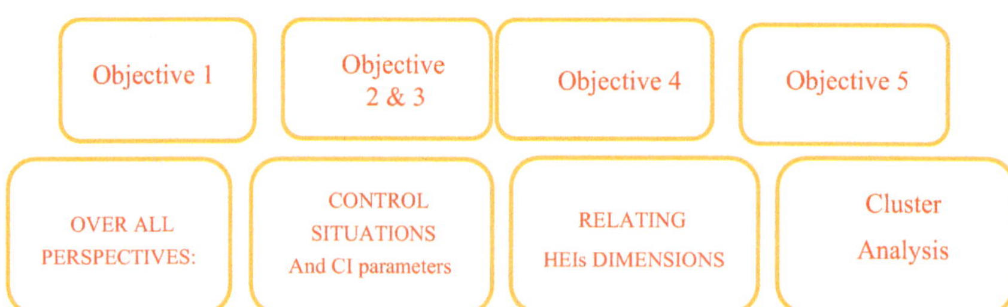

Fig. 1 Quantitative techniques for data computation

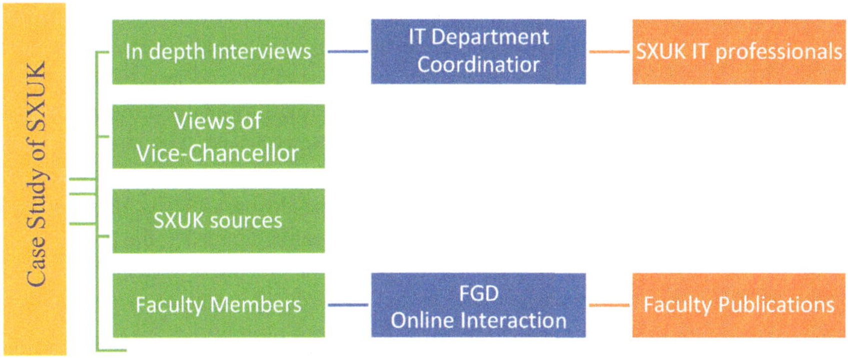

Fig. 2 Case study design

3.6 *SXUK Case Study Process*

Merriam [22] argued that case study plays a significant role in adding to the prevailing knowledge in terms of the contextual issues associated with a case. The objective of case study is to have a comprehensive perspective of the organizations in terms of their responses toward knowledge of ICT and CI applications in their teaching–learning process. The case study of St. Xavier's University, Kolkata, provides ample opportunities to study the role of ICT tools and CI applications in their teaching–Learning process during the pandemic. Figure 2 indicates the case analysis tools used for collecting information about the university.

4 Research Findings and Discussion

The research findings of the current research have received responses from 143 respondents (out of 200), which signifies a response rate of 71.5%. It has been observed that the obtained value of reliability using Cronbach's alpha (0.936) is highly satisfactory, which signifies the overall strength of 61 items of the research construct. The sixty-one aspects used in the research have been validated, examined, and applied to study the relationship among the identified aspects, factors relating to them and the cluster closeness.

4.1 *Teaching–Learning Context During Covid-19*

The objective 1 was to study the overall influence and nature of relationships among the identified aspects. When we are using Pearson's correlation test to establish the findings of the aspects, we need to also understand the role of learning and teaching gaps existing during the Covid-19 and the lockdown of Higher Educational Institutes (HEIs). The present work has revealed more insights on the pandemic influence and its damages to the educational institutes in West Bengal. The Focused Group Discussion (FGD) with selected faculties online has enabled the researcher to examine the context in which the teaching–learning is placed. The insights drawn have indicated that the Covid-19 has paralyzed the active participation of students in Higher Educational Institutes. The context analysis of closure of HEIs has given rise to several student-related issues. The researcher has ranked in order, the problems of students in terms of their learning during the pandemic closure of HEIs. The student mindset during the pandemic period oriented toward video games, long hours of engagement with social media and spending time with mobile.

4.2 Content Development Orientation

The context analysis has enabled the teaching faculties of HEIs to discover newer way of instructing students with technology-enabled interventions. Based on the contextual issues, faculties of HEIs are using content development orientation to prepare teaching–learning modules, online curriculum design tools and instructional methods to bridge the learning gap among the students. The content development orientation has enhanced to promote innovative and creative solutions to enable students to be active in their learning process and respond positively.

In mean value ranking, Table 3 indicates that curriculum assessment having mean of (4.02) is the leading aspect among HEIs.

HEIs in West Bengal during the pandemic have undertaken the survey of how students are able to understand the online education and assessment. HEIs have introduced curriculum assessment during the pandemic at two levels, namely individual and group levels. HEIs are using curriculum assessment as a tool to evaluate individuals with individual focused examinations and assignments. The group also is assigned to specific topics for group discussion and group learning. Curriculum assessment in HEIs is having threefold process, namely the phase 1 is having pre-assessment strategies to know the position of the learner, phase 2 helps to identify the leaner's response during the learning process, phase 3 indicates the post-learning assessment of students and how teaching–learning impacting on them to develop their intellectual quotient.

Table 3 Curriculum design in HEIs

	N	Mean	Std. deviation
Curriculum assessment	143	4.02	0.726
Curriculum design	143	3.90	0.705
Curriculum implementation	143	3.86	0.810
Curriculum review	143	3.85	0.927

Table 4 The ICT context in HEIs

	N	Mean	Std. deviation
ICT skills	143	4.24	0.778
ICT dependency	143	4.13	0.786
ICT lesson plan	143	4.06	0.748
ICT application	143	3.99	0.796
ICT adaptation	143	3.97	0.769

4.3 ICT Technology Strategies in HEIs

Table 4 gives an overview of faculties in HEIs who are technology-driven and actively involved in teaching–learning process during pandemic lockdown. The present mode of learning is being halted. The alternative way out is to use online platforms for teaching–learning. Faculties in HEIs have adopted ICT Skills. The mean value of Table 4 ranks ICT skill (Mean 4.24) and ICT dependency (Mean 4.13) as top ICT practicing elements among the faculties in HEIs. It has been observed that many HEIs in West Bengal are found to be using ICT skill development strategies to help the faculty members to understand the need of enhancing themselves with ICT skills and applications in their curriculum designing and implementation.

From the table, it has been observed that the faculties of HEIs are more prone to use ICT skills in the context of teaching–learning process. The ICT skills include technology-oriented teaching–learning process. It has been observed that there is a growing techno savvy mindset of faculty members, and they are trying to use digital platforms for instructional purposes. The mean values in Table 4 indicate that faculties are getting acquainted with ICT skill in teaching–learning paradigm. On the other hand, it has been found that HEIs are struggling to use ICT adaptation as it has low mean value of (3.97). It indicates that there is a provision for ICT skill integration and application but there is less accountability to ICT adaptation to the large extent.

4.4 "Big Five" Strategies

The objective 1 was to study the nature of relationship between the different identified aspects used in technology-enabled teaching–learning paradigm of HEIs in West Bengal. It is also to examine how an aspect of technology-enabled teaching strategy is having linked statistically significant with other aspects. Faculties in HEIs in West Bengal are using the identified aspects that are having significant influence on the teaching–learning of faculty members. This objective 1 shows how the technology-enabled aspects are interrelated to influence the context of Faculty teaching and learning. To establish the nature of relationship among the aspects, researcher has used Pearson's correlation to determine the relationship. These aspects are having strong significant values of correlation coefficient (r).

In the context of current research, one aspect of technology-enabled teaching–learning is being statistically correlated with other 61 variables that are used by faculties in HEIs. The relationship of one aspect (Variable) is to be strategically significant in the context of technology-enabled learning and teaching in HEIs, if it has statistically significant relationship ($r > 0.6$) with a greater number of aspects in HEIs paradigm.

In comparing Table 4 with Table 5, we could discover the unifying element of curriculum assessment and co-assessing which are common to both. The overarching aspect of co-assessing is having statistically significant correlation with 51 aspects of technology-enabled teaching and learning components along with computational intelligence, deep learning (DL), natural language processing (NLP), and data visualization (DV).

Faculties of HEIs have maneuvered ICT application into their teaching and learning. Co-assessing has become central to faculties to be familiar with and try to use its tools and techniques to instruct students online. The second aspect is ICT Skills, having 48 aspects which connect the faculties to learn and disseminate the information, lesson input, and insights to the students effectively. It has been observed during the ZOOM-based interview with teachers of HEIs that the ICT skills are vital for teachers to share their common problems, strategies, and resources to empower students to learn effectively.

The third aspect of big five strategies is CI application in HEIs. The CI application has statistically correlated with 48 aspects. It has been observed that CI application has a greater relationship with data mining, data security, and data visualization relating to data analysis through CI applications. HEIs are prone to use CI application for the benefit of the faculties who can learn the basics of CI application and be aware of CI application in teaching–learning process. Additionally, B-Schools in the research have used CI application to enhance marketing analysis, tracking human resource performance, and financial allocation process and motivate students to enhance CI application knowledge process and integrating it as a Business Management Solutions The fourth aspect is reflective thinking which is the hallmark of teaching–learning process. Reflective thinking is having 48 aspects of correlation with identified aspects of HEIs. Reflective thinking is having positive correlations with cognitive and emotional development, student growth orientation, curriculum designing and implementation. The faculties of HEIs have voiced that teaching–learning process during the pandemic addressed to promote reflective thinking as a

Table 5 "Big five" strategies

Co-assessing	51
ICT skills	48
CI application	48
Reflective thinking	48
Online simulation	46

foundational tool to enhance the growth of cognitive elements in students and help them to become reflective thinkers. The final aspect is online simulation is having 46 aspects correlated with other identified aspects.

Faculties of B-Schools have voiced that online simulation helps students to be creative and innovative in solving cases and propose solutions to problem presented. The faculties of B-Schools use online simulation for students to develop team working skills, their capability to take decisions and increasing the performance of the students.

4.5 Technology-CI Adapted Teaching–Learning Strategies

The objective 2 of the current research is to examine the strategic relationship between HEI variables in control situation like different Higher Educational Institutes (HEIs) and experience of establishment. The objective is to study the overall influence of identified aspects along with four types of HEIs and their interrelation. Role of years of experience in technology-adapted teaching–learning plays a vital role to shape the teaching–learning process.

Years of Experience in Technology-Adapted Teaching–Learning

The years of experience plays a vital role in adopting technology in teaching and learning. The years of experience of the faculties in HEIs are considered for the correlation analysis to study the impact on them. It is to understand how faculties with more than 10 years of experience adopt in comparison with faculties with less than 10 years of experience in technology-adapted teaching and learning as well as HEIs themselves in adopting ICT skills and CI-based applications.

Table 6 shows the correlation analysis and how one aspect of technology-adapted teaching–learning establishes relationship with other aspects in HEIs. The statistical significance of first aspect, namely ICT application, is having 38 aspects relational among HEIs with experience of teaching–learning more than 10 years of establishment. HEIs with 10 years experience are more prone to use ICT application, curriculum planning, online team learning, and curriculum organization of the content of teaching–learning. These aspects have strong correlations with other

Table 6 HEIs having more than 10 years of establishments

	Statistical significance
ICT application	38
Curriculum planning	37
CI awareness	37
Curriculum review	36
Online simulation	36
Cognitive development	36

Table 7 Years of experience less than 10 years

	Statistical significance
ICT skill	30
Curriculum organization	29
Team sharing	29
Student mentoring	28
Teacher skills	27

aspects used in the study. It has been observed that ICT application is the sole focus of HEIs and adopts various sources to enhance online mode of communication and to ensure smooth teaching–learning experience. The second aspect is curriculum planning having 37 aspects being correlated with. Curriculum planning is important in the context of teaching–learning process during the pandemic crisis and to enhance the learning of students and orienting them toward cognitive development process. The third aspect is computational intelligence awareness having 37 aspects being correlated with other aspects. HEIs are having CI awareness to use the components of CI in their teaching–learning process. HEIs are enhanced with CI-based applications to help the IT team to develop CI-based solutions for the effectiveness of teaching–learning strategies with outcomes.

Years of Experience Less Than 10 Years

In Table 7, we are trying to examine how one aspect is Statistically Corelated with other aspects in the current research. The findings of Table 7 indicate that the aspect of ICT Skill is having Statistical significance with other thirty aspects covered in the current research. The Correlation of ICT Skill with thirty aspects is having highest association. Thus, we could conclude that HEIS with less than 10 years of establishments are more prone to use ICT Skills as their top priority. The aspects of Curriculum Organization and Team Sharing are having equal number of Statisticall significance with twenty nine aspects respectively. HEIs with less than 10 years use Student mentoring in the third place and followed by Teacher Skills in the final place. The teacher skills in third place signify the importance of developing teacher skills like competency, cognitive skills and language skills.

4.6 *Higher Educational Institutes Wise*

Affiliated Collages in Content Management

The first group of HEIs is affiliated collages. The aim is to identify the dominant areas of teaching–learning paradigms that are operating very strongly.

Table 8 reveals that curriculum is the sole focus of the affiliated collages in the current research. Affiliated collages have integrated curriculum assessment strategies and enabled the faculties to design lessons during the pandemic crisis. Curriculum

Table 8 Content management

	N	Mean	Std. deviation
Curriculum assessment	105	4.01	0.753
Curriculum design	105	3.91	0.735
Curriculum review	105	3.89	0.891
Curriculum implementation	105	3.83	0.860

assessment strategies are developed along with curriculum design of the teaching–learning process. The faculties in affiliated collages are to use curriculum assessment strategies to evaluate the level of students during the learning process. Curriculum assessment strategies are enhancing the growth and development of the students, and it contributes to their cognitive and emotional development positively. Curriculum implementation scores the lowest mean value in Table 8, and it indicates that affiliated collages have lower score of curriculum implementation with online teaching.

Teaching–Learning Strategies

The current research was aiming to understand the strategies for teaching–learning of affiliated collages. It has been observed that affiliated collages are designing their curriculum with team learning concepts. Onboarding of students and faculties during the online interaction has shaped the teaching–learning process.

Affiliated collages have adopted teaching–learning strategies like co-learning which was ranked first in Table 9. It reveals that faculties are promoting co-learning as strategic option to help the students and learn together. The curriculum designing is aimed to introduce the idea of co-developing of lessons, cases, and insights. The online platform is helping faculties to create an atmosphere of learning and creating interaction among students positively.

Universities in Teaching–Learning Management

The teaching–learning system in universities are focusing more on faculties and their orientations and helping them to onboard online education system. The faculties of the universities in the current research have voiced that the importance was given for ICT skill upgradation and application in the context of teaching–learning.

Table 10 reveals that faculties are oriented toward ICT application in teaching–learning process. Faculties are found to be motivated in using ICT applications in

Table 9 Strategies for teaching–learning

	N	Mean	Std. deviation
Co-learning	105	4.06	0.818
Co-developing	105	4.05	0.870
Co-designing	105	4.04	0.940
Co-assessing	105	3.98	0.796
Co-researching	105	3.92	0.997
Co-inquiring	105	3.89	1.022

Table 10 Faculty orientation

	N	Mean	Std. deviation
Teacher mindset	4	4.75	0.500
Teacher organizing	4	4.50	0.577
Teacher knowledge	4	4.25	0.957
Teacher skills	4	4.25	0.500
Teacher learning	4	4.00	0.816

their teaching. Teacher mindset toward ICT and CI awareness is ranked as the top mean value. Teacher mindset of the faculties is oriented toward ICT skill development which is positive. It has been observed in the data that teacher learning is found to be the lower score in Table 10, and focus must be on learning.

Faculty Team Dynamics

During the pandemic, universities have enhanced faculties to work in teams to share the burden of the workload and make the learning as team-based approach and team learning model.

Table 11 indicates that the team evaluation has the highest score. Team evaluation is having mean score of 4.25, one of the teaching–learning strategies that enhance students to work in online model team-based learning. Team evaluation is another form of enhancing faculties to work in teams and do the curriculum designing and implementing learning strategies.

The faculties of the universities in the research have indicated that team-based approach to teaching and learning is important during the pandemic so that we could work in groups and enhance teaching online with creativity and innovative simulation and lesson plans. It has been observed that team-based evaluation has twofold process, namely firstly, faculties could evaluate their teaching strategies along with online simulation and case studies and the effectiveness of their teaching online, and secondly, it is also to examine the learning outcomes of the students online. The last mean score value is 3.75 of team planning. This is the indication that the team planning is managed poorly by the faculties.

B-Schools

In the current research, B-Schools are concerned with data management during the pandemic to use them for teaching–learning process along with data management strategies.

Table 11 Faculty team dynamics

	N	Mean	Std. deviation
Team evaluation	4	4.25	0.500
Team communication	4	4.25	0.500
Team sharing	4	4.25	0.500
Team planning	4	3.75	0.500

Table 12 Data information

	N	Mean	Std. deviation
Data mining	10	3.70	1.160
Data visualization	10	3.00	1.491
Data economy	10	2.90	1.524
Data security	10	2.90	1.197

Table 12 indicates that data management is sole focus of B-Schools to use the information for the teaching–learning process. The data mining tops the table of mean value. B-Schools are giving due importance to data mining and using the data to generate new information with the CI application and techniques. B-Schools are also using the data visualization process to understand the trend in students pursuing MBA programs graphically.

The graphical representation of the data helps B-Schools to analyze the intake of students and adopt strategies to increase admission.

Strategic Thinking Design

B-Schools in the current research have used strategic thinking design to develop the skill of students and help them to adopt analytical thinking in learning process with learning outcomes.

Table 13 indicates the mean value of the strategic thinking aspects. B-Schools are using analytical thinking having mean value of 3.90 as a learning tool to help the students to think creatively while they are online. The online teaching pedagogy of B-Schools aims to enable students to think analytically and use case study to foster reflective and design thinking to benefit the students in articulating their thinking process and convert the process into learning outcomes.

Technical Institutes in ICT Skill Adoption

The introduction of ICT tools and techniques in HEIs is positive. During pandemic crisis, the use of ICT has become central focus of technical institutes in the current research.

The role of ICT has gained the momentum in teaching–learning process with outcome-based and knowledge creation interventions. Table 14 indicates that Technical Institutes in West Bengal are using ICT Skills (ranks with 4.21) and application

Table 13 Strategic thinking

	N	Mean	Std. deviation
Analytical thinking	10	3.90	0.876
Group discussion	10	3.90	1.287
Case study	10	3.70	0.949
Reflective thinking	10	3.60	0.843
Design thinking	10	3.30	1.160
Online simulation	10	3.10	1.197

Table 14 ICT skill orientation

	N	Mean	Std. deviation
ICT skills	24	4.21	0.415
ICT application	24	4.13	0.612
ICT dependency	24	4.00	0.511
ICT adaptation	24	4.00	0.590
ICT lesson plan	24	3.92	0.504

Table 15 Teaching–learning process

	N	Mean	Std. deviation
Co-developing	24	4.13	0.850
Co-designing	24	4.00	1.022
Co-Researching	24	3.92	0.974
Co-learning	24	3.87	0.992
Co-assessing	24	3.83	0.917
Co-inquiring	24	3.71	1.042

of ICT skills in teaching–learning process and motivating faculties to use the skills of ICT knowledge and adopt them to teach online effectively with outcome-based learning. It aims to develop ICT orientation among HEIs.

Teaching–Learning Process

Technical institutes in the current research have used teaching–learning process as strategic advantage to empower students to collaborate in curriculum development and implementation process. Table 15 indicates that technical institutes have given priority to teaching–learning process and outcome-based educational inputs. During the Pandemic, HEIs have used a collaborative method to involve students as Co-creators in the learning process. In ranking of aspects related to Teaching-Learning Process, Co-Developing ranks first in the Table 15 with the Pearson's Correlation value 4.13, followed by Co-designing (4.00) and so on. Thus, the findings have indicated that Students are collaborators in their learning process with teachers in designing their curriculum and its development. The collaborative learning would enhance to reduce learning gaps and enable students to be active participants in their learning than passive spectators in learning.

4.7 CI Awareness and Application in HEIs

The objective 3 is to study the usage and the application of computational intelligence in HEIs. Artificial intelligence (1) is dominating all the sectors of business, education, and military. Zawacki-Richter et al. [23] have indicated that there is a sharp growth of 43% in AI usage and AI-based applications in education. Computational intelligence is part of AI and plays an important role in education and its applications. The current research has explored the concepts of CI in HEIs and how HEIs in West Bengal are using CI in their teaching–learning process.

Affiliated Collages and CI Interface

CI-based application is emerging need of the educational institutes. AI- and CI-based applications are used widely in manufacturing industry and other sectors, particularly in educational sector.

Table 16 indicates the role of CI in affiliated collages of the current research. CI awareness is the top mean value among affiliated collages. It has been observed that affiliated collages are disseminating CI-based awareness among the faculties, administrators, and IT departments to create database and CI tools and techniques could be applied. The mean value of CI designing is the second position which helps the affiliated collages to design their CI-based applications to enhance their data management.

Significance of CI Aspects

The paired samples' correlations are used in the present study to understand the correlation between threefold process indicators. The pair sample correlations are indicating that affiliated collages have positive correlations in all the three, but the levels of correlation are bare minimum. In Table 17, it has been observed that CI application in the context of students and their learning paradigm is gaining momentum. There is correlation between CI application to enhance their learning process. The correlation of CI awareness and institutional CI applications are moving at slow pace and minimum interaction. The pair 3 seems to be higher valued at the institutional level of CI application with the development students.

Table 16 CI-based application

	N	Mean	Std. deviation
CI Awareness	105	4.08	1.016
CI Designing	105	3.47	1.271
CI Application	105	3.23	1.416

Table 17 Significance of CI aspects

		N	Correlation	Sig
Pair 1	CI awareness and institutional	105	0.187	0.056
Pair 2	CI designing and instructional	105	0.385	0.000
Pair 3	CI application and student	105	0.501	0.000

Table 18 Relationship between HEIs with CI

HEIs		CI awareness	CI designing	CI application
Universities	Mean	4.50	3.75	3.75
	N	4	4	4
	Std. deviation	0.577	0.957	0.957
Total	Mean	4.50	3.75	3.75
	N	4	4	4
	Std. deviation	0.577	0.957	0.957

Table 19 B-Schools and CI knowledge

	N	Mean	Std. deviation
CI awareness	10	3.60	1.265
CI application	10	2.80	1.317
CI designing	10	2.70	1.160

Universities and Their CI Awareness

In the current research, comparing mean is used to understand the influence of CI components on universities. It is to examine how universities can adopt CI-based application for the effectives of teaching–learning process and administration of CI application in ERP system. Table 18 indicates that the comparison of universities in applying CI tools and techniques to structure CI awareness among HEIs in West Bengal, and it is found to be using CI tools.

B-Schools and CI Knowledge

CI knowledge and application in Business Schools are important and significant to enhance Business Intelligence. Business Intelligence is emerging as a core element to use it for analyzing market driven data and propose business solutions (Table 19).

B-Schools are using CI-based approach to teaching marketing, human resource and finance. Table 19 indicates that B-Schools in the current research have CI awareness as it tops the table with 3.60. B-schools have used CI application to the extent to create a new knowledge and information about resources like Market share, Human Resource Audit and Financial trends.

Role of CI in Teaching–Learning Process

The secondary sources and Focused Group Discuss with faculties have indicated that B-Schools are prone to use CI applications in Teaching–Learning Process to help the students to use CI in understanding Business with clarity and coherence (Fig. 3).

B-Schools in Figure have used CI-based applications to help the students and to make them realize the importance of CI-based analysis of Management subjects like Marketing, Human Resource etc.

The Teaching–Learning Pedagogy in Business Schools uses customer intelligence as a tool to enhance students to study and relate the marketing information of the

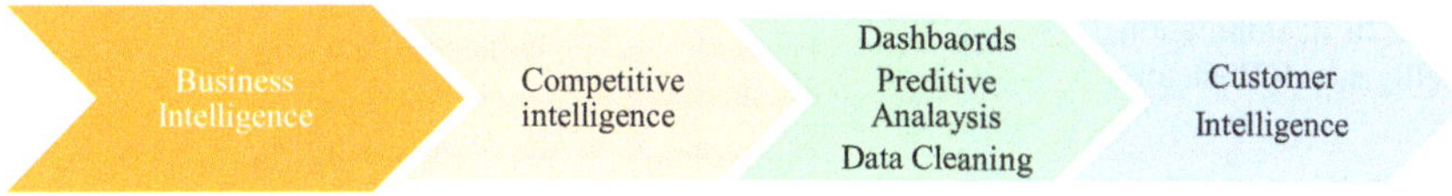

Fig. 3 Role of CI in teaching–learning process

product, customer choice, customer loyalty, and delight. It enables the students to use customer intelligence and apply real-time cases to track customer preferences and choices in shaping market orientation-Schools are using customer intelligence as a tool to help the students to analyze the real-time cases and to collect the data to study the demographic, psychological, and personalized marketing orientation. The students of B-Schools are streaming customer data to understand the real-time customer experience. The use of CI application in the context of tracking employees and their performance is through dashboards and their applicability in evaluating employees. This is additional knowledge given to students. The role of faculties is remarkable in shaping business intelligence-based approach in learning.

4.8 Computational Intelligence-ICT Factors Confluence

The objective 3 is to extract the different dimensions (factors) of technology-enabled teaching and learning aspects comprising of 61 aspects. This is to extract factors by using factor reduction along with 61 aspects. Results of factor analysis reveal that the 61 aspects converged into 9 factors which have been considered as dimensions of technology-enabled teaching and learning factors. It can be observed that the values of Cronbach's alpha of all the technology-enabled teaching–learning dimensions are greater than 0.60. We have obtained very high value for the first dimension (0.928); also, high values up to sixth dimensions also signify higher values (greater than 0.8). This shows the strength of the factor scores. The first factor accounts for 48.5% of variance explained and comprises 9 aspects. On the basis of the aspects that comprise the factor, the factor has been named *curriculum technology factor* having construct reliability 0.928. The *Curriculum technology* factor is related to internal aspects of Google Meet, ZOOM, CISCO, NEYON, OPENSIS, and their usage. The observation during the interview has helped the researcher to understand how the faculties have used digital platforms for the instructional purpose and trying to communicate with their students. These digital classrooms have given space for creativity to display content and enable faculties to deliver online lectures and class discussions (Table 20).

The second factor is named as *Team Learning Orientation* and comprises of seven aspects, namely *team communication, team resources, team learning*. HEIs have oriented them to do. It has been observed that the Covid-19 has impacted faculties to share their ideas, learnings, and teaching resources on digital platforms and share

Table 20 Computational intelligence-ICT factors

S. No.	Factors orientation	Dimension	Construct reliability
1	Curriculum technology	9	0.928
2	Team-learning orientation	7	0.880
3	CI-driven	7	0.892
4	Data-driven	6	0.891
5	Learning pyramid	6	0.860
6	Teaching impact	5	0.817
7	Competency development	4	0.805
8	Collaborative learning	4	0.743
9	Teaching impact factor	3	0.690

their class information on technology mode of communication. It has become easier to share and communicate in organizing classes and class notes.

The third factor is *Computational Intelligence Driven* having seven aspects, namely *Queriumand **Quizle,**Edmodo, Kahoot, TalentLMS, Class-Marker, Bigbluebutton, and Teacher Ease. In* the ZOOM-based Interview with faculties of HEIs, we have observed many facilities are familiar with Querium and **Quizlet** as a digital platform to conduct interactive classes and share information.

The faculties in HEIs are using CI-driven mechanisms to increase the participation of students in real-time problem-solving cases. CI-driven HEIs are organizations who are using CI-driven aspects linked with digital assessment system, predictive analysis, listening, and sensing technologies. The teaching–learning system in HEIs is using CI-driven platforms to strategize effective learning outcomes with CI components. The fourth dimension is *data driven* which helps HEIs are to create data archives for maintenance of data information received from faculties and students. The combination of CI and data-driven components is to enhance the profile of the students, faculty profiles, data visualization of HEIs, and data security of HEIs cloud management with CI significance. The fifth factor is *Learning Pyramid.* The *Learning Pyramid factor* involves the process of learning steps, namely Remember, Understand, Apply, Analyze, Evaluate, and Create. These steps are used for effective implementation of online learning. The CI plays vital role in creating learner's assessment of skills and knowledge. The sixth factor is named as *Competency Development.* The *Competency Development* factor is associated with cognitive skills, creative skills, and interpersonal skills. These aspects are to enable faculties to give attention while they are using online platforms for their learning purposes. It has enabled them to evaluate how each faculty is using one's skills. The seventh factor is *Collaborative Learning* which creates a common platform for teaching–learning paradigm and enables faculties to use *Collaborative Learning* as a methodology to enable students to be active in their learning process. It has been observed that HEIs are using computational model to create new learning environments and adopting new strategies to help the students to onboard online effectively. The computational method of learning shapes the faculties to teach creatively with innovative ways and students are engaged in a collaborative learning way. The final factor is the *Teaching Impact factor* is related to focus on the development of students, while faculties go online for instruction. It has been observed that the faculties are making more efforts to coach and mentor students by attending to them. Online mentoring and coaching of individuals students have an impact in online teaching–learning process.

4.9 CI-Based HEIs Cluster Membership

In addressing the fourth objective of this research work, faculties in HEIs have been grouped based on commonalities with the help of cluster analysis. Researcher has carried out hierarchical clustering for faculties in HEIs followed by K-Means clustering to form clusters. As part of hierarchical clustering researcher has examined the dendrograms with respect to faculties in HEIs. From the dendrogram, two for faculties in HEIs could be identified.

Subsequently, K-means clustering is chosen to recognize cluster membership. The number of clusters in each of the clusters has been obtained from the results of K-means clustering, and these have been exhibited in Table 21.

Outstanding CI-Based HEIs

The first cluster is named as *Outstanding CI-based HEIs.* In this cluster, the faculties in HEIs adequately focus on the teaching competencies developed through technology-enabled teaching and learning along with CI-based application in education. Higher emphasis has been observed in faculties of HEIs who use curriculum technology, skill-building, assessment technology tools, development of specific coaching and mentoring, and the faculties are becoming techno savvy in learning ICT tools and techniques to engage students digitally with more online creativity (Fig. 4).

Table 21 CI-based HEIs cluster formation

Cluster	1	12.00
	2	43.00
	3	35.00
	4	53.00
Valid		143.00

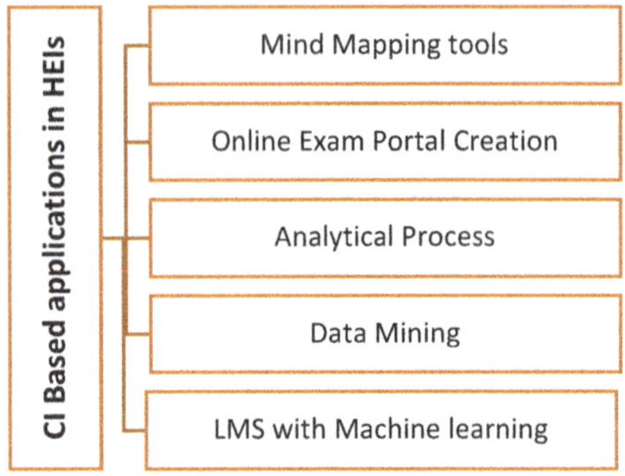

Fig. 4 Computational intelligent web-enabled education model

The CI-based education model addresses real-world applications and computer-based learning environment. Many facilities in HEIs have voiced that CI-based educational strategies are enhancing learners to be oriented toward outcomes. Outstanding CI-based HEIs are prone to use CI application and data-driven interface solution for effective learning. Outstanding CI-based HEIs enable facilities to create smart-content strategies to enhance the transparency of teaching–learning. It has been observed that the use of intelligent coaching system is the CI application which helps the faculties to reduce failures and maximize the outcomes of learning. The figure indicates that the HEIs in these clusters are using various CI- and ICT-based tools to enhance teaching–learning outcomes. The mind mapping tools are used to provide cognitive and intellectual development spaces for their students and to develop a comprehensive understanding of analytical thinking process and propose solutions. HEIs are using the interface of LMs with machine learning components. The CI-based HEIs are using *Thinkseter math* as a CI applied educational tool to track the performance of the students. This cluster of 12 HEIs is using special algorithms in CI applications to create assessments of the performance of the students. It has been observed that the twelve HEIs of the cluster 1 have used machine learning, CI applications, data visualization and ICT skills to become effective in creating smart-content components and assess the progressive nature of the performance of the students. These HEIs are also using CI-based designing and applications for creating online portal for admission process, conducting online examinations which is protected by CI applications and publishing results and tracking payment methods to increase financial viability.

High Performing CI-Based HEIs

The second cluster having 43 HEIs is named as high performing CI-based HEIs. A significant number of faculties as well as HEIs fall under this cluster. The current research has emphasized on some specific technology-enabled and CI-based teaching–learning aspects that are practiced by faculties. Faculties in this cluster largely get acquittance with medium level of learning from online digital platforms and birdbrained with technology-based education model purposes. These HEIs are

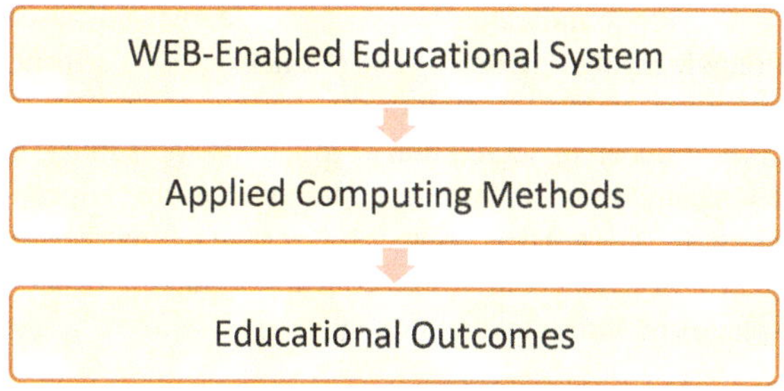

Fig. 5 Setting for web-based education in HEIs

concentrating computing methods to enhance their learning management system with outcomes (Fig. 5).

The Covid-19 has a positive impact on faculties to go online using digital platforms to teach students virtually and enabled them to learn at Home. HEIs are high performing due to the application of CI components, data structure, and visualization methods, and it enhances organizational effectiveness in teaching–learning paradigm, tracking students' progress effectively. The Fig. 5 shows the computational intelligence process is being used in HEIs in the current research. The computational intelligence process is beginning with web-enabled educational system tools development through algorithms and fuzzy logic-oriented integration and their application to make online education strategies effective in teaching and learning. The application of computing methods and tools using data visualization helps in educational outcomes.

Moderate CI-Based HEIs

The cluster three having 35 HEIs in the current research is using Information and commination technology (ICT). It has been observed that that the moderate CI-based HEIs are more prone to use ICT-enabled teaching–learning methods to design and create lesson plans using ICT tools (Fig. 6).

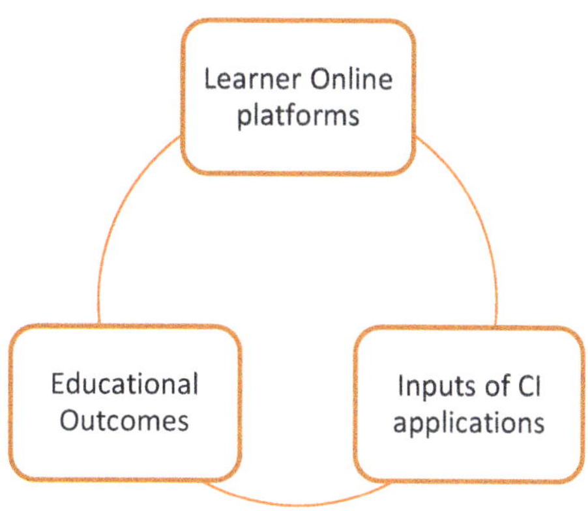

Fig. 6 Architecture of educational web programming

The Fig. 6 indicates the process of learner-CI-based applications to create educational learning outcomes. The learner online platforms supports LMS orientation to empower students to create collaborative learning outcomes.

It has been observed that productivity tools like Google Docs, Edpuzzle, Educreations, and Slide-Poll are used to create online education effective and collaborative learning. These HEIs are using machine learning-based applications to track performance of students in online education than interested in using CI components in all spheres of student development.

Stunted CI-Based HEIs

The final cluster having 53 HEIs are using ICT and CI-based application sparingly. These HEIs are moving slowly from offline to online with minimum engagement and investment on learning management system. There are colleges both in rural and semi-urban areas which are facing investment problems of using online educational system which needs more investment to make online portal and web-enabled solutions for teaching and learning processes.

Figure 7 indicates that the interaction of ICT tools and educational content in this cluster is minimum. There is an integration process of educational content development, using online faculty orientation with specific apps and learners' outcomes. It has been observed that the onboarding of faculties in this cluster needs motivation to go online confidently and use online platform for teaching–learning process.

Thus, the data analysis has given an orientation to understand how Higher Educational Institutes in West Bengal are faring in adopting ICT tools and techniques to modernize their educational system and enhance their teaching–learning process during the pandemic with outcome-based interventions.

Fig. 7 Offline-to-online orientation process

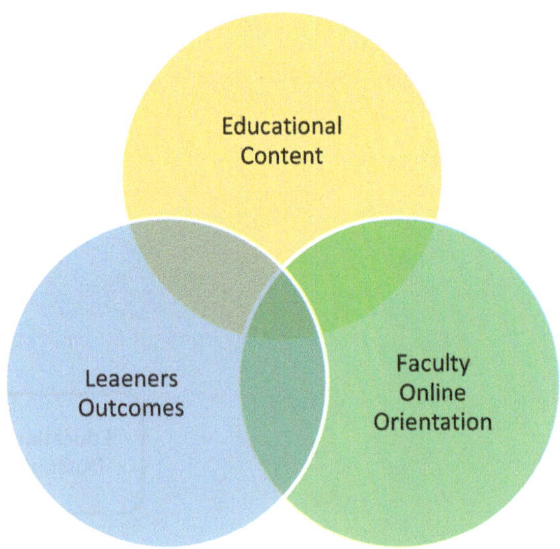

Thus, the research findings have indicated that HEIs in West Bengal are prone to use ICT tools and techniques along with CI-based applications for the instructional purpose and other management related programs. It has been observed that the cluster analysis has shown the close association of HEIs in terms of their practice and applications.

5 Case Organization: SXUK

5.1 Introduction

St. Xavier's University, Kolkata (SXUK), is run by Jesuits of Calcutta Province. It was established with SXUK Act passed in the State Assembly, West Bengal. Dr. Fr. John Felix Raj, SJ along with St. Xavier's College, Kolkata Alumni, has envisioned an institute that would serve the people of Bengal in Higher Education with vision and values of Ignatian Heritage. The birth of SXUK is the cumulative efforts of Jesuits, alumni, and benefactors.

5.2 Historical Millstones of SXUK

Dr. Fr. John Felix Raj, SJ was the pioneer and instrumental to initiate the project of establishing St. Xavier's University, Kolkata (SXUK). The process of establishment of SXUK is shown in Fig. 9. It was a great achievement for Jesuits in West Bengal that St. Xavier's University Kolkata Act is passed in West Bengal Assembly on December 15th, 2016 [24] (Fig. 8).

The Vice-Chancellor in his interview has explained "The Chief Minister, Ms. Mamata Banerjee, The Education Minister, Dr. Paratha Chatterjee, The Chairman and CEO of Arcelor Mittal and Mrs. Usha Mittal, Mr. Lakshmi Niwas Mittal,, The Chancellor Rev. Fr. Jeyaraj Veluswamy, S.J., The Vice-Chancellor Rev. Dr. John Felix Raj, S.J., The Rector of SXC, Dr. Fr. Dominic Savio, S.J, and several other dignitaries were present for the occasion" [25].

5.3 SXUK Organogram

St. Xavier's University has its own organogram with functional areas of management of the university. The functional management has the combination of diverse background people with vast experiences of having lived in educational arena. The organogram of SXUK is given a bird view of how SXUK functions and shows

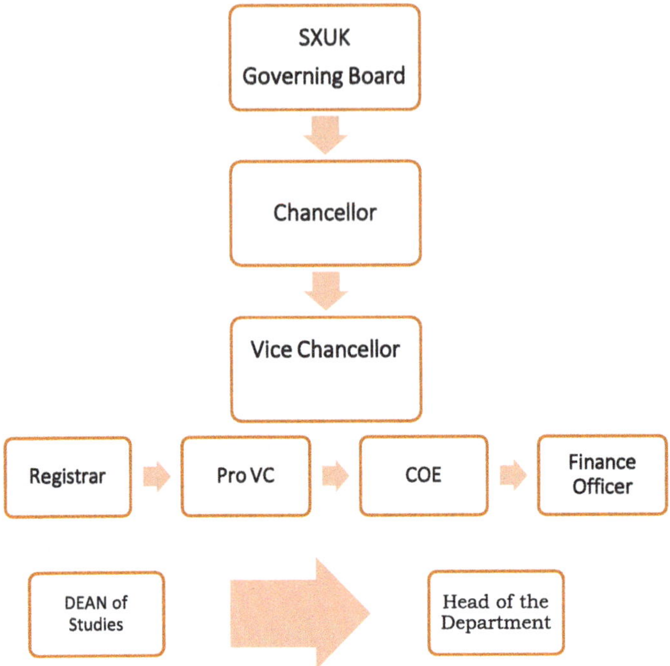

Fig. 8 SXUK organogram

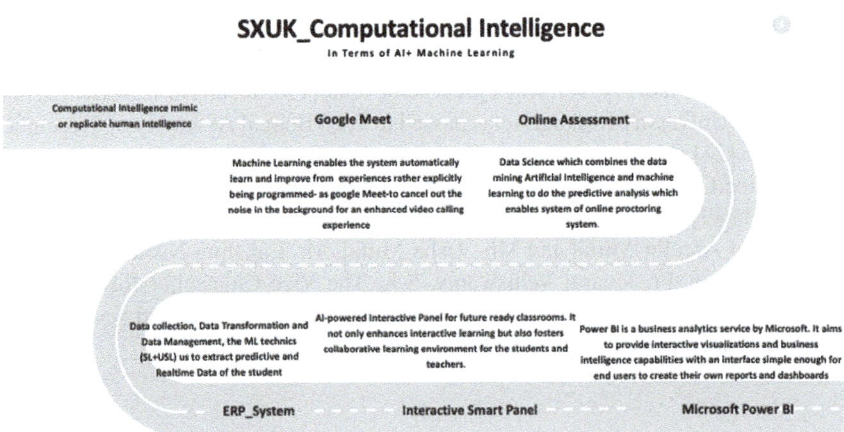

Fig. 9 SXUK model of CI interface

its accountability. The accountability and the decision-making process take place simultaneously.

5.4 *AI-CI Interface Strategies for SXUK*

The age of digitalization rules the world and its functions. We are in the era of Alexa Amazon, Apple Siri, and Google voice assistants which is the direction of our lives today and enabling us to be become technocracy. In this scenario, the arrival of artificial and computational intelligence is using mathematical algorisms to advance business, education, and other spheres of the planet.

In this case study, we are going to explore how AI-CI interface works in the context of SXUK and how SXUK has used AI-CI into their system to benefit the students and the faculties. Figure 11 has indicated the process of SXUK CI model using Google Meet with new features added upon, ERP system including payment of fees and hostel leave applications, and interactive smart panel used for online collaborative learning with group-based interactive learning outcomes (Fig. 10).

CI-Based Applications in SXUK

AI-computational intelligence is the main domain that shapes various aspects of intelligence, namely logical reasoning, learning, problem solving, decision making, and perception orientation. The utilization of machine learning approach is to use the system through computational approach rather than using through programming approach. In the domain of Higher Educational Institutes, it has been observed that the educational data mining (EDM) and learning analytics (LA) are used, where AI-CI-big data process will be used to increase the relevance modernized digital education platform in all the three levels.

Instructional Strategy 1: AI-Based Interactive Solution

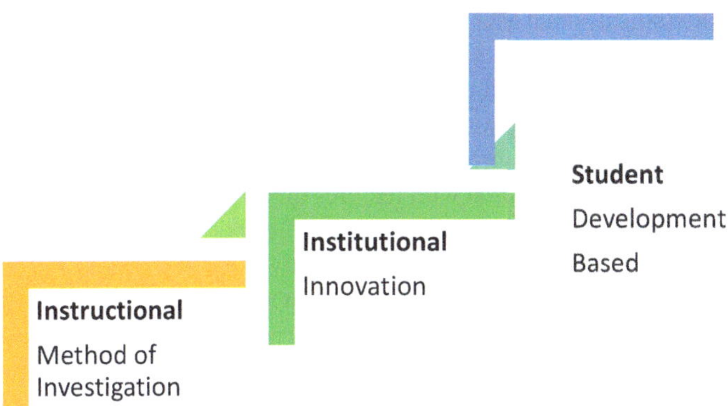

Fig. 10 Application of AI-CI-based intervention

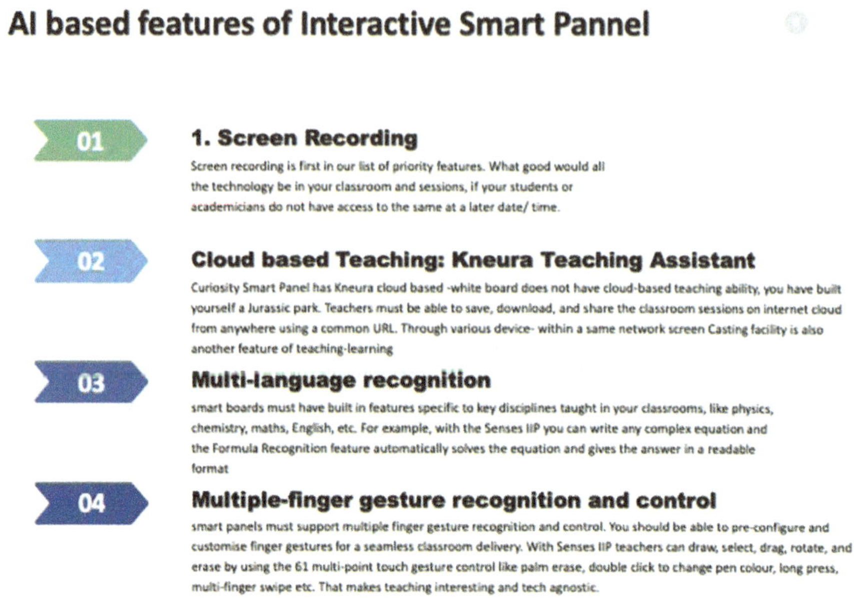

Fig. 11 AI-based interactive solution

Sangsawang [26] has indicated that instructional design framework for education through media interventions in the teaching–learning process. Instructional level applications consist of creation of pedagogical systems capable of addressing the individual learner's capability and progress. Such software monitors students' academic progress and deploys course contents customized for individual students. One of the most popular AI-based systems is the intelligent tutoring systems (ITS). SXUK has developed a model of instruction design of education in Fig. 11. Instructional strategies are developed with pandemic arrest of offline education mode, and they are to be effective in conducting online interactive planning and implementation.

This figure indicates that SXUK has installed interactive smart panel to introduce online teaching–learning. This panel is AI-enabled applications to help the faculties to teach students remotely with interactive features.

Faculties during the pandemic were unable to use cases, mathematical formulas, and other platforms. With the introduction of the interactive panel, faculties are able to use *AI*-powered *interactive panel* with features that would enhance screen recording, multi-language recognition group sharing of information, student–teacher connect, and my cloud options to use the portal for effective online digital transformation of knowledge. SXUK has interactive panels to assist the students, faculties, and visitors to share the knowledge in a platform. The instructional design orientation of AI-based solution has enabled faculties to make teaching–learning process effective and interactive. This has made a deep impact on the learners to be active in online class.

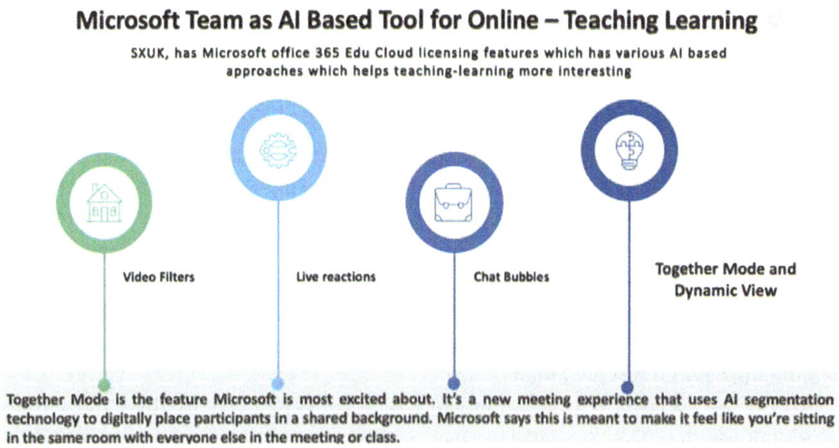

Fig. 12 AI applications-based learning process

Instructional Strategy 2: Teaching–Learning AI-Based Applications in SXUK

SXUK has devised students' support applications. It deals with the implementation of student's support systems by utilizing the strength of machine learning. Microsoft Team is part of Microsoft Edu cloud license package being subscribed by the university. During the pandemic situation, this application has given AI-based features to integrate in the teaching–learning process. The Microsoft App for online teaching–learning has been shown in Fig. 12. Chatbot is another mobile-based application that has been introduced by SXUK. During the pandemic, students are using Chatbots application to establish char conversation with teachers to clarify doubts, lesson outcomes, and effectiveness of learning.

The impact of using AI-based application for teaching–learning is remarkable and has success stories in SXUK. The instructional paradigm shift from offline to online has not an inch difference in teaching–learning opportunities. The AI supported model of applications in SXUK is to develop speech recognition makes noise suppression sound much more achievable during the calling of students to teacher and teacher to the students with clarity of inputs. The faculties in SXUK are using the feature of AI and the Microsoft Graph to provide voice assistance. It has been noted that the various features involving AI-Microsoft cloud, use of whiteboard and camera detection of students are applied during the meeting hours. This is the specialty of the feature that has enabled our faculties to onboard online with more information-related content presentation. Faculties of SXUK have used the time slots to conduct the class hours and help the students to use their mobiles to log in.

Institutional Strategy 3: CI-Based Online Examination Portal in SXUK

Institutional level applications are developed to automate administrative function of the education institutions which can include various functions like recruitment, students' admission and enrollment, timetabling, and attendance tracking. SXUK

Institutional level applications are actively using 'enrollment analytics' by harnessing the power of machine learning to gauge the prospective student's interest level in joining their respective courses. SXUK also uses two other applications, namely payment gate way ERP system and online examination portal.

These two are being developed using CI-based applications and features relating to ERP system to handle the fee information and tracking the payment system based on paid and non-paid situation. Online assessment tool has been adopted by SXUK for conducting online examination. This tool has the feature of face recognition and anomaly voice recognition which helps the students to write online examination free from error and duplicity. The online assessment system in SXUK has the application of CI-based. It has ensured the administration that the CI features used in online examination portal has benefited.

This is the SXUK CI-AI based model which is the pathway to direct the activity of SXUK online. This model describes various usability of various tools which helps online teaching–learning effectively and efficiently. This is model of automated dashboard Microsoft tool which helps Edu cloud administrator to track down the activity and analytics of all Microsoft applications.

Thus, the case study of SXUK has been a motivating experience to study and to understand the nature of ICT-based teaching–learning in the context of Higher Education. The outcomes of the case analysis of SXUK have indicated that there is a lot of scope in applying CI- and ICT-based interventions in teaching–learning process. SXUK has been adapting newer technologies in CI and ICT tools to enhance online educational system of the university and reach out to the students. The arrival of Covid-19 has opened new opportunities for SXUK to analyze the need of ICT-CI interventions and apply those mechanisms to empower faculties to assist students in their teaching–learning process along with instruction module (Figs. 13 and 14).

6 Conclusion

The current research has come to end of the road of the survey of ICT- and CI-based application in teaching and learning processes. The current research has given a new orientation to the Higher Educational Institutes (HEIs), in West Bengal. Though many HEIs have not gone to online mode of communication with students before the lockdown, the Covid-19 has impacted on HEIs in West Bengal to utilize the online mode of instruction to help students and encourage faculties of HEIs to incorporate digital learning mechanisms in their teaching patterns. The objectives of the current research have contributed toward the understanding of using ICT tools in teaching–learning as well as CI-based applications. The online teaching–learning platforms have opened new doors to impart outcome-based education and help the students to become co-designers in learning environment. One of the major outcomes of the current research is that the objectives have been used to analyze the overall influence and nature of relationships among the identified aspects of ICT tools. It is also to examine how an aspect of technology-enabled teaching strategy is having linked

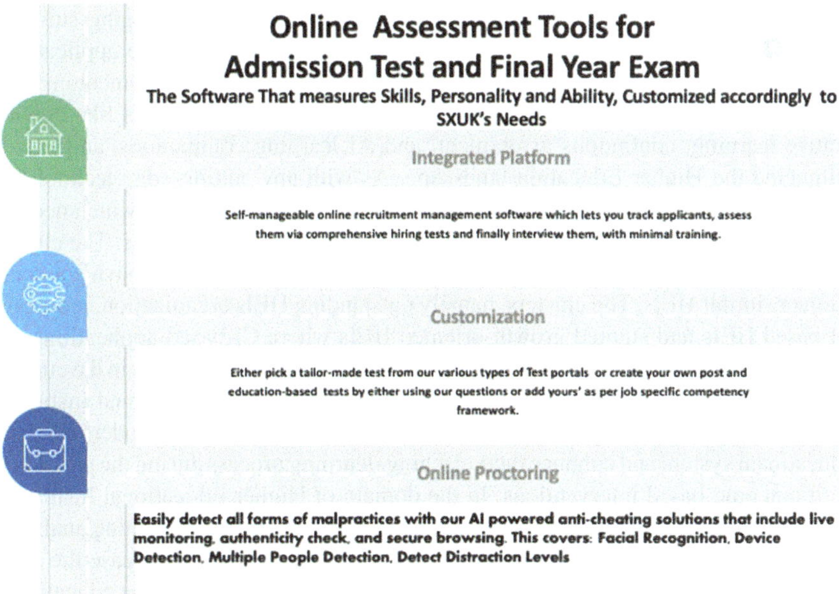

Fig. 13 CI-based online examination model

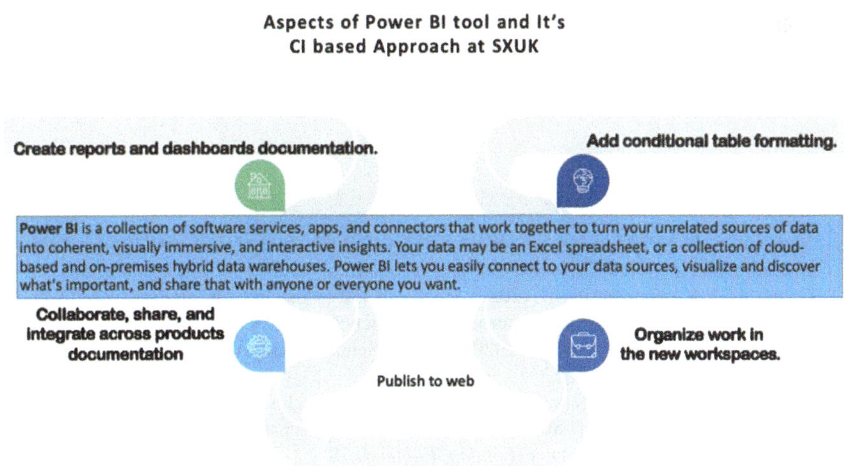

Fig. 14 BI-CI interface recognition

statistically significant with other aspects. Faculties in HEIs in West Bengal are using the identified aspects that are having significant influence on the teaching–learning of faculty members.

The pandemic reality has led HEIs to think newer ways of engaging students online. The outcomes of the current research have indicated that the applications of CI in HEIs and their management are favorable and gaining momentum in a large scale. The future of AI-CI is very exciting, with learning tools like collaborative learning, continuous assessment, and AI learning companions, and it will reimagine the Higher Education landscape. As with any cutting-edge technology, there are certain serious issues of ethics, data privacy, and singularity, which need to be monitored and addressed to do away with unintended consequences. The cluster analysis has shown Higher Educational Institutes into groups that are having association or similar HEIs. The clusters, namely outstanding HEIs organization, moderate CI-based HEIs and stunted growth-oriented HEIs where CI-based applications are found to be new insights drawn from current research. The data analysis in the current research has given an orientation to understand how Higher Educational Institutes in West Bengal are faring in adopting ICT tools and techniques to modernize their educational system and enhance their teaching–learning process during the pandemic with outcome-based interventions. In the domain of Higher Educational Institutes, it has been observed that the educational data mining (EDM) and learning analytics (LA) are the areas where AI-CI-big data process will be used to increase the relevance modernized digital education platform in all the three levels. The educational transformative developments in AI-CI interface in SXUK have helped the administration to evolve CI-based programs and to shape the future of SXUK in promoting online teaching–learning. Thus, the use of AI-CI components in HEIs is crucial to their teaching–learning process and enable them to adopt newer applications in CI and ICT tools and enhance growth and development of students.

References

1. Marshall, A. L., & Wolanskyj-Spinner, A. (2020). *COVID-19-challenges and opportunities for educators and generation Z learners*. Paper presented at the Mayo Clinic Proceedings.
2. Cohen, J., & Kupferschmidt, K. (2020). Countries test tactics in 'war' against COVID-19. In: American Association for the Advancement of Science.
3. Burgess, S., & Sievertsen, H. H. (2020, April 1). Schools, skills, and learning: The impact of COVID-19 on education. *Vox*.
4. Nicola, M., Alsafi, Z., Sohrabi, C., Kerwan, A., Al-Jabir, A., Iosifidis, C., Agha, M., & Agha, R. (2020). The socio-economic implications of the coronavirus pandemic (COVID-19): A review. *International Journal of Surgery (London, England)* 78.
5. Rundle, A. G., Park, Y., Herbstman, J. B., Kinsey, E. W., & Wang, Y. C. (2020). COVID-19–related school closings and risk of weight gain among children. *Obesity*.
6. Sintema, E. J. (2020). Effect of COVID-19 on the Performance of Grade 12 Students: Implications for STEM Education. *Eurasia Journal of Mathematics, Science and Technology Education, 16*(7), em1851.
7. Crawford, J., Butler-Henderson, K., Rudolph, J., & Glowatz, M. (2020). COVID-19: 20 countries' higher education intra-period digital pedagogy responses. *Journal of Applied Teaching and Learning (JALT), 3*(1).
8. Sahu, P. (2020). Closure of universities due to coronavirus disease 2019 (COVID-19): Impact on education and mental health of students and academic staff. *Cureus, 12*(4).

9. Ozili, P. K. (2020). Covid-19 pandemic and economic crisis—The Nigerian experience and structural causes. *Available at SSRN 3567419*.
10. Cao, W., Fang, Z., Hou, G., Mei Han, Xu, X., Dong, J., & Zheng, J. (2020). The psychological impact of the COVID-19 epidemic on college students in China. *Psychiatry Research*.
11. Chick, R. C., Clifton, G. T., Peace, K. M., Propper, B. W., Hale, D. F., Alseidi, A. A., & Vreeland, T. J. (2020). Using technology to maintain the education of residents during the COVID-19 pandemic. *Journal of Surgical Education*.
12. Parul, P. (2020). Big and small stories from India in the COVID19 plot: Directions for a 'Post Coronial' Psychology. *Integrative Psychological and Behavioural Science,* 1–26.
13. Huang, G. B., Cambria, E., Toh, K. A., Widrow, B., & Xu, Z. (2015). New trends of learning in computational intelligence. *IEEE Computational Intelligence Magazine, 10*(2), 16–17
14. Mame Omar Diop, & Tarush J. (2020). COVID-19 crisis sheds light on the need for a new education model. *Education Times*.
15. Lu, J., Behbood, V., Hao, P., Zuo, H., Xue, S., & Zhang, G. (2015). Transfer learning using computational intelligence: A survey. *Knowledge-Based Systems, 80*, 14–23
16. Hanne, T., & Dornberger, R (2020). Adapting the teaching of computational intelligence techniques to improve learning outcomes. In *New trends in business information systems and technology* (pp. 113–129). Springer.
17. Williamson, B. J. (2020). New digital laboratories of experimental knowledge production: Artificial intelligence and education research. *London Review of Education*.
18. Yunanto, A. A., Herumurti, D., Rochimah, S., & Kuswardayan, I. (2019). English education game using non-player character based on natural language processing. *Procedia Computer Science, 161*, 502–508
19. Salem, A. B. M., & Nikitaeva, A. Y. (2019). Knowledge engineering paradigms for smart education and learning systems. In *2019 42nd International Convention on Information and Communication Technology, Electronics and Microelectronics (MIPRO)* (pp. 1571–1574). IEEE. (2019, May).
20. Santos, J. R. A. (1999). Cronbach's alpha: A tool for assessing the reliability of scales. *Journal of extension, 37*(2), 1–5
21. Nunnally, J. C (1978). *Psychometric theory* (2nd ed.). McGraw-Hill.
22. Merriam, S. B. (1988). *Case study research in education: A qualitative approach*, 1–248.
23. Zawacki-Richter, O., Marín, V. I., Bond, M., & Gouverneur, F. (2019). Systematic review of research on artificial intelligence applications in higher education–where are the educators?. *International Journal of Educational Technology in Higher Education, 16*(1), 1–27.
24. Rev. Dr. J. Felix Raj, S. J (2017). St. Xavier's univerity annual report. Retrieved from SXUK, Newtown, Kolkata
25. Rev. Dr. J. Felix Raj, S. J. (2020). Technology in St. Xavier's university, Kolkata /Interviewer: D. Mourlin K, Xavier Bsuiness School (XBS).
26. Sangsawang, T. (2015). Instructional design framework for educational media. *Procedia-Social and Behavioral Sciences, 176*, 65–80.

COVID-19: Virology, Epidemiology, Diagnostics and Predictive Modeling

Dheeraj Gunwant, Ajitanshu Vedrtnam, Sneh Gour, Ravi Deval, Rohit Verma, Vikas Kumar, Harshit Upadhyay, Shakti Sharma, Balendra V. S. Chauhan, and Sawan Bharti

Abbreviations

ACE2	Angiotensin-converting enzyme 2
AH	Absolute humidity
ARDS	Acute respiratory distress syndrome
BCG	Bacillus Calmette–Guérin
CFR	Case fatality rate
COVID-19	Coronavirus disease
MERS-CoV	Middle East respiratory syndrome
NAAT	Nucleic acid amplification test
NACO	National AIDS control organization

D. Gunwant
GET Group of Institutions-Faculty of Technology, Bazpur, Uttarakhand, India

D. Gunwant · A. Vedrtnam (✉) · S. Gour · R. Deval · V. Kumar · H. Upadhyay · S. Bharti
Invertis University, Bareilly, Uttar Pradesh 243001, India
e-mail: ajitanshu.m@invertis.org

R. Deval
e-mail: ravi.d@invertis.org

V. Kumar
e-mail: vikas.k@invertis.org

S. Bharti
e-mail: sawan.k@invertis.org

A. Vedrtnam
Universidad de Alcalá, Alcalá, Spain

R. Verma · S. Sharma
Donau- Ries Klinikum, Donauwörth 86609, Germany

B. V. S. Chauhan
Department of Mechanical Engineering, Invertis University, Bareilly 243001, Uttar Pradesh, India

M. Niranjanamurthy et al. (eds.), *Intelligent Data Analysis for COVID-19 Pandemic*, Algorithms for Intelligent Systems, https://doi.org/10.1007/978-981-16-1574-0_9

NTEP	National Tuberculosis Elimination Programme
qRT-PCR	Reverse transcription polymerase chain reaction
R0	Reproduction number
RBD	Receptor-binding domain
RNA	Ribonucleic acid
RSV	Respiratory syncytial virus
SARS-CoV	Severe acute respiratory syndrome
SARS-CoV-2	Severe acute respiratory syndrome coronavirus-2
SEM	Scanning electron microscopy
SEIR	Susceptible-exposed-infected-recovered
SHERLOCK	Specific high-sensitivity enzymatic reporter unlocking
SIR	Susceptible-infected-removed
SIRD	Susceptible-infected-recovered-dead
SOFA score	Sequential organ failure assessment score

1 Introduction

China reported the World Health Organization (WHO) about a series of pneumonia cases in Wuhan city in December 2019 and subsequently WHO declared the outbreak as 'public health emergency of international concern' [1]. The causes of outbreak were reported as unknown, which speedily spread to other areas of China and all over the world. WHO has confirmed SARS-CoV-2 as a pandemic and termed it as COVID-19 [2]. Coronavirus family of viruses was first reported in 1930 in form of a severe respiratory infection in household chickens. The coronavirus in human was affirmed in 1960 from the nasal fluids of volunteers collected at the common cold unit of Salisbury, UK. These viruses consist of genetic material encased in an envelope covered with 'club'-like structures composed of protein, giving them crown-like appearance and thus, named corona, derived from the Latin word used for crown. SARS-CoV-2 is highly infective with higher transmissibility but lower mortality rate as compared to SARS-CoV and MERS-CoV. SARS-CoV and SARS-CoV-2 have stake 79.6% sequence identity, similar entry receptors and identical acute respiratory syndromes [3]. The typical diameter of virus ranges between 60 and 200 nm with clubs of length approximately 20 nm [4]. Figure 1 shows the SEM image of human coronavirus.

The coronavirus transmits from human to human through droplets [5] and remain alive on fomites for different durations [6]. Infection transmits through surfaces as the humans have natural tendency of touching mouth, eyes or nose by their infected hands unknowingly after touching the fomites [7]. The non-pharmaceutical interventions such as public awareness, reduction in contact rates, case isolation, intensive contact tracing, and social distancing are followed by different countries for combating COVID-19 as vaccine was not developed by July, 2020 [8]. The closure of universities and other places of socializing enabling flattening the COVID-19 infected

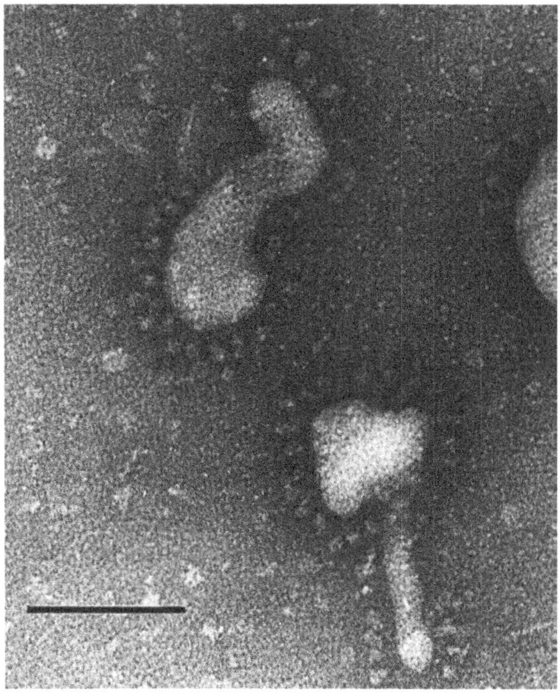

Fig. 1 Particles of human coronavirus grown in human fibroblast cells [4]

curve [9]. The basic reproduction number (R0) value in Wuhan decreased from 2.35 to 1.05 within 1-week post implementation of the travel restrictions [10] and by the end of April, 2020, the Wuhan was declared corona free with a very few cases. However, these social measures could be a temporary solution in practice, and there is an urgent need of developing vaccines and therapies for SARS-CoV-2 for mitigating the global socio-economic losses [11]. The growth of pandemic around globe was modeled using a susceptible-infected-removed (SIR) model. It was predicted that there would be up to 900 million infected individuals globally by the time pandemic ceases in absence of significant counter measures [12]. The effects of incubation period, R0 and countermeasures on the growth pattern of COVID-19 in Italy, South Korea, and Iran along with the possible time taken to control the COVID-19 have been estimated [13–15]. A susceptible-infected-recovered-dead (SIRD) model was reported for predicting the spread dynamics of COVID-19 in France, Italy and China indicated equal recovery rate but different infection rates in Italy and China [16]. However, the variation in predicted and actual data could be due to strict implementation of lockdown in China as compared to Italy and France, different social fabric and different childhood vaccination measures. In addition to a generalized SEIR model [17], the modified SIR model was also reported [18]. The authors have forecasted COVID-19 spread in Brazil [19], Australia [20], South Korea [21] and African countries [22]. The phenomenological models were reported for forecasting the short-term (five consecutive days) COVID-19 spread [23–28]. Artificial intelligence can assist in fighting COVID-19 by populace screening, clinical assistance, warning and instructions about the disease control. Machine intelligence techniques can be a very useful tool as they can assist in tracking the virus spread, spotting the patients at high risk, assisting in real-time governing of this disease, and by in examining patient's record; the machine intelligence techniques can prognosticate the mortality risk.

Table 1 describes the scope and findings of the selected article on COVID-19 with an Indian perspective published in 2020.

This chapter consists summary of published evidences on virology, epidemiology and spread dynamics modeling of COVID-19. The measures taken for mitigating the effect of pandemic along with the current line of treatment were also discussed.

2 Virology of SARS-CoV-2

The novel SARS-CoV-2 virus possibly has zoonotic origin and partially resembles with MERS-CoV and SARS-CoV pathologically and clinically. It was reported that the average size of virus and average surface projections are 70–80 nm and 15 $\pm$ 2 nm, respectively [43]. This enveloped virus contains the largest known genome of single-stranded positive-sense RNA [44]. The similarity between genome sequence of SARS-CoV-2 and SARS-CoV present in bats, SARS-CoV and MERS-CoV is 89%, 82% and 50%, respectively [45]. It was reported that the pangolins have genome sequence 85.5–92.4% identical with the SARS-CoV-2 and suspected to be the intermediate carrier of the virus [46]. However, bat or snake origin of SARS-CoV-2 was also speculated as intermediate carriers [47]. The open seafood market of Wuhan, China, was considered as the breeding ground for SARS-CoV-2 due to the selling of dead and alive doubted intermediate carriers, and zeroth COVID-19-infected patient belongs to this market [48]. However, the conspiracy theories from USA, Germany, Australia, Russia and UK media reports point out that the virus might be a product of genetic engineering and it was spread deliberately with unscrupulous intentions. However, researchers from Scripps Research Institute claimed that the identified origin of the SARS-CoV-2 was through natural selection process rather than genetic engineering. The investigations of the receptor-binding domain (RBD) revealed significantly higher chances of attachment between human ACE2 and the spike protein of virus mainly enhanced due to natural selection process. Their study indicated the possible spillover of SARS-CoV-2 from high-population-density animal species. It was suspected that the bats and Malaya Pangolins, illegally imported into the Guandong province of China, were infected with coronavirus which might have mutated due to natural selection and finally reached humans. Further, the Wuhan wet market was considered significant in widespread transmission of SARS-CoV-2 [49]. In April 2020, the Chinese authorities have decided to scrutinize academic research article dealing with origin of COVID-19 due to political reasons [50].

Table 1 Scope and findings of the selected article on COVID-19 focusing an Indian perspective published in 2020

S. No.	Scope	Findings	References
1	Studying the effects of limited movement of human beings due to pandemic on the air quality index of 22 Indian cities	During 16th March, 2020 and 14th April, 2020 up to 43% reduction in PM2.5, PM10, CO, and NO_2 in India with negligible increase of 17% in O_3 and minor change in SO_2were reported as compared to previous years. In North, East, Central and Western India the air quality index reduced up 44%. In addition to this, there was a countrywide approximately 52% reduction in the mean excessive risk of PM was also registered. Model studies reveal up to 33% increase in the PM2.5 under conditions of unfavorable meteorology	[29]
2	Discussion on the proposed protocol, dosage, sample collection, frequency of monitoring for use of Lopinavir/Ritonavir against COVID-19 in India	Based on the evidences of effectiveness of Lopinavir/Ritonavir in COVID-19, the Indian Council for Medical Research has allowed these drugs for treating patients in India. Lopinavir/Ritonavir can be administered (taken through mouth or injected d) in prescribed dosage to symptomatic patients. The administration must commence before the onset of severe symptoms in patients including high cases such as those aged >60 years and with comorbidities (hypertension, compromised immunity, diabetes mellitus, chronic lung disease or renal failure). If found effective, the spectrum of drug use can be extended via randomized control trial design for future use	[30]
3	Suggestions on an operative approach for ending the COVID-19 spread in India	General Indian population is unaffected by the danger of COVID-19 pandemic mainly due to their poor economic status. It is high time that Indians realize the severity and work in synchrony with government to stop the community spread. The government should also develop confidence in its people and fulfill their basic requirement in this harsh time. The organized sector employees can contribute toward alleviating financial problems of people working in unorganized sectors. The public distribution system should be used effectively to provide food to the downtrodden. Such governmental actions will surely motivate common Indians to follow social distancing, isolation, etc. Government should also facilitate the front-line corona warriors (doctors, medical staff, police personnel, janitors, etc.) and with proper personal protection equipment (PPE) kits, masks and alcohol-based hand sanitizers	[31]

(continued)

Table 1 (continued)

S. No.	Scope	Findings	References
4	Convalescent plasma as potential treatment option in India for COVID-19	Five critical patients in China were administered the convalescent plasma 10–22 days after being admitted. After, the treatment with plasma, antiviral drugs (Lopinavir, interferon, Favipiravir etc.) and mechanical ventilation their medical condition improved and all were discharged 51–55 days after admission. Convalescent plasma therapy has limited potential in combating the COVID-19 pandemic and in India also, patients recovering can be harvested for collecting antibodies loaded plasma. Recently, ICMR has given approval to start trial of this therapy at SCTIMST, Kerala	[32]
5	Modeling study and prediction of COVID-19 transmission dynamics in Indian context. Insight into efficacy of lockdown under different recovery rates	Spread of pandemic in India was studied using mathematical modeling approach. Effect of lockdown was investigated using model and found to play crucial role in restricting the number of infected Indian population. However, sudden discovery of hidden infected individuals can lead to steep increase in infected individuals, easily overwhelming the country's healthcare sector. It is also observed that in place of multiple phased lockdowns, a single lockdown would be more beneficial in Indian context	[33]
6	Exploring the potential pathway for increasing the qRT-PCR testing capability for COVID-19 in India	A 24 h working model can be implemented in existing laboratories across India and testing rates as high as 40,464 tests/per day can be achieved. The testing capacity can be easily ramped using the machines available in NACO and NTEP. By implementing these steps and procurement of sophisticate machines along with deployment of more workforce and improved transportation facilities can enhance testing capacity up to 1.5–2 times and push the testing rates to 100,000–120,000 tests/day	[34]
7	Exploring the possibility of India becoming the next COVID-19 type epidemic	Coronaviruses and other viruses carried by bats can infect humans specially living in rural areas of India via spill over through animals such as camels, goats, pigs, poultry, etc. through saliva, fecal matter and body fluids. Bats can directly infect fruits which when consumed by human beings can transmit virus in them. By this way, even vegetarians can get infection which are normally considered unaffected from animal borne viruses. Being the second most populous country with almost 17% of world population residing in it, India is at the brink of any epidemic outbreak. Any outbreak would easily get deteriorated due to pollution and deforestation along with poor health infrastructure	[35]

(continued)

Table 1 (continued)

S. No.	Scope	Findings	References
8	Survey of parameters of mental health in the Indian people during COVID-19	A total of 662 individuals participated in a survey of which most had a medium awareness level about COVID-19 Most of the participants were willing to follow government guidelines regarding isolation, social distancing and quarantine. About 80% were paranoid and more than 72% reported need for masks, hand sanitizers, etc. Various issues such as sleeping difficulties, paranoia and social media distress were observed in the participants. Study concluded that >80% individuals needed immediate counseling and healthcare support and intensification of awareness spreading is a must in order to reduce distress	[36]
9	Steps on how India can transcend from containment to community mitigation for flattening the contracted individuals curve	Present national strategy of containment is implemented for diseases with small growth rate. As the growth rate increases, the containment of complete population will become more and more difficult. Therefore, community mitigation steps such as closure of schools and mass gatherings are crucial for ironing out the curve of infected population. A peaked curve means large number of cases within short duration of time leading to overburdened healthcare infrastructure. Various steps suggested are: social distancing, use of personal protection equipment, home isolation when sick for up to 14 days, taking care of vulnerable population groups such as elderly, infants, pregnant women and those with comorbidities and expanding testing rates and capacity for treatment	[37]
10	Study of outbreak of COVID-19 pandemic in India up to 30th March, 2020 and predictions for number of infected in forthcoming two weeks using modeling approach	Modeling study evaluated using root mean squared log error (RMLSE) reached 1.52 and 1.75 for SEIR and regression models, respectively. On the other hand, RMLSE between these two models was 2.01 along with the R0 value equal to 2.02. It is speculated that infected cases may reach 5000–6000 within the forthcoming two weeks. This short-term modeling study can be optimized to predict the transmission pattern in India in long run, enabling government to actively plan beforehand	[38]

(continued)

Table 1 (continued)

S. No.	Scope	Findings	References
11	Assessment of 21-day lockdown in three states Delhi, Tamil Nadu and Maharashtra, as well as overall India by SEIR model extension	A novel model was presented which includes effect of lockdown and variation of transmission among symptomatic and asymptomatic cases. Based on daily data of reported cases in three states (Maharashtra, Tamil Nadu and New Delhi) and modeling study it is concluded that 21-day lockdown is insufficient for curbing the pandemic spread in Maharashtra. Instead, high number of super-spreaders would deteriorate the condition in Maharashtra; however, New Delhi as well as Tamil Nadu may see decrease in cases as well as deaths. The transmission can be effectively restricted by extensive survey and lockdown in infected areas, while relaxing of restriction in other areas	[39]
12	Insights into the use of hydroxychloroquine for treatment of COVID-19 in India	Despite recommendation from ministry of health and family welfare government of India, role of hydroxychloroquine remains suspicious as a credible treatment option for COVID-19. Few in vitro studies report antiviral effect of hydroxychloroquine and chloroquine but still in the absence of any peer-reviewed research article, the treatment efficiency of these drugs against is doubtful. The patients being administered chloroquine of hydroxychloroquine must be explained the risks involved. It is also suggested that clinical outcomes are well documented to record any evidence of collateral damage, adverse effects, etc.	[40]
13	Assessing the network structure of COVID-19 and current testing strategy in India	With transmission rate of 0.43 in India and daily growth rate mainly concerned with individuals returning back from foreign countries, this could be an artifact in India's testing strategies. In India, testing only foreign returned and their close contacts appears that the testing strategy is biased. This indicates that actual problem of pandemic has not been confronted by governmental agencies yet. At this time, there is need to systematically enhance the testing capacities in India so that actual course of pandemic can be understood in a better way	[41]
14	Exploring the efficacy of measures such as travel restrictions and quarantine symptomatic individuals in delaying the local outbreaks of COVID-19 in India through mathematical modeling	The cumulative incidences will be reduced by 62% if 50% symptomatic patients are quarantined within 3 days of symptoms development, R0 of 1.5 and zero infectiousness in asymptomatic infections. However, the cumulative incidences would be reduced by just 2% if R0 is 4.0 and 50% of asymptomatic patients are infectious. There would be delay in introduction of virus into community if port-of-entry-based restrictions are imposed on the entry of travelers with suggestive clinical manifestations. If the virus starts spreading within community, the symptomatic cases must be quarantined to curb the transmission. Robustness of healthcare infrastructure would play important role in deciding the course of COVID-19 in India	[42]

The binding capability of SARS-CoV-2 S-Protein with angiotensin-converting enzyme 2 (ACE2) is up to 10–20 times greater as compared to the SARS-CoV. ACE2 is an enzyme present on the cells of vital organs, and its function includes monitoring the blood pressure [51]. ACE2 being a trans-membrane protein serves as the gateway for viruses into the cells. The cells having ACE-2 and TMPRSS2 are more susceptible for entry of SARS-CoV-2 [52]. ACE2 increases the production of vasodilator angiotensin as a counter-measure to the viral attack on lungs. A study on mice has reported decrease in ACE2 levels following coronavirus attacks leading to severe lung damage [53]. Table 2 presents a summary of selected articles published on epidemiology and virology of SARS-CoV-2. The predicted values of R0, incubation period and case fatality rate (CFR) for SARS-CoV-2 are reported considerably in the literature [54–69].

3 Diagnostics and Current Line of Treatment of Coronavirus Disease-2019 (COVID-19)

An urgent need is felt to develop methods for restricting the spread of the ongoing pandemic. The common symptoms reported by mild as well as moderate patients range from dry cough, pyrexia, headache, nasal blockage, pain in joints, myalgia, and arthralgia. Patients report difficulty in breathing accompanied by hypoxemia in the second week of illness. Unattended patients may subsequently suffer from acute pneumonia and difficulty in eating or drinking [44]. ARDS was indicated in both the lungs during pathological findings of severe patients (10–20% cases) [44, 76]. The maximum incubation period ranges from 1 to 14 days which in most cases lies between 3–7 days [44].

The qRT-PCR as well as next-generation sequencing is being used to detect viral sequences from nasal and throat swab of patients for diagnosis of SARS-CoV-2. For high efficiency, nucleic acid test paper has been successfully developed which provides rapid results. CRISPR/Cas13-based SHERLOCK (specific high-sensitivity enzymatic reporter unlocking) technology has been released for SARS-CoV-2 detection. Block chain and artificial Intelligence technology coupled with CT imaging is in clinical practice which can provide 96% diagnostic accuracy. Short turnaround time assays such as serological antibody testing are also valuable [76–78]. Figure 2 shows the mechanism of COVID-10 infection in human body and immune response.Please note that figures are renumbered to maintain sequential order. Please check and confirm.The renumbered Figs. are in sequential order and correct.

COVID-19 has given a limited time to study or understand the disease before it has accounted for tremendous social and economic loss. Normally, a vaccine goes through various stages in development, namely testing stage, preclinical trials, clinical development (human trials), regulatory review and approval before launching mass production. These stages usually take a long time and are aimed to regulate

Table 2 Summary of selected articles published in 2020 on epidemiology and virology of SARS-CoV-2

Epidemiology and virology			
S. No.	Scope	Finding	References
1	Review of present situation of pandemic in terms of causatives, pathogenesis, immune responses, epidemiology, diagnosis, treatment options, etc.	SARS-CoV-2 is an enclosed single-stranded RNA-based virus belonging to beta coronaviruses family similar to SARS-CoV and MERS-CoV. Although zoonotic, primary transmission occurs via human to human contact mainly affecting the adult population especially with comorbidities. Effective binding with human ACE2 appears to be the most favorable entry point for virus into human beings. Infected individuals show symptoms, viz. pyrexia, dyspnea, fatigue and dry cough. Radio diagnosis shows ground glass opacities in lungs. In the absence of drugs, effective management and isolation combined with oxygen therapy and secondary bacterial treatment	[70]
2	Insights into the COVID-19 pandemic and what can be gained from SARS and MERS	Highlighted genomic similarity and bat origin among SARS-CoV-2, SARS-CoV and MERS-CoV. COVID-19 is more severe than predecessors due to high R0 due to high binding ability of S-protein with human ACE2, incubation period and much higher fatality in comorbid patients. Pathology of COVID-19 resembles predecessors in terms of respiratory and gastroenteral symptoms. Possible treatment options till the vaccination are developed include chloroquine, remdesivir, tocilizumab and convalescent plasma infusion. In absence of a sure-shot treatment, hand hygiene, isolation, quarantine, masks, social distancing and cluster containment remain only preventive measures	[3]
3	Review of published literature on COVID-19 transmission mechanism and possible options for treatment in context cardiovascular findings	Coronaviruses consist of the protein nucleocapsid (N) enveloping the virus RNA and facilitating interaction between it and the three proteins—Spike (S) protein responsible for interaction between virus and receptor, membrane (M) protein and envelope (E) protein, responsible for fusion. It uses ACE2 as the entry point. Between 7–28% of the hospitalized patients of COVID-19 were presented with cardiac injury. Mostly were comorbid with diabetes and hypertension, etc. Cardiac arrest has also been reported as a major cause of mortalities in COVID-19 patients. Presence of ACE2 increases the possibility of heart muscles being directly affected by the viral load	[71]

(continued)

Table 2 (continued)

Epidemiology and virology			
S. No.	Scope	Finding	References
4	Overview of coronaviruses in broad sense with special focus on SARS-CoV-2 in terms of molecular biology, epidemiology, diagnostics as well as treatment options and laboratory findings	A total of 12,000 cases on 2nd Feb 2020 increased four times to 88,400 on 1st March 2020 and doubled to 167,500 on 15th March 2020. CoV are spherical-shaped viruses, around 125 nm in size with spikes resembling club giving it the typical crown shape. These are characterized by the names α, β and γ as per serological patterns. SARS-CoV is approximately 80% similar to SARS-CoV genome and 96% similar to bat coronavirus. Out of the first 1091 patients in China, just 1.9% visited the Wuhan seafood market and up to 72.3% have come in contact with Wuhan residents. This indicates the human-to-human contact to be prominent means of transmission. Up to 88.7% patients developed fever while treatment in hospitals	[72]
5	Systematic review of epidemiology, diagnosis as well as prognosis and treatment protocols for COVID-19	Model studies indicate up to 10 times better capability of binding ability between SARS-CoV-2 and ACE2 of humans making it more dangerous than its predecessors. Exact mechanism of interaction with human cells and organ failure remains to be discovered. Various estimates of R0 indicate values ranging 2.0–3.0 which is lower than MERS-CoV. SARS-CoV-2 shares genomic sequence with bat (96%) and pangolins (99%) making them potential spillover agents. Neurological manifestations, ocular surface infection (viral RNA in eye secretion), impaired renal, liver and heart functions in addition to lung damage have also been reported in some patients	[73]
6	Review of published data on COVID-19 patients suffering from gastrointestinal infection (GI) symptoms	During SARS and MERS outbreaks, about 76% and 25% patients reportedly developed diarrhea due to GI and abdominal pain. It was later discovered that the SARS-CoV replicated effectively inside small as well as large intestines. RNA of the virus was also discovered from liver of SARS patients. In case of SARS-CoV-2, around 20% patients out of more than 4000 reported symptoms of GI such as pain in abdomen, diarrhea, nausea and vomiting. About 50% patients tested positive viral RNA in their feces. In another study on cohort of 200 individuals, around 50% displayed symptoms of GI. At present literature does not cover various aspects of GI in COVID-19 patients. Detailed and systematical model study must be undertaken to investigate the presence of GI in such patients	[74]

(continued)

Table 2 (continued)

Epidemiology and virology			
S. No.	Scope	Finding	References
7	Study of epidemiology of COVID-19 was studied in 2143 infected children in China analytically	Retrospective analytical of a 2143 children (of which 731 were confirmed positive and 1412 were suspected) with median age 7 years was conducted. The subjects all aged less than 18 years were identified on the basis of predefined criterion based on pathological and radiographic reports. Infants were observed to be at higher risk of infection and al children displayed an early rapid increase in the disease followed by gradual and steady decrease. Almost all the children exhibited mild symptoms with critical cases around 5.9%. This might be due to proper care taking in household settings, lower ACE2 (binding sites of SARS-CoV-2) levels, and exposure to common cold and flu in winter season	[75]

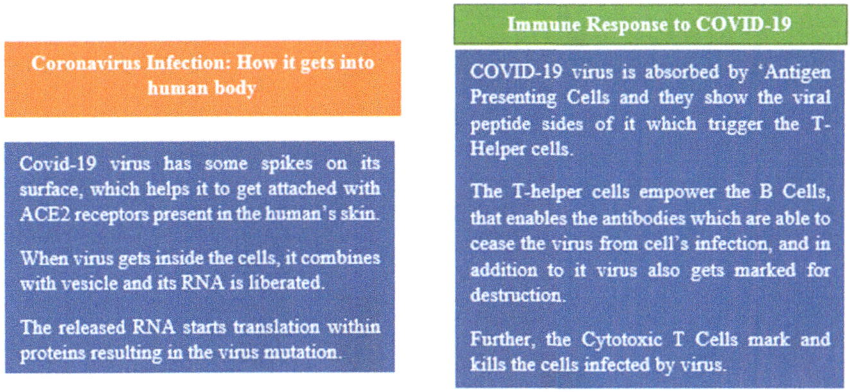

Fig. 2 Mechanism of COVID-19 infection in human body and immune response

the efficacy and safety of the vaccine for human use and avoidance of serious long-term side effects. Nevertheless, to address this ongoing pandemic there are several vaccines already in developmental stage across the world, most being either in first stage or waiting for human trial, while few are already under human trial. Besides the time constraint, another challenge in vaccine development stems from the existence of various human variants of coronaviruses and diversified affected populations. To engineer a vaccine absolutely compatible for various populations and races in different continents, under a never-seen-before time pressure remains a dream yet to come true.

With the number of cases rising, the WHO had approved 54 different vaccine trials undergoing in different countries to curtail the progression and spread by mid-April 2020. These vaccines are classified under 3 categories—'live vaccines', 'inactivated vaccines' and 'gene technique vaccines' and are being developed with the help of findings from Cure Vac (Germany), Novavax (USA), University of Queensland (Australia) and University of Oxford (UK), where University of Oxford (UK) has begun the human trials. In comparison to traditional vaccines, RNA-based vaccines are rapid and economical, which, in such pandemic conditions, could be a major advantage [52]. RNA-based vaccines have high potency, low manufacturing costs, short production cycle and safe administration [79]. RNA-based vaccines use mRNA that stimulates the immune system as they are translated to antigenic molecules [52]. Clinical trials of SARS-CoV-2 mRNA vaccine (mRNA-1273, encoding S protein) developed by Moderna are expected to be conducted on 20–25 registered medically fit individuals by April 2020 [79]. With time lag of 28 days, two doses of mRNA vaccine will be given to subject for immunogenicity assessment [52]. Figure 3 shows the proportion of vaccines in development around the world reported in the open sources and scientific articles by April 2020. Figure 4 shows summary of types of vaccines in development for COVID-19.

DNA vaccines are considered to be more effective and stable than the mRNA vaccines with simultaneous risk of vector integration and host genome mutation. The Pennsylvania-based INOVIO has accelerated the testing of INO-4800, which is

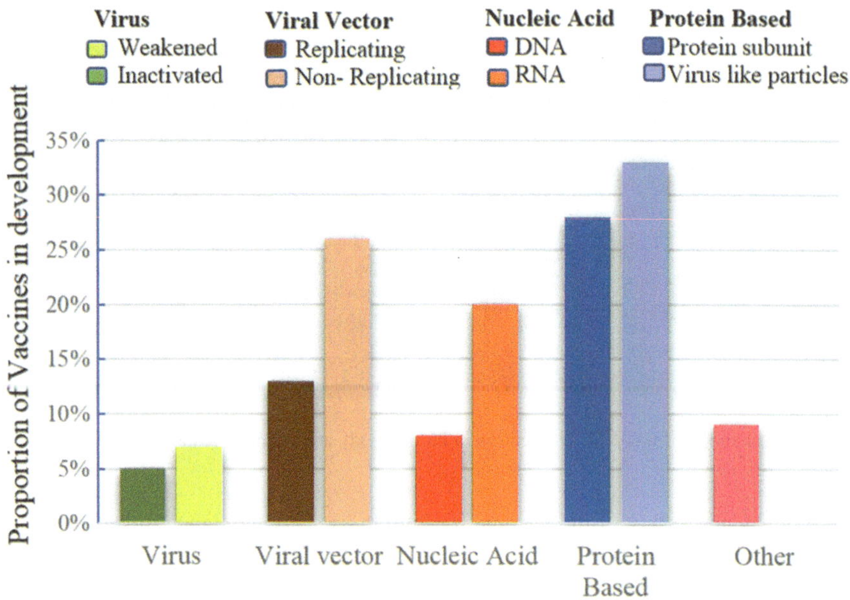

Fig. 3 Proportion of vaccines in development around the world reported in the open sources and scientific articles by April 2020

a potential DNA vaccine for COVID-19. The vaccine is in preclinical phase right now and will enter the clinical phase soon. The European Commission has supported CureVac for DNA vaccine they have proposed.

In the line of treatment in patients of COVID-19, chloroquine or its variant hydroxychloroquine, an antimalarial drug has proven effective in shortening the disease course during treatment in China. Hydroxychloroquine is also efficient in combating rheumatoid arthritis-related inflammation as well as lupus erythematous [80]. Hydroxychloroquine renders the ACE-2-SARS-CoV-2 interaction less efficient [78, 52, 81] and elevates the endosomol pH value, thus making it difficult for virus to infuse into host cell. It interferes with the glycosylation of the receptors of virus [82]. French researchers have reported complete attrition of viral load in nasopharyngeal samples of 70% of patients treated with hydroxychloroquine in comparison with the control samples [83]. The results were yet more motivating as all the patients administered a mix of azithromycin and hydroxychloroquine showed negative PCR and were cured virologically within 6 days of treatment. However, some side effects are also connected with the use of hydroxychloroquine and chloroquine which include poor vision, giddiness, GI and even cardiac arrest in some cases [84]. Other drugs such as Remdesivir, Atazanavir, Saquinavir and Formoterol are also under clinical trials and can be introduced as treatment [78]. Drug repurposing can also be employed for reducing the time and cost related to development of novel drugs. Repurposing of available trusted and safe drugs can significantly lower the time requirement in development of novel drug which is the current need. The spike (S) protein of the

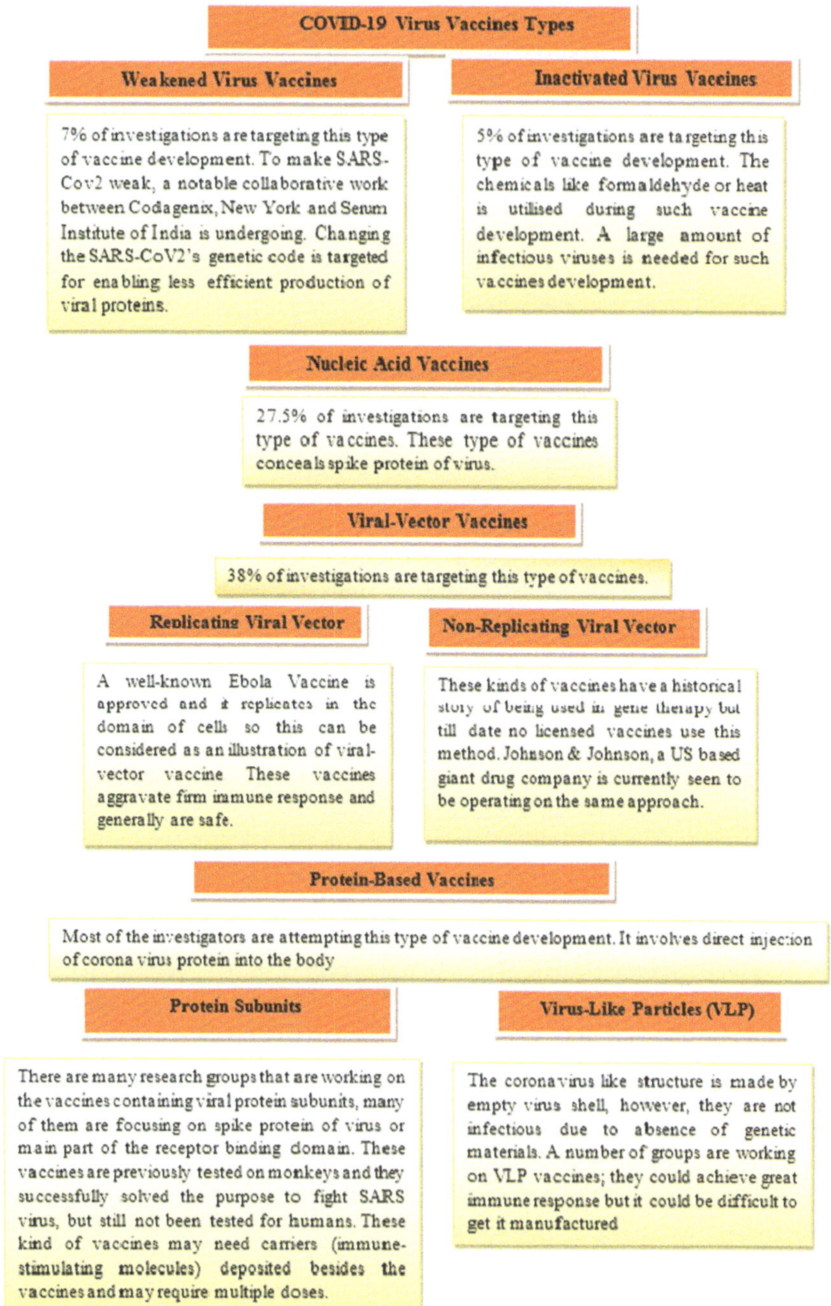

Fig. 4 Summary of types of vaccines in development for COVID-19

SARS-CoV-2 appears to be the most tempting target right now; efforts are also being directed toward targeting other components such as papain-like protease and helicase in the SARS-CoV-2 virus along with it [85]. To limit the COVID-19 pandemic, a passive immunization can also be considered [50]. For the neutralization of virus, immunotherapy by antibodies would be better if they are collected from fully recovered patients of that geographical area [86]. The main shortcoming of these treatments is that they be given before initiation of viral replication before the onset of humoral response [86]. A ray of hope appears from the convalescent plasma therapy in which a predetermined quantity of blood from recovered patients is used to extract plasma and is subsequently transfused into active patients so that antibodies can attack and annihilate the viral load. A convalescent plasma treatment regime given to five patients in China has resulted in motivating results. Transfusion showed antipyretic effect and decrease in sequential organ failure assessment score (SOFA score) [87–89]. In India, the states of Delhi and Kerala have been granted the approval on a convalescent therapy treatment protocol in patients, whereas Tamil Nadu and Gujarat states have applied for permission allowing trials of plasma therapy. Although effective, convalescent plasma is not completely free from risks such as infections resulting from transfusion, viz. HIV, hepatitis B and C viruses, syphilis, etc. In addition to these, patients may suffer from problems, such as chills and anaphylactic reactions and even acute lung injury in some cases [84]. Although the vaccine development is in early stage, a remarkable progress in research has been made from complete genome sequencing to the beginning of SARS-CoV-2 vaccine clinical trials. As many as six Indian companies are also contributing toward the global efforts of vaccine development for restricting the transmission of this fatal disease [90]. Prolonged global efforts are now required to unravel questions about novel corona virus including its virulence, transmissibility and sources of infection [91].

It was reported that Bacillus Calmette–Guérin (BCG) vaccination policy of a country may have positive correlation with reduction in COVID-19 morbidity and mortalities [92]. Countries without universal BCG policy reported significantly higher number of COVID-19 cases till March 21, 2020. Iran, where BCG policy was introduced in 1984 (leaving population above 36 years to be prone to pandemic) reported 19.7 deaths per million due to COVID-19. On the other hand, Japan, where the policy was introduced in 1947 and Brazil where BCG policy was introduced in 1920, reported a mere 0.28 and 0.0573 deaths per million, respectively. China implemented BCG vaccination policy in 1950, yet it has reported a high number of cases. This might be attributed to the disbanding and weakening of TB prevention agencies during the decade of Cultural Revolution from 1966–1976. More recent study on correlation between BCG vaccination and number of COVID-19 cases exhibits significant positive effect of vaccination on limiting the number of cases in countries with universal BCG policy [93]. Out of the total 178 countries considered, 131 are currently having BCG vaccination policy. While countries with such policy reported just 38.4 cases and 4.28 deaths per million populations; those without any such policy reported a huge 358.4 cases and 40 deaths per million populations. Such correlation might be the result of immunological benefits of BCG vaccine. Table 3 presents summary of selected research papers on diagnostics and current line of treatment.

Table 3 Summary of review articles on diagnostics and current line of treatment published in 2020

Diagnostics and current line of treatment			
S. No.	Scope	Finding	References
1	Systematic review articles published on efficiency and efficacy chloroquine related drugs from commencement of COVID-19 up to 1st March 2020	Significantly reduced viral replication tendency has been reported with standard dosing of chloroquine due to its effective absorption in lung tissues. In absence of contraindications, a dose of 200 mg, 300 mg or 500 mg chloroquine phosphate can be administered to patients exhibiting moderate to mild symptoms two times in a day for a maximum 10 days. Substantial proof exists reinforcing the efficacy of chloroquine-based drugs in treating COVID-19 patients in the absence of any sure-shot treatment. However, intense care must be exercised and changes in pathological reports of patients must be properly correlated	[94]
2	Evaluation of convalescent plasma as treatment option for COVID-19 patients through published clinical evidences	Convalescent plasma is the blood component recovered from patients who have recovered from and developed antibodies against a particular infectious disease. Convalescent plasma, which has been reported to be safe and effective in other infectious diseases, is yet to prove so in case of COVID-19. Many trials are underway in order to evaluate the efficacy of such treatment in several countries. If administered within 14 days (shortly after symptoms are visible), convalescent plasma may drastically reduce the viral load in patients. China has reported significant improvement in clinical symptoms in 9 of its seriously ill patients within 3 days of transfusion. Standard protocols need to be developed for identification of donors, processing of blood, testing, serological assaying and adjustment of dosage	[95]
3	Presently available treatment options of COVID-19 are reviewed with insight into their action mechanism, efficacy and safety	Remdesivir has shown motivating results improving the clinical reports of a patient in USA and protect human cell lining in China. It has been shown to decrease the mortality rate of critical patients requiring and not requiring invasive ventilation to 18% and 5% respectively. Another drug, Favipiravir originally developed for HIV, affects the viral RNA genome of SARS-CoV-2 by retarding its replication capability. Patients transfused with convalescent plasma have also showed improvement due to restricted inflammatory response and symptomatic conditions. Other options include blocking of virus S protein binding with ACE2 and use of recombinant human ACE2 are being investigated. Hydroxychloroquine has also been demonstrated to reduce the viral load significantly. Various immunity enhancers are also being tested clinically for efficacy against the SARS-CoV-2	[96]

(continued)

Table 3 (continued)

Diagnostics and current line of treatment			
S. No.	Scope	Finding	References
4	Potential application of IoT for the diagnosis and treatment of COVID-19	At present, the concept of Internet of things (IoT) means the use of local networks and internet for establishing seamless between human beings and things such as sensors, machines, etc. IoT can be used for locating patients, monitoring, planning & management, statistical analysis in a secure and private manner. Other applications include answering queries, linkage between patient and doctor, diagnosis and referrals. An application named nCapp, developed based on this technology, is being used for swift generation of database based upon predefined data and questionnaires and categorized individuals as suspected, suspicion and confirmed. Also, the patients are automatically classified in categories such as mild, moderate and serious. Further, by establishing effective linkage between medical professionals and experts, it helps in providing timely treatment to infected people	[97]
5	Review of published literature with focus on virology of SARS-CoV-2, epidemiology, diagnostics and treatment of COVID-19	After the complete genome sequence of SARS-CoV-2 became available on 10th January 2020, several developments have been reported in the field of rapid diagnosis and testing. However, seeing the pace of advancement of pandemic, the dependability and sensitivity of these tests remains under question. The tests results are affected by the sample type. Samples from throat swabs were demonstrated to carry significantly less amount of viral load as compared to sputum. The rT-PCR test remains gold standard as rapid antibody which detect the presence of antibodies in any individual tests have smaller accuracy and therefore limited role in diagnosis of COVID-19. In addition to this, around 30% patients from a cohort reportedly did not develop enough neutralizing antibodies indicating the need of proper testing of convalescent plasma before transfusion	[98]

(continued)

Table 3 (continued)

Diagnostics and current line of treatment			
S. No.	Scope	Finding	References
6	Review of general features, pathogenesis, diagnosis, treatment of COVID-19 based upon present knowledge regarding SARS and MERS	COVID-19 patients exhibit fever, cough, fatigue, myalgia and normal or reduced leukocyte counts along with evidence of pneumonia in radiography. These being identical to SARS as well as MERS give us a fair understanding of diagnosis of COVID-19. The main cause of death in patients reporting during early outbreak is ARDS which is a common event in SARS and MERS also. ARDS is caused by the uncontrolled storming of lungs with inflammation causing cytokines and chemokines leading to hyper-activation of immune system and multiple organ failure resulting in death. The diagnosis is based upon clinical manifestations, nucleic acid detection, CT scanning, immune identification technology, ELISA and blood culture. Auxiliary examinations are compulsory as they provide demarcating infected and non-infected individuals	[99]
7	Review of published literature regarding COVID-19 virus-based as well as host-based treatment options	Presently, two formulations Favilavir and Remdesivir are being used in China for treating COVID-19 patients. While Favilavir is used in symptomatic treatment of COVID-19, and Remdesivir has displayed motivating results by restricting the SARS-CoV and MERS-CoV earlier. The drug is known for early termination of RNA transcriptase inhibiting virus replication capability. Chloroquine and hydroxychloroquine are other options that have shown good results in inhibiting SARS-CoV and SARS-CoV-2 in an in vitro study. Hydroxychloroquine is better equipped to fight against SARS-CoV-2 and therefore is being administered in COVID-19 patients in the USA. Canadian researchers have already developed a SARS-CoV-2 virus like particle which can be used to trigger the immune response in humans	[100]

(continued)

Table 3 (continued)

Diagnostics and current line of treatment			
S. No.	Scope	Finding	References
8	Evaluation of chest CT scan in diagnosis of COVID-19. Comparison of CT scan of SARS-CoV-2-infected individuals with the other viruses	Fifty-one confirmed cases of COVID-19 aging between 26 and 83 years and two patients of adenovirus aged 58 and 66 years were considered for the study. COVID-19 affected all five lobes of lungs in 74.5%, both lower lobes in 15.7%, right lower lobe in 5.9% and left upper and right lower lobes in 2% patients. CT images displayed prominently ground glass opacities along with COVID-19 lesions. Adenovirus-infected patients also displayed similar radiographic findings. CT scanning showed huge potential a standard diagnosis tool with just 3.9% instances of misdiagnosis in cases of COVID-19. Early diagnosis can significantly reduce the spread of pandemic as the patients can be timely isolated or quarantined. However, CT cannot be employed for identifying different viruses as there is small difference between the CT images of patients infected with viruses of different families	[101]

Table 4 gives the summary of main drugs that are being used for treatment of COVID-19 along with the specific reasons and side effects [42, 78, 80–82, 84, 98, 99].

4 Comparison of Population Distribution of India, USA and Spain

It is evident the spread of COVID-19, specifically the CFR depends on age of patient considerably [102]. Figure 5 shows the population distribution of India, USA and Spain prepared based on available data [103]. India is second highest populated country and every 5th person of world belongs to India [104]. India has largest number (greater than 9%) of people in the age group 10–14, and the general bulge in distribution lies ranging from 5–9 to 20–24 years with a median age of 28.1 years. This implies that 50% of Indian population is below 28.1 years of age and has higher immunity to fight pandemics. On the other hand, population distribution for USA bulges at age group 40–44 years with a median age of 38.1 years. This implies that 50% population is below above 38.1 years and hence more prone to reduced immunity and susceptible to pandemics, whereas Spain, with a median age of 42.7 years and population distribution bulge at 25–29 years, has considerably high population prone to the severe effects of pandemic. The population pyramid of these countries shown in Fig. 6 reflects the same. India has an expansive population pyramid dome which has a broader base signifying that most of the people are in their youth age. Such expansive pyramid symbolizes high birth rates and high fertility rates. Although the fertility rate has come down from 6 in 1955 to 2.2 in the year 2020, it is still higher than USA (1.779) and Spain (1.354). USA has a relatively constrictive population pyramid with a smaller population in lower age group. On the other hand, Spain has a highly constrictive pyramid indicative of very low birth rates and very small population within lower age groups. As indicated by initial patient data, elderly patients are more prone to the fatal nature of COVID-19. As a matter of fact, the mortality rate in patients aged $\geq$80 years was up to 14.8%, while, in case of patients having age $<$ 40 years, mortality rate was only 0.2. Old -aged patients were already suffering from problems such as diabetes, cardiovascular, hypertension, various respiratory disorders and cancer. Therefore, such population pyramid indicates higher number of population prone to pandemics.

Role of contact matrix is vital in understanding the interaction among various age groups in a country within different settings (home, school, work, etc.). They present a systematic pictorial insight into the possible spread of a disease within different age groups of a country or region. Figure 7 shows the contact matrices for India, USA and Spain [105]. The dark diagonal line shows the strong bonding between persons of same age. On the other hand, light off-diagonal positions signify the interaction between persons of different age groups within same family (grandparents and grandchildren). It is evident from the contact matrix of India that owing to its

Table 4 Summary of main drugs (with reasons and side effects) being used for treating COVID-19 patients

S. No	Medicine	Reason	Side-effect
1	Chloroquine and Hydroxychloroquine	Chloroquine is a broad spectrum antiviral drug efficient in treating rheumatoid arthritis-related inflammation as well as lupus erythematous, which is shown to enhance endosomol pH preventing fusion of host cell and virus. It prevents glycosylation of SARS-CoV cell by interfering with its receptors Hydroxychloroquine shows higher potency than chloroquine and is known to inhibit cytokine storm due to SARS-CoV-2 in the patients	• Serious irregularity in heartbeats, which may lead to cardiac failure • Weak pulse • Prolonged use may cause damaged retina • Nausea • Digestive disorders • Ventricular tachycardia
2	Azithromycin	High in vitro activity against the Ebola virus. High potency in treating severe respiratory tract infection, skin infection as well as sexually transmitted diseases. It enhances the efficiency of hydroxychloroquine in treating COVID-19. Combination capable of replacing Remdesivir for treatment of patients	• Irregularity of heart beats • Liver problems • Tiredness and debility • Loss of appetite
3	Remdesivir	Most promising antiviral drug for treating SARS-CoV-2. Shows broad spectrum potency against assorted viruses including SARS-CoV and MERS-CoV. Works by replacing RNA polymerase enzyme thus inhibiting virus replication Despite high in vitro activity, application is limited by possible adverse effects	• Nausea • Vomiting • Hemorrhage • Hepatic toxicity • Respiratory failure • Skin discoloration • Low platelets, RBCs, albumin and potassium

(continued)

Table 4 (continued)

S. No	Medicine	Reason	Side-effect
4	Atazanavir	Belongs to protease inhibiting class of drugs and primarily used for preventing and treating HIV/AIDS. Works by restricting protease activity leading to growth of new viruses with faulty proteins rendering them unable to infect host cells. This leads to reduced viral load in host body. Artificial studies have shown Atazanavir to possess high binding ability to multiple coronavirus components as well as inhibitory characteristics against SARS-CoV-2. Tests are underway and conclusive results expected soon	• Increased bilirubin in blood (Jaundice) • Vomiting • Nausea • Decrease in heart rate • Pain in muscles • Insomnia • Pain in abdomen
5	Teicoplanin	Belonging to glycopeptides class of drugs, Teicoplanin shows efficacy in preventing entry of Ebola, SARS-CoV and MERS-CoV viruses into cytoplasm as well as inhibitory action on viral transcription and replication. Teicoplanin is known to inhibit host cell's cathespin L and cathespin B which facilitate the cleavage of viral glycoprotein allowing it to meet RBD and subsequent release into host cell cytoplasm. These findings favor the role teicoplanin, and its derivatives can play in treating cathespin-L-dependent viruses	• Maculopapular/erythematous rashes • Drug-related fever
6	Tipranavir	Belongs to protease inhibiting class of drugs used with ritonavir or antiretroviral for treating HIV infection. Capable of inhibiting viral replication in case patient is resistant to other protease-inhibiting drugs	• Diabetes mellitus • Hepatitis • Intracranial hemorrhage • Increased triglycerides and cholesterol
7	Cefditoren	A cephalosporin antibiotic with broad-spectrum activity against pathogens (gram positive as well as gram negative bacteria), used for treating variety of conditions such as pneumonia, acute bacterial infection and chronic bronchitis. The drug is stable against hydrolysis and works by reducing IL6 &K L6 which in turn reduces inflammation in lungs as well as epithelial damage	• Severe stomach pain • Fever • Swollen glands • Rash and itching • Bloody and watery diarrhea • Yellow skin • Dark colored urination

(continued)

Table 4 (continued)

S. No	Medicine	Reason	Side-effect
8	Indinavir	Inhibits protease and used in treatment of HIV/AIDS. Virus may become drug resistant if exact dosage is not monitored. Its lower water solubility may lead to formation of crystals which may be avoided by increasing water intake. Experimental studies on SARS-CoV-2 receptors indicate the binding capability of Indinavir lying between tipranavir and atazanavir	• Changes in metabolism • Increased bilirubin level (yellowing of skin) • Abdominal pain • Nausea • Changes in body shape • Formation of renal stones and abnormalities
9	Ritonavir/Lopinavir	Lopinavir, identified in the year 1998, is known as a treatment of HIV which works by restricting the protease and boosting antiviral activity. This drug, combined with oseltamivir, has been successfully used for treating COVID-19 patients suffering from pneumonia Ritonavir restricts enzymatic activity in liver and intestines associated with metabolism of protease inhibition with small dosages of drugs. In effect, ritonavir boosts the function of lopinavir in reducing HIV infection in human body	• Diarrhea • Headache • Nausea • Stomach dysfunction • Insomnia • Changed sense of taste
10	Telbivudine	Telbivudine falls in class of drugs identified as hepatitis B virus nucleoside reverse transcriptase inhibitors is primarily used for treating chronic hepatitis B virus. It leads to the chain termination by replacing virus DNA restricting replication of virus	• Fatigue • Headache • Dizziness • Stomach dysfunction and pain • Insomnia • Cough and throat • Joint and back pain, muscle pain • Fever and rashes

(continued)

Table 4 (continued)

S. No	Medicine	Reason	Side-effect
11	Ribavirin	Ribavirin is abroad spectrum antiviral agent used for treating respiratory syncytial virus (RSV) as well as hepatitis C infection. It effectively inhibits growth of RNA- and DNA-based viruses. Even if the replication is incompletely restricted, the replication of nucleic acid is done with reduced fidelity resulting in random mutations in virus DNA and hence decreased viability. Ribavirin has shown motivating in vitro activity on the first SARS-CoV-2 viral strain from sample of lung fluid of earliest of patients in China	• Chills or shaking • Headache • Dizziness • Stomach dysfunction and pain • Feeling irritable • Flu-like symptoms • Muscle pain • Mood swings • Vomiting and loss of appetite
12	Tocilizumab	One of the primary reasons of the fatal nature of COVID-19 has been identified as increased concentration of inflammatory cytokines. Research suggests the IL-6 to be the main cytokines responsible causing lung inflammation. Tocilizumab is one of the earliest IL-6 blockers being used for treatment of rheumatoid arthritis. As far as COVID-19 is concerned, out of 21 patients who received tocilizumab along with other antivirals, 20 showed reduced body temperature and respiratory function improvement within two weeks of treatment. No adverse effects of drugs were observed in patients	• Urinary tract infection (UTI) • Runny/stuffy nose, [G] • Itching, • Pain in sinus, • Sore throat, • Headache, • Mild stomach cramps, • Dizziness,
13	Ivermectin	Researchers at the Monash University of Australia have reported effective action of well-known antiparasite drug ivermectin against the SARS-CoV-2 in in vitro studies. Results of many clinical trials are awaited to test the efficacy and safety as far as COVID-19 is concerned	• Tiredness • General weakness • Stomach ache • Vomiting • Diarrhea

(continued)

Table 4 (continued)

S. No	Medicine	Reason	Side-effect
14	Darunavir	Darunavir is another trusted protease inhibitor antiretroviral drug for treating of HIV. In vitro studies conducted in China have indicated blocking the replication of SARS-CoV-2. Molecular docking studies suggest effective binding of darunavir with papain like viral protease	• Headache • Rashes and pain in abdomen • Nausea • Change in body shape • Diarrhea
15	Interferon Alpha-2b	Interferons are class of protein released as a response to virus entry and are capable of inhibiting its replication. Researchers at University of Texas observed indirect antiviral effect of interferon alpha against SARS-CoV-2 in a laboratory study. Interferon treatment resulted in up to 10,000-fold reduction in virus titer in host cells. Similar study in China reported reduction in time of viral shedding and lowering of inflammatory cytokine IL-6 in moderate patients of COVID-19 receiving interferon alpha-2b. Studies suggest that interferon treatment at an early stage of disease might reduce the viral load, lesser IL-6 production and better recovery rate	• Fever, chills, breathing trouble • Cough with mucous • Increased heart rate • Numbness and weakness • Loss of coordination, slurry speech • Vision problems • Light headedness
16	Favipiravir	Favipiravir has been typically used for the treatment of all three types of influenza. It inhibits the replication of rhinovirus; the primary working mechanism being inhibition of virus RNA polymerase. It also shows antiviral action against a variety of RNA viruses that are known to infect humans. Studies on small cohorts of COVID-19 patients are conclusive that treatment with favipiravir resulted in improvement in CT scans with reduction in viral load over shorter period of time. The drug is being used in few countries and under trial in many others including India	• May harm the fetal growth in pregnant women

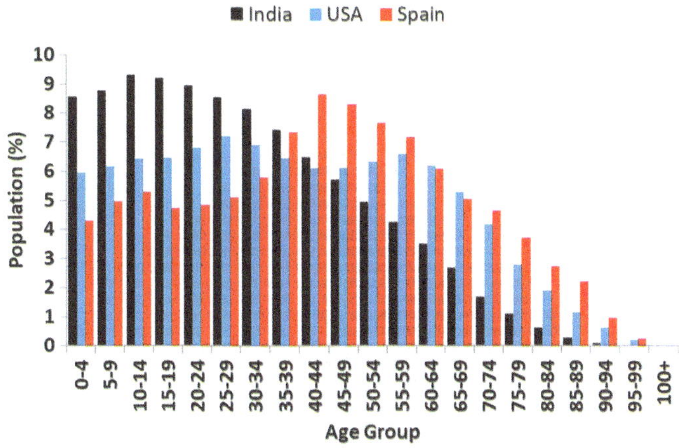

Fig. 5 Distribution of population (%) in India, USA and Spain with age group

complex family structure in which most of the rural families live as joint family and are therefore, much susceptible to pandemic in comparison with USA and Spain which show weaker off-diagonal locations (see Fig. 7).

In the work setting, all three countries have dark central locations indicating high level of interaction between persons of different age groups at workplace. This implies more homogenous contact among persons of different age groups in workplace and hence more uniform transfer of disease among persons who were safe in their respective homes. The diagonal elements in school setting in India are more prominent as compared with USA and Spain. This might be due to higher density of students in the schools inherently owing to the higher population. On the other hand, across the group interaction in school setting displays weaker locations indicating small interaction between teachers and students. Similarly, at other locations also the interaction among same age groups in India is significantly stronger than USA and Spain mainly due to the high population density. This implies that the general risk of catching the pandemic is significantly higher in India as compared to USA and Spain. However, people in both USA as well as Spain are also susceptible to the pandemic if they visit the locations such as marketplace, tourist spots, theater, gyms, restaurants.

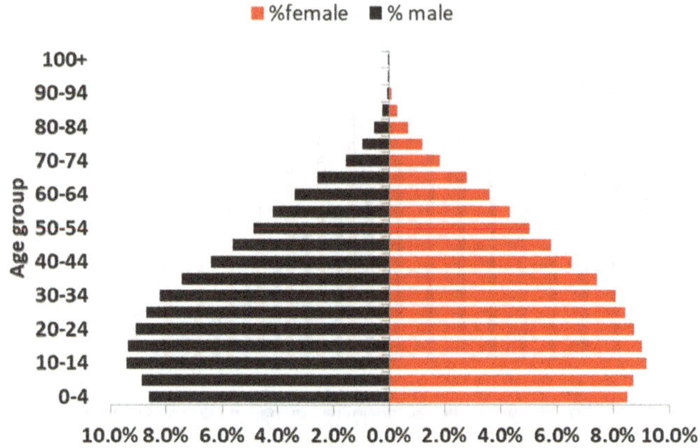

(a) India

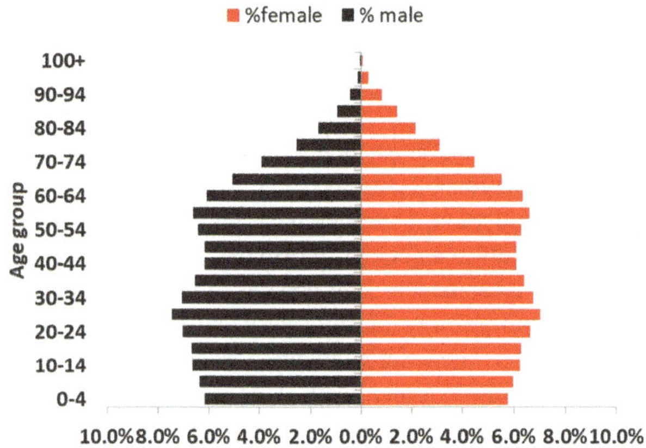

(b) USA

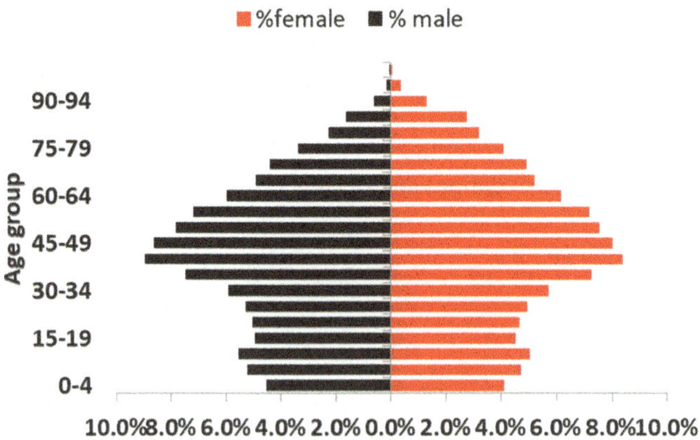

(c) Spain

Fig. 6 Population pyramid for India, USA and Spain

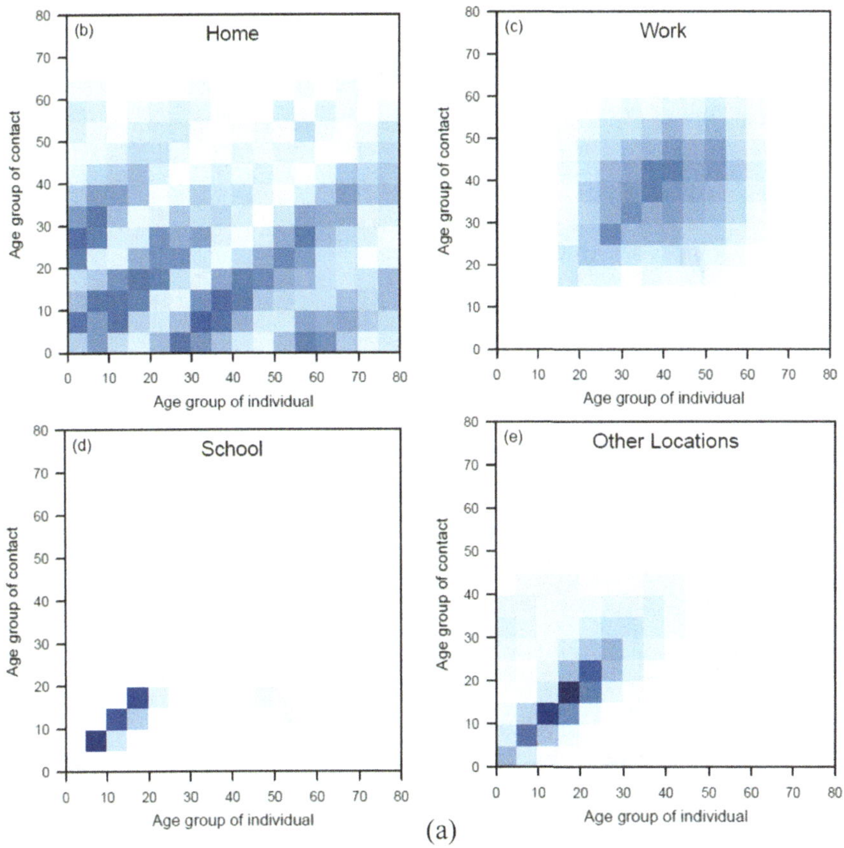

Fig. 7 Contact structures of **a** India, **b** USA and **c** Spain

Indian government has taken strict actions to curb the transmission of COVID-19 by implementation of nationwide lockdown, closure of academic institutions, government and private offices, marketplaces, cinema halls, public transport and even the religious places. It is worth mentioning that for the first time in 167 years, the largest employer of India, the Indian railways withdrew their services completely. In addition to this, the age structure of India comprising of a higher percentage of citizens in lower age groups translated into the late onset of COVID-19 in India which is evident from Fig. 8 showing the time taken by USA, Spain and India to cross first 5000 cases in logarithmic scale. It is evident that the rate of growth in India is significantly lower than USA and Spain. First case was reported on 30th January, 22nd January and 1st February in India, USA and Spain, respectively. It has taken 56 and 42 days, respectively, in USA and Spain to cross first 5000 cases. On the other hand, India took 69 days to cross the 5000 cases mark since the first case was reported. Relatively lower testing rate of India as compared to USA and Spain could be justified by the fact that ratio of infected individual out of number of tests in lower in India [58].

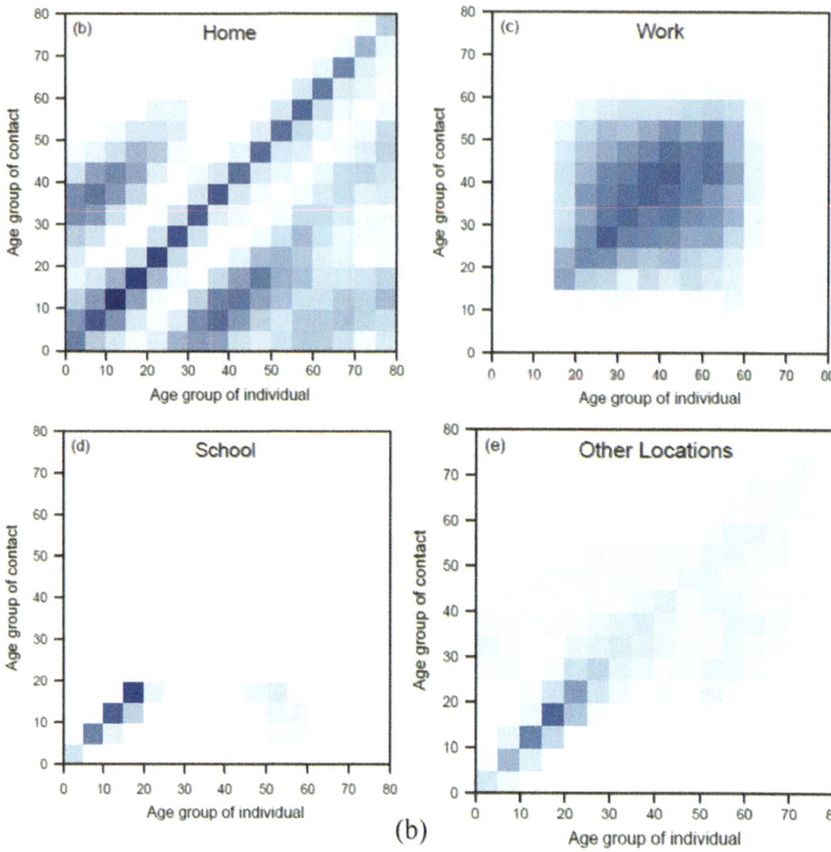

Fig. 7 (continued)

5 Mathematical Modeling

The standard SIR model has been employed for modeling the transmission dynamics of pandemic in India. The Indian population was segregated into three partitions, namely Susceptible (S), Infected (I) and Removed (R). These divisions were expressed as function of time, where S (t) is the number of susceptible population at the time t, I (t) is the number of infected population at the time t and R (t) is the number of removed individuals at time t. An individual may either recover (develop immunity) or may die. In both cases, they will not be able to affect the end results and therefore considered 'removed'. The rate of exchange of population between the compartments was simulated through differential Eq. (1):

$$\frac{dS}{dt} = -\beta SI$$

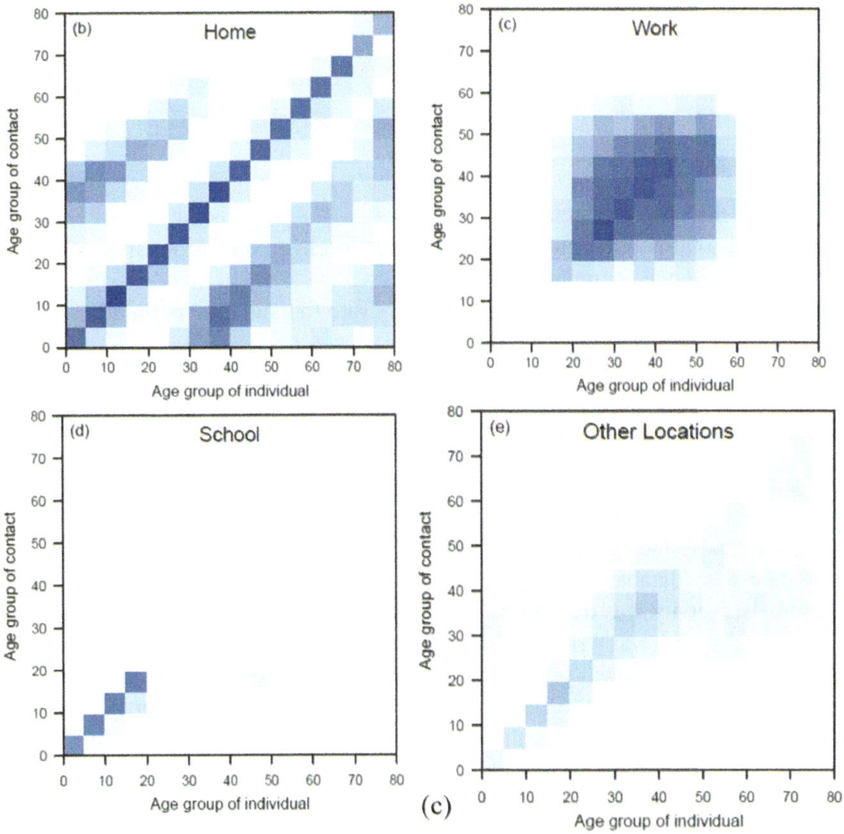

Fig. 7 (continued)

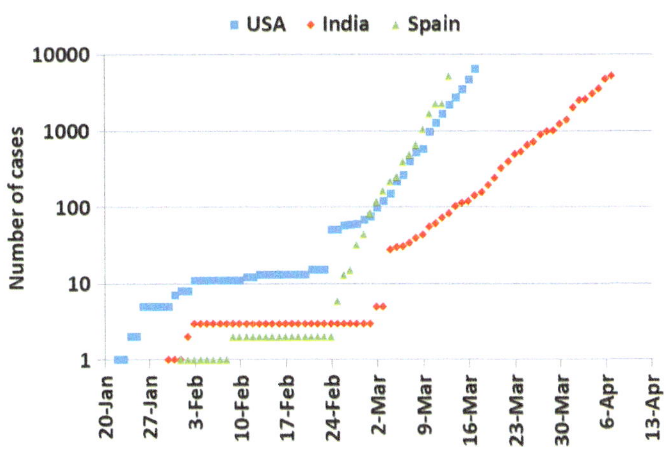

Fig. 8 Number of days taken to reach 5000 confirmed cases of COVID-19

$$\frac{dI}{dt} = \beta SI - \alpha I$$
$$\frac{dR}{dt} = \alpha I$$
$$N = S + I + R \tag{1}$$

where, β is the rate of infection and $\alpha = \frac{1}{\text{No. of days to recover}}$ is the rate of recovery, N being the total population and S, I, R are respective populations in susceptible, infected and removed compartments.

R0 is related to infection rate (β), recovery rate (α) and total population (N) by the relation:

$$R0 = \frac{\beta N}{\alpha} \tag{2}$$

The parameter R0, conceptualized by [106], and named by [107], is defined as the expected number of secondary infections appearing from an infected individual in a wholly naïve (susceptible) population over the course of the disease.

A date-wise database of reported cases of COVID-19 prepared by the John Hopkins University was used in the present work [108]. In order to implement the SIR model, a macro was written in Microsoft excel application and day wise progress of COVID-19 in India was predicted from the day of first confirmed case, i.e., 30th January 2020 onward. It is well known that the patients can be of either symptomatic or asymptomatic in nature. As the number of tests conducted in India still stands small in comparison with the population, the number of asymptomatic cases cannot be determined with certainty. Therefore, we have considered all the cases to be symptomatic; however, this reduces the severity of pandemic [11]. The total population of India was considered as 1,340,000,000 (134 Crores), and infected population was 1 (first confirmed case of India reported in Kerala state on 30th January 2020). Initial removed (recovered or dead) population was taken to be 0. The time of recovery was decided to be 3 weeks (21 days) based on published reports [109, 110]. The prediction was made for different value of R0 as given in Table 5. First of all, the value of R0 was adjusted for fitting it into the actual number of cases reported up to April 16, 2020, and corresponding value of β was calculated from Eq. (2). These cases were reported during the lockdown. If lockdown would not have been imposed, the scenario would have been much tragic. The studies have indicated that the R0 lies between 1.5 and 4.9 [42]. Therefore, it was attempted to predict the advance of COVID-19 by taking the value of R0 equal to 4.0 and 4.5, respectively, which were important for understanding the effect of lockdown and social distancing as well as cluster containment strategies employed by the government.

The model was subsequently run for forthcoming 8 months till end of November and the transmission dynamics of the pandemic was obtained. Figure 9 shows the comparison between actual and predicted number of cases in India till April 16, 2020. The close agreement between predicted values at (R0 value of 3.80) and actual cases is remarkable. For example, prediction shows about 15,329 cases as on April

16, 2020. Whereas, on same date, actual number of cases reported were 13,430. Model predicts that at this rate and in absence of strict measures, there will be about 88,500 cases in India till April end and about 3,760,000 cases till May end. These are very large numbers for a developing country like India and seem to overwhelm the already burdened healthcare facilities. However, such figures may not come up in reality as whole country is working toward flattening the curve through measures such as lockdown, cluster containment and social distancing. We expect that these

Table 5 Initial compartmental sizes and values of other parameters employed in the SIR model

S. No.	Parameter	Value
1	Initial susceptible population S(0)	1,340,000,000 (134 crores)
2	Initial infected population I(0)	1 (as on 30th January, 2020)
3	Initial removed population R(0)	0
4	Basic reproduction number, R0	3.80, 4.00, 4.50
5	Recovery rate, α	1/21 (21 days being time for recovery)
6	Rate of infection, β	Calculated using Eq. (2)

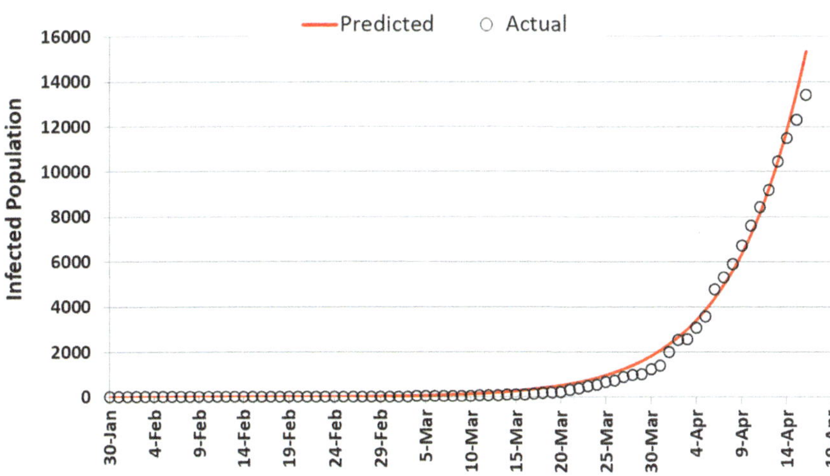

Fig. 9 Agreement between the model and actual reported cases of COVID-19 in India (actual and predicted for R0 = 3.80)

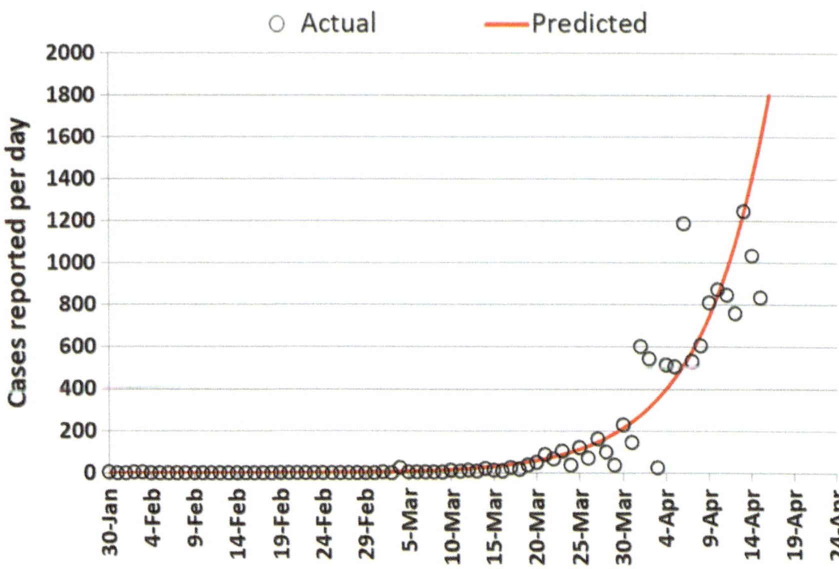

Fig. 10 Number of cases reported per day (actual and predicted)

figures shall come down significantly by the end of lockdown. In addition to this, there would be gradual decay in the pandemic over the period of time.

This is evident from the Fig. 10 showing predicted and actual daily increase in number of cases reported in India. The prediction goes very well with actual cases till March 25, 2020, after which the actual data shows scattering. This might be due to non-uniformity of cases being reported in India due to varying levels of stringency in strategies of various states of the country. Also, the effect of lockdown and containment measures is also quite evident. For example, on April 15, 2020 prediction shows up to 1600 new cases than April 14, 2020, whereas the actual increase in number of cases was just 835. A total of 17 districts of the country have not reported any new COVID-19 case since last 28 days as on 29th April, 2020 [111]. Also, not a single new case has been reported in 325 districts of the country out of the total 736 districts till April 16, 2020. The model indicates presence of huge number of asymptomatic patients in the population. In order to check the sensitivity of model, actual number confirmed cases were compared with the predicted number of infected individuals till 5th May, 2020.

Figure 11 displays the comparison between actual reported cases, predicted number of cases for R0 values equal to 3.5, 3.55 and 3.8. Actually reported confirmed cases as on 5th May, 2020 stood at 49,400. At R0 value of 3.8, the model predicts total number of infected individuals to be 165,290. This is quite high in comparison with actual cases and exhibits the scenario if there was no preventive action (social distancing, lockdown, cluster containment, etc.) against the pandemic in country. At R0 of 3.5, the predicted infected individuals are 48,914 which is just 0.9% lower than the actual number of cases. It is understandable that not all infected can be confirmed

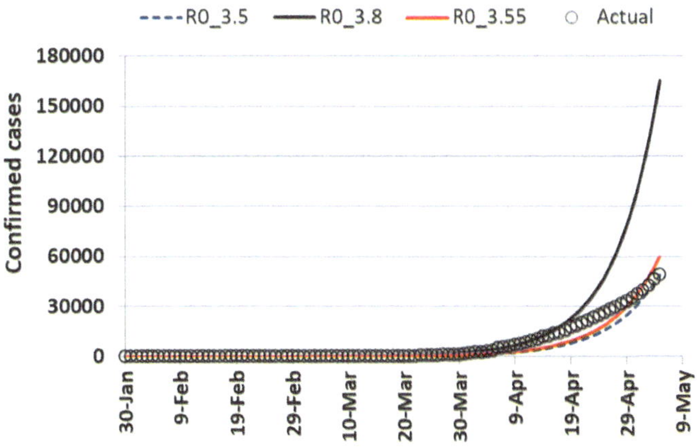

Fig. 11 Comparison between the model and actual reported cases of COVID-19 in India (actual and predicted for R0 = 3.50, 3.55 and 3.80) till 5th May, 2020

as many of them being asymptomatic and remaining unreported on a given date. At R0 value of 3.55, the predicted cases are 59,984 being about 20% higher than the actual value. Therefore, it can be stated that R0 value of 3.55 justifies the prediction of symptomatic as well as asymptomatic cases existing in India as on 5th May, 2020.

To put things in right perspective, we altered the value of R0 to 4.50 and 5.00 in order to predict advance of COVID-19 in relatively pessimistic scenarios. The time frame was selected to coincide with the occurrence of these incidents, i.e., March 25, 2020 to April 16, 2020. Figure 12 shows the predicted and actual number of cases reported in India within the considered time frame in logarithmic scale. It is clear that the predicted number cases are in excellent agreement with actual numbers for

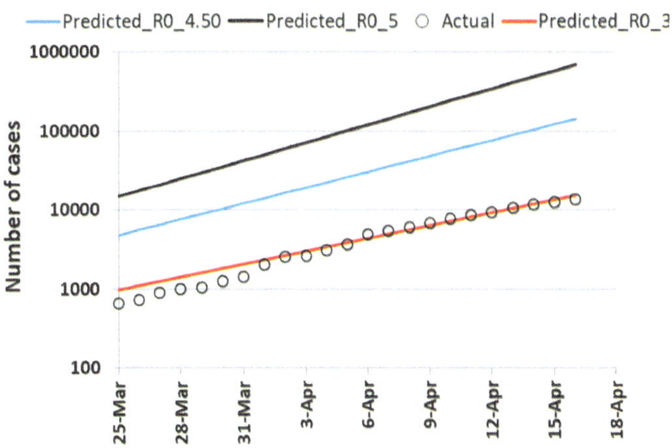

Fig. 12 Number of cases reported (actual and predicted) between March 25, 2020 and April 16, 2020

R0 equal to 3.80. This implies that during this timeframe, the R0 was approximately 3.80. As per media reports, very systematic and strict containment actions were taken by the government to restrict the transmission the pandemic after these incidents. In the absence of such strict measures, the R0 which is a function of infection rate (β) could have jumped to higher values. Due to demographics of India, a small increase in R0 to 4.5 could have pushed the number of confirmed cases to around 142,000 on April 16, 2020. Similarly, an R0 value of 5 could have escalated number of cases to 676,000 on April 16, 2020.

It is well known that the healthcare facilities are not sufficient to cater such huge population. Presently, India is having allopathic doctor to population ratio of 1:10, 926 which is much lower than 1:1000 recommended by the WHO [57]. Indian healthcare sector evolved from the Bhore committee report of 1946 and is based on three-tier healthcare systems. The main strategy before 1980s was to encourage more and more health providers to be on government payroll so that health facilities may be delivered to the lower middle class of country. However, shortage of top-end medical devices and professionals in government hospitals has resulted in the emerging of private sector as the key player in Indian healthcare sector [58]. In the public sector, there are 25,778 hospitals having a total number of 713,986 beds as on year 2019. Out of these, about 40% beds are available in hospitals situated in rural and 60% beds are available in hospitals situated in urban locations [59]. For COVID-19 patients, mechanical ventilation is the last service which is employed for revival of a dying patient. India is presently having approximately 40,000 ventilators which are negligible vis-à-vis the huge population base. The requirement of healthcare facilities was predicted if the pandemic takes its toll on India in its current pace. As per Indian Council of Medical Research, about 80% the total patients have no or mild symptoms. About 15% of those infected transform into severe cases and require hospitalization and around 5% need critical care. However, the doubling rate in India has increased from 3.4 before lockdown to 7.5 days during April, 2020, shows positive effect of social measures taken by Indian government. This fact can't be neglected the states where testing rate is high red zones are more.

6 Concluding Remarks

COVID-19 has become a menace for the mankind and has claimed more than 586,845 precious lives by July 16, 2020. The novel SARS-CoV-2 is probably zoonotic nature which gained its present form after several mutations within animals (Malaya pangolins or bats) before transmitting to human domain via spill-over. The SARS-CoV-2 has excellent binding ability with ACE2 present on vital organs such as lungs, heart, arteries and kidneys. The modeling in literature estimated R0 of COVID-19 varies from 1.5–3.77.

Researchers are working toward development of vaccine, and several trials are at various stages of testing by July 2020. The convalescent plasma therapy, which is an unconventional yet attractive line of treatment, was reported potential in treating the patients of COVID-19. BCG vaccination has been also reported effective by researchers. In addition to this, drug repurposing may also present a viable defense against COVID-19. Researchers should attempt repurposing of potential drugs using modeling tools. In absence of vaccination, social distancing and lockdown are the only discernible ways to avoid contracting the virus.

A comparison of demographics and contact structure of the USA, Spain and India revealed higher rate of propagation in USA in comparison with India. India has about 50% of population below 28.1 years of age as compared to 38.1 years in USA and 42.7 years in Spain. Thus, India has reported better recovery rate. We implemented a simple model to study the course of the pandemic in India. Fitting the SIR model to actually reported cases in India, R0 of 3.80 was estimated. The actual and predicted daily increase in patients show that these two are in agreement with each other with the constituted model.References [112] are given in the list but not cited in the text. Please cite them in text or delete them from the list.The reference [112] can be deleted.

References

1. Zhu, N., Zhang, D., Wang, W., Li, X., Yang, B., Song, J., Zhao, X., Huang, B., Shi, W., Lu, R., & Niu, P. (2020). A novel coronavirus from patients with pneumonia in China, 2019. *New England Journal of Medicine*.
2. WHO home page https://www.euro.who.int/en/health-topics/health-emergencies/coronavirus-covid-19/news/news/2020/3/who-announces-covid-19-outbreak-a-pandemic. Accessed 10 April, 2020.
3. Xie, M., & Chen, Q. (2020). Insight into 2019 novel coronavirus—an updated interim review and lessons from SARS-CoV and MERS-CoV. *International Journal of Infectious Diseases*.
4. McIntosh, K., & Peiris, J. S. M. (2009). Coronaviruses. In *Clinical virology*, (3rd edn, pp. 1155–1171). American Society of Microbiology.
5. World Health Organization and World Health Organization. (2020). Report of the WHO-China joint mission on coronavirus disease 2019 (COVID-19).
6. Kampf, G., Todt, D., Pfaender, S., & Steinmann, E. (2020). Persistence of coronaviruses on inanimate surfaces and their inactivation with biocidal agents. *Journal of Hospital Infection, 104*(3), 246–251.
7. Kwok, Y. L. A., Gralton, J., & McLaws, M. L. (2015). Face touching: A frequent habit that has implications for hand hygiene. *American Journal of Infection Control, 43*(2), 112–114.
8. Ferguson, N., Laydon, D., Nedjati Gilani, G., Imai, N., Ainslie, K., Baguelin, M., Bhatia, S., Boonyasiri, A., Cucunuba Perez, Z. U. L. M. A., Cuomo-Dannenburg, G., & Dighe, A. (2020). Report 9: Impact of non-pharmaceutical interventions (NPIs) to reduce COVID19 mortality and healthcare demand.
9. Bayham, J., & Fenichel, E. P. (2020). Impact of school closures for COVID-19 on the US health-care workforce and net mortality: A modelling study. *The Lancet Public Health*. https://doi.org/10.1016/S2468-2667(20)30082-7
10. Kucharski, A. J., Russell, T. W., Diamond, C., Liu, Y., Edmunds, J., Funk, S., Eggo, R. M., Sun, F., Jit, M., Munday, J. D., & Davies, N. (2020). Early dynamics of transmission and control of COVID-19: A mathematical modelling study. *The Lancet Infectious Diseases*. https://doi.org/10.1016/S1473-3099(20)30144-4
11. Singh, R., & Adhikari, R. (2020). Age-structured impact of social distancing on the COVID-19 epidemic in India. arXiv preprint arXiv:2003.12055.

12. Li, L., Yang, Z., Dang, Z., Meng, C., Huang, J., Meng, H., Wang, D., Chen, G., Zhang, J., Peng, H., & Shao, Y. (2020). Propagation analysis and prediction of the COVID-19. *Infectious Disease Modelling, 5*, 282–292. https://doi.org/10.1016/j.idm.2020.03.002
13. Choi, S., & Ki, M. (2020). Estimating the reproductive number and the outbreak size of COVID-19 in Korea. *Epidemiology and Health, 42*. https://doi.org/10.3946/kjme.2015.27.2.87
14. Sjödin, H., Wilder-Smith, A., Osman, S., Farooq, Z., & Rocklöv, J. (2020). Only strict quarantine measures can curb the coronavirus disease (COVID-19) outbreak in Italy, 2020. *Eurosurveillance, 25*(13), 2000280.
15. Ghaffarzadegan, N., & Rahmandad, H. (2020). Simulation-based estimation of the spread of COVID-19 in Iran. medRxiv. https://doi.org/10.1101/2020.03.22.20040956
16. Fanelli, D., & Piazza, F. (2020). Analysis and forecast of COVID-19 spreading in China, Italy and France. *Chaos, Solitons and Fractals, 134*, 109761. https://doi.org/10.1016/j.chaos.2020.109761
17. Peng, L., Yang, W., Zhang, D., Zhuge, C., & Hong, L. (2020). Epidemic analysis of COVID-19 in China by dynamical modeling. arXiv preprint arXiv:2002.06563
18. Calafiore, G. C., Novara, C., & Possieri, C. (2020) A modified SIR model for the COVID-19 contagion in italy. arXiv preprint arXiv:2003.14391
19. Bastos, S. B., & Cajueiro, D. O. (2020). Modeling and forecasting the Covid-19 pandemic in Brazil. arXiv preprint arXiv:2003.14288
20. Chang, S. L., Harding, N., Zachreson, C., Cliff, O. M. & Prokopenko, M. (2020). Modelling transmission and control of the COVID-19 pandemic in Australia. arXiv preprint arXiv:2003.10218
21. Nesteruk, I. (2020). Estimations of the coronavirus epidemic dynamics in South Korea with the use of SIR model. Preprint. ResearchGate.
22. Gilbert, M., Pullano, G., Pinotti, F., Valdano, E., Poletto, C., Boëlle, P. Y., d'Ortenzio, E., Yazdanpanah, Y., Eholie, S. P., Altmann, M., & Gutierrez, B. (2020). Preparedness and vulnerability of African countries against importations of COVID-19: a modelling study. *The Lancet, 395*(10227), 871–877. https://doi.org/10.1016/S0140-6736(20)30411-6
23. Roosa, K., Lee, Y., Luo, R., Kirpich, A., Rothenberg, R., Hyman, J. M., Yan, P., & Chowell, G. (2020). Real-time forecasts of the COVID-19 epidemic in China from February 5th to February 24th, 2020. *Infectious Disease Modelling, 5*, 256–263. https://doi.org/10.1016/j.idm.2020.02.002
24. Hellewell, J., Abbott, S., Gimma, A., Bosse, N. I., Jarvis, C. I., Russell, T. W., Munday, J. D., Kucharski, A. J., Edmunds, W. J., Sun, F., & Flasche, S. (2020). Feasibility of controlling COVID-19 outbreaks by isolation of cases and contacts. *The Lancet Global Health*. https://doi.org/10.1016/S2214-109X(20)30074-7
25. Prem, K., Liu, Y., Russell, T. W., Kucharski, A. J., Eggo, R. M., Davies, N., Flasche, S., Clifford, S., Pearson, C. A., Munday, J. D., & Abbott, S. (2020). The effect of control strategies to reduce social mixing on outcomes of the COVID-19 epidemic in Wuhan, China: a modelling study. *The Lancet Public Health*. https://doi.org/10.1016/S2468-2667(20)30073-6
26. Gupta, S., Raghuwanshi, G. S., & Chanda, A. (2020). Effect of weather on COVID-19 spread in the US: A prediction model for India in 2020. *Science of The Total Environment*, 138860. https://doi.org/10.1016/j.scitotenv.2020.138860
27. Chatterjee, K., Chatterjee, K., Kumar, A., & Shankar, S. (2020). Healthcare impact of COVID-19 epidemic in India: A stochastic mathematical model. *Medical Journal Armed Forces India*. https://doi.org/10.1016/j.mjafi.2020.03.022
28. Vega, D. I. (2020). Lockdown, one, two, none, or smart. Modeling containing COVID-19 infection. A conceptual model. *Science of the Total Environment*, 138917. https://doi.org/10.1016/j.scitotenv.2020.138917
29. Sharma, S., Zhang, M., Gao, J., Zhang, H., & Kota, S. H. (2020). Effect of restricted emissions during COVID-19 on air quality in India. *Science of the Total Environment, 728*, 138878. https://doi.org/10.1016/j.scitotenv.2020.138878

30. Bhatnagar, T., Murhekar, M. V., Soneja, M., Gupta, N., Giri, S., Wig, N., & Gangakhedkar, R. (2020). Lopinavir/ritonavir combination therapy amongst symptomatic coronavirus disease 2019 patients in India: Protocol for restricted public health emergency use. *Indian Journal of Medical Research, 151*(2), 184. https://doi.org/10.4103/ijmr.IJMR_502_20
31. Krishnakumar, B., & Rana, S. (2020). COVID 19 in INDIA: Strategies to combat from combination threat of life and livelihood. *Journal of Microbiology, Immunology and Infection.* https://doi.org/10.1016/j.jmii.2020.03.024
32. da Silva, J. A. T. (2020). Convalescent plasma: A possible treatment of COVID-19 in India. *Medical Journal, Armed Forces India.* https://doi.org/10.1016/j.mjafi.2020.04.006
33. Arti, M. K., & Bhatnagar, K., Modeling and predictions for COVID 19 Spread in India. *ResearchGate.*
34. Gupta, N., Bhatnagar, T., Rade, K., Murhekar, M., Gangakhedkar, R. R., Nagar, A., & ICMR COVID Team. (2020). Strategic planning to augment the testing capacity for COVID-19 in India. *Indian Journal of Medical Research, 151*(2), 210. https://doi.org/10.4103/ijmr.IJMR_1166_20
35. Minhas, S. (2020). Could India be the origin of next COVID-19 like epidemic? *Science of The Total Environment*, 138918. https://doi.org/10.1016/j.scitotenv.2020.138918
36. Roy, D., Tripathy, S., Kar, S. K., Sharma, N., Verma, S. K., & Kaushal, V. (2020). Study of knowledge, attitude, anxiety and perceived mental healthcare need in Indian population during COVID-19 pandemic. *Asian Journal of Psychiatry*, 102083. https://doi.org/10.1016/j.ajp.2020.102083
37. Varghese, G. M., & John, R. (2020). COVID-19 in India: Moving from containment to mitigation. *Indian Journal of Medical Research, 151*(2), 136. https://doi.org/10.4103/ijmr.IJMR_860_20
38. Pandey, G., Chaudhary, P., Gupta, R., & Pal, S. (2020). SEIR and regression model based COVID-19 outbreak predictions in India. arXiv preprint arXiv:2004.00958
39. Sardar, T., Nadim, S. S., & Chattopadhyay, J. (2020). Assessment of 21 days lockdown effect in some states and overall India: A predictive mathematical study on COVID-19 outbreak. arXiv preprint arXiv:2004.03487
40. Rathi, S., Ish, P., Kalantri, A., & Kalantri, S. (2020). Hydroxychloroquine prophylaxis for COVID-19 contacts in India. *The Lancet Infectious Diseases.* https://doi.org/https://doi.org/10.1016/S1473-3099(20)30313-3
41. Sahasranaman, A., & Kumar, N. (2020). Network structure of COVID-19 spread and the lacuna in India's testing strategy. Available at SSRN 3558548. https://doi.org/10.2139/ssrn.3558548
42. Mandal, S., Bhatnagar, T., Arinaminpathy, N., Agarwal, A., Chowdhury, A., Murhekar, M., Gangakhedkar, R. R., & Sarkar, S. (2020). Prudent public health intervention strategies to control the coronavirus disease 2019 transmission in India: A mathematical model-based approach. *The Indian journal of medical research, 151*(2–3), 190. https://doi.org/10.4103/ijmr.IJMR_504_20
43. Prasad, S., Potdar, V., Cherian, S., Abraham, P., Basu, A., & Team INN. (2020). Transmission electron microscopy imaging of SARS-CoV-2. *The Indian Journal of Medical Research, 151*(2–3), 241. https://doi.org/10.4103/ijmr.IJMR_577_20
44. Zhou, M., Zhang, X., & Qu, J. (2020). Coronavirus disease 2019 (COVID-19): A clinical update. *Frontiers of Medicine*, 1–10.
45. Chan, J. F. W., Kok, K. H., Zhu, Z., Chu, H., To, K. K. W., Yuan, S., & Yuen, K. Y. (2020). Genomic characterization of the 2019 novel human-pathogenic coronavirus isolated from a patient with atypical pneumonia after visiting Wuhan. *Emerging Microbes and Infections, 9*(1), 221–236. https://doi.org/10.1080/22221751.2020.1719902
46. Lam, T. T. Y., Shum, M. H. H., Zhu, H. C., Tong, Y. G., Ni, X. B., Liao, Y. S., Wei, W., Cheung, W. Y. M., Li, W. J., Li, L. F., & Leung, G. M. (2020). Identification of 2019-nCoV related coronaviruses in Malayan pangolins in southern China. *BioRxiv.* https://doi.org/10.1038/s41586-020-2169-0

47. Ji, W., Wang, W., Zhao, X., Zai, J., & Li, X. (2020). Cross-species transmission of the newly identified coronavirus 2019-nCoV. *Journal of Medical Virology, 92*(4), 433–440. https://doi.org/10.1002/jmv.25682
48. Chen, N., Zhou, M., Dong, X., Qu, J., Gong, F., Han, Y., Qiu, Y., Wang, J., Liu, Y., Wei, Y., & Yu, T. (2020). Epidemiological and clinical characteristics of 99 cases of 2019 novel coronavirus pneumonia in Wuhan, China: A descriptive study. *The Lancet, 395*(10223), 507–513. https://doi.org/10.1016/S0140-6736(20)30211-7
49. Andersen, K. G., Rambaut, A., Lipkin, W. I., Holmes, E. C., & Garry, R. F. (2020). The proximal origin of SARS-CoV-2. *Nature Medicine, 26*(4), 450–452. https://doi.org/10.1038/s41591-020-0820-9
50. https://edition.cnn.com/2020/04/12/asia/china-coronavirus-research-restrictions-intl-hnk/index.html?utm_term=link&utm_content=2020-04-12T18%3A06%3A56&utm_source=fbCNN&utm_medium=social
51. Wrapp, D., Wang, N., Corbett, K. S., Goldsmith, J. A., Hsieh, C. L., Abiona, O., Graham, B. S., & McLellan, J. S. (2020). Cryo-EM structure of the 2019-nCoV spike in the prefusion conformation. *Science, 367*(6483), 1260–1263. https://doi.org/10.1126/science.abb2507
52. Rabi, F. A., Al Zoubi, M. S., Kasasbeh, G. A., Salameh, D. M., & Al-Nasser, A. D. (2020). SARS-CoV-2 and coronavirus disease 2019: What we know so far. *Pathogens, 9*(3), 231. https://doi.org/10.3390/pathogens9030231
53. Imai, Y., Kuba, K., & Penninger, J. M. (2008). The discovery of angiotensin-converting enzyme 2 and its role in acute lung injury in mice. *Experimental Physiology, 93*(5), 543–548. https://doi.org/10.1113/expphysiol.2007.040048
54. Pan, X., Chen, D., Xia, Y., Wu, X., Li, T., Ou, X., Zhou, L., & Liu, J. (2020). Asymptomatic cases in a family cluster with SARS-CoV-2 infection. *The Lancet Infectious Diseases, 20*(4), 410–411. https://doi.org/10.1016/S1473-3099(20)30114-6
55. Liu, Y., Gayle, A. A., Wilder-Smith, A., & Rocklöv, J. (2020). The reproductive number of COVID-19 is higher compared to SARS coronavirus. *Journal of Travel Medicine*. https://doi.org/10.1093/jtm/taaa021
56. Li, Q., Guan, X., Wu, P., Wang, X., Zhou, L., Tong, Y., Ren, R., Leung, K. S., Lau, E. H., Wong, J. Y., & Xing, X. (2020). Early transmission dynamics in Wuhan, China, of novel coronavirus–infected pneumonia. *New England Journal of Medicine*. https://doi.org/10.1056/NEJMoa2001316
57. Yang, Y., Lu, Q., Liu, M., Wang, Y., Zhang, A., Jalali, N., Dean, N., Longini, I., Halloran, M. E., Xu, B., & Zhang, X. (2020). Epidemiological and clinical features of the 2019 novel coronavirus outbreak in China. *medRxiv*. https://doi.org/10.1101/2020.02.10.20021675
58. Shen, M., Peng, Z., Xiao, Y., & Zhang, L. (2020). Modelling the epidemic trend of the 2019 novel coronavirus outbreak in China. *bioRxiv*. https://doi.org/10.1016/j.xinn.2020.100048
59. Wu, J. T., Leung, K., & Leung, G. M. (2020). Nowcasting and forecasting the potential domestic and international spread of the 2019-nCoV outbreak originating in Wuhan, China: A modelling study. *The Lancet, 395*(10225), 689–697. https://doi.org/10.1016/S0140-6736(20)30260-9
60. Deb, S., & Majumdar, M. (2020). A time series method to analyze incidence pattern and estimate reproduction number of COVID-19. arXiv preprint arXiv:2003.10655.
61. Ranjan, R. (2020). Predictions for COVID-19 outbreak in India using epidemiological models. *medRxiv*. https://doi.org/10.1101/2020.04.02.20051466
62. Backer, J. A., Klinkenberg, D., & Wallinga, J. (2020). Incubation period of 2019 novel coronavirus (2019-nCoV) infections among travellers from Wuhan, China, 20–28 January 2020. *Eurosurveillance, 25*(5), 2000062.
63. Park, J. E., Jung, S., & Kim, A. (2018). MERS transmission and risk factors: a systematic review. *BMC Public Health, 18*(1), 574. https://doi.org/10.1186/s12889-018-5484-8
64. Huang, C., Wang, Y., Li, X., Ren, L., Zhao, J., Hu, Y., Zhang, L., Fan, G., Xu, J., Gu, X., & Cheng, Z. (2020). Clinical features of patients infected with 2019 novel coronavirus in Wuhan, China. *The Lancet, 395*(10223), 497–506. https://doi.org/10.1016/S0140-6736(20)30183-5

65. Onder, G., Rezza, G., & Brusaferro, S. (2020). Case-fatality rate and characteristics of patients dying in relation to COVID-19 in Italy. *JAMA, 323*(18), 1775–1776. https://doi.org/10.1001/jama.2020.4683
66. Yuan, J., Li, M., Lv, G., & Lu, Z. K. (2020). Monitoring transmissibility and mortality of COVID-19 in Europe. *International Journal of Infectious Diseases*. https://doi.org/10.1016/j.ijid.2020.03.050
67. Wang, L., Li, J., Guo, S., Xie, N., Yao, L., Cao, Y., Day, S. W., Howard, S. C., Graff, J. C., Gu, T., & Ji, J. (2020). Real-time estimation and prediction of mortality caused by COVID-19 with patient information based algorithm. *Science of the Total Environment*, 138394. https://doi.org/10.1016/j.scitotenv.2020.138394
68. Wangping, J., Ke, H., Yang, S., Wenzhe, C., Shengshu, W., Shanshan, Y., Jianwei, W., Fuyin, K., Penggang, T., Jing, L., & Miao, L. (2020). Extended SIR prediction of the epidemics trend of COVID-19 in Italy and compared with Hunan, China. *Frontiers in Medicine, 7*, 169.
69. Khafaie, M. A., & Rahim, F. (2020). Cross-country comparison of case fatality rates of COVID-19/SARS-COV-2. *Osong Public Health and Research Perspectives, 11*(2), 74. https://doi.org/10.3389/fmed.2020.00169
70. Harapan, H., Itoh, N., Yufika, A., Winardi, W., Keam, S., Te, H., Megawati, D., Hayati, Z., Wagner, A. L., & Mudatsir, M. (2020). Coronavirus disease 2019 (COVID-19): A literature review. *Journal of Infection and Public Health*. https://doi.org/10.1016/j.jiph.2020.03.019
71. Atri, D., Siddiqi, H. K., Lang, J., Nauffal, V., Morrow, D. A., & Bohula, E. A. (2020). COVID-19 for the cardiologist: A current review of the virology, clinical epidemiology, cardiac and other clinical manifestations and potential therapeutic strategies. *JACC: Basic to Translational Science*. https://doi.org/10.1016/j.jacbts.2020.04.002
72. Kaul, D. (2020). An overview of coronaviruses including the SARS-2 coronavirus—Molecular biology, epidemiology and clinical implications. *Current Medicine Research and Practice*. https://doi.org/10.1016/j.cmrp.2020.04.001
73. Wang, L. S., Wang, Y. R., Ye, D. W., & Liu, Q. Q. (2020). A review of the 2019 novel coronavirus (COVID-19) based on current evidence. *International Journal of Antimicrobial Agents*, 105948. https://doi.org/10.1016/j.ijantimicag.2020.105948
74. Ding, S., & Liang, T. J. (2020). Is SARS-CoV-2 also an enteric pathogen with potential fecal-oral transmission: A COVID-19 virological and clinical review. Gastroenterology. https://doi.org/10.1053/j.gastro.2020.04.052
75. Dong, Y., Mo, X., Hu, Y., Qi, X., Jiang, F., Jiang, Z., and Tong, S. (2020). Epidemiological characteristics of 2143 pediatric patients with 2019 coronavirus disease in China. *Pediatrics*. https://doi.org/10.1542/peds.2020-0702
76. Jin, Y., Yang, H., Ji, W., Wu, W., Chen, S., Zhang, W., & Duan, G. (2020). Virology, epidemiology, pathogenesis, and control of COVID-19. *Viruses, 12*(4), 372. https://doi.org/10.3390/v12040372
77. Mashamba-Thompson, T. P., & Crayton, E. D. (2020). Blockchain and artificial intelligence technology for novel coronavirus disease-19 self-testing. https://doi.org/10.3390/diagnostics10040198
78. Rismanbaf, A. (2020). Potential treatments for COVID-19: A narrative literature review. *Archives of Academic Emergency Medicine, 8*(1).
79. Zhang, J., Zeng, H., Gu, J., Li, H., Zheng, L., & Zou, Q. (2020). Progress and prospects on vaccine development against SARS-CoV-2. *Vaccines, 8*(2), 153. https://doi.org/10.3390/vaccines8020153
80. Gao, J., Tian, Z., & Yang, X. (2020). Breakthrough: Chloroquine phosphate has shown apparent efficacy in treatment of COVID-19 associated pneumonia in clinical studies. *Bioscience Trends*. https://doi.org/10.5582/bst.2020.01047
81. Liu, C., Zhou, Q., Li, Y., Garner, L. V., Watkins, S. P., Carter, L. J., Smoot, J., Gregg, A. C., Daniels, A. D., Jervey, S., & Albaiu, D. (2020). Research and development on therapeutic agents and vaccines for COVID-19 and related human coronavirus diseases. https://doi.org/10.1021/acscentsci.0c00272

82. Badyal, D. K., & Mahajan, R. (2020). Chloroquine: Can it be a novel drug for COVID-19. *International Journal of Applied and Basic Medical Research, 10*(2), 128. https://doi.org/10.4103/ijabmr.IJABMR_141_20
83. Gautret, P., Lagier, J. C., Parola, P., Meddeb, L., Mailhe, M., Doudier, B., Courjon, J., Giordanengo, V., Vieira, V. E., Dupont, H. T., & Honoré, S. (2020). Hydroxychloroquine and azithromycin as a treatment of COVID-19: results of an open-label non-randomized clinical trial. *International Journal of Antimicrobial Agents*, 105949. https://doi.org/10.1016/j.ijantimicag.2020.105949
84. Zhao, Q., & He, Y. (2020). Challenges of convalescent plasma therapy on COVID-19. *Journal of Clinical Virology, 127*, 104358. https://doi.org/10.1016/j.jcv.2020.104358
85. Cherian, S. S., Agrawal, M., Basu, A., Abraham, P., Gangakhedkar, R. R., & Bhargava, B. (2020). Perspectives for repurposing drugs for the coronavirus disease 2019. *Indian Journal of Medical Research, 151*(2), 160.
86. Roback, J. D., & Guarner, J. (2020). Convalescent plasma to treat COVID-19: Possibilities and challenges. *JAMA, 323*(16), 1561–1562. https://doi.org/10.1001/jama.2020.4940
87. Shanmugaraj, B., Siriwattananon, K., Wangkanont, K., & Phoolcharoen, W. (2020). Perspectives on monoclonal antibody therapy as potential therapeutic intervention for Coronavirus disease-19 (COVID-19). *Asian Pacific Journal of Allergy and Immunology, 38*(1), 10–18.
88. Jawhara, S. (2020). Could Intravenous immunoglobulin collected from recovered coronavirus patients protect against COVID-19 and strengthen the immune system of new patients? *International journal of molecular sciences, 21*(7), 2272. https://doi.org/10.3390/ijms21072272
89. Shen, C., Wang, Z., Zhao, F., Yang, Y., Li, J., Yuan, J., Wang, F., Li, D., Yang, M., Xing, L., & Wei, J. (2020). Treatment of 5 critically ill patients with COVID-19 with convalescent plasma. *JAMA, 323*(16), 1582–1589. https://doi.org/10.1001/jama.2020.4783
90. Economic times home page https://economictimes.indiatimes.com/industry/healthcare/biotech/pharmaceuticals/six-indian-companies-working-on-covid-19-vaccine-many-challenges-in-finding-a-preventive-experts/articleshow/75160500.cms?from=mdr. Accessed 20 April, 2020.
91. Ahn, D. G., Shin, H. J., Kim, M. H., Lee, S., Kim, H. S., Myoung, J., Kim, B. T., & Kim, S. J. (2020). Current status of epidemiology, diagnosis, therapeutics, and vaccines for novel coronavirus disease 2019 (COVID-19). 313–324. https://doi.org/10.4014/jmb.2003.03011
92. Miller, A., Reandelar, M. J., Fasciglione, K., Roumenova, V., Li, Y., & Otazu, G. H. (2020). Correlation between universal BCG vaccination policy and reduced morbidity and mortality for COVID-19: An epidemiological study. *MedRxiv*. https://doi.org/10.1101/2020.03.24.20042937
93. Hegarty, P. K., Kamat, A. M., Zafirakis, H., & Dinardo, A. (2020). BCG vaccination may be protective against Covid-19. Preprint.
94. Cortegiani, A., Ingoglia, G., Ippolito, M., Giarratano, A., & Einav, S. (2020). A systematic review on the efficacy and safety of chloroquine for the treatment of COVID-19. *Journal of Critical Care*. https://doi.org/10.1016/j.jcrc.2020.03.005
95. Brown, B. L., & McCullough, J. (2020). Treatment for emerging viruses: convalescent plasma and COVID-19. *Transfusion and Apheresis Science*, 102790. https://doi.org/10.1016/j.transci.2020.102790
96. Zhang, J., Xie, B., & Hashimoto, K. (2020). Current status of potential therapeutic candidates for the COVID-19 crisis. *Brain, Behavior, and Immunity*. https://doi.org/10.1016/j.bbi.2020.04.046
97. Bai, L., Yang, D., Wang, X., Tong, L., Zhu, X., Zhong, N., Bai, C., Powell, C. A., Chen, R., Zhou, J., & Song, Y. (2020). Chinese experts' consensus on the internet of things-aided diagnosis and treatment of coronavirus disease 2019 (COVID-19). *Clinical eHealth, 3*, 7–15. https://doi.org/10.1016/j.ceh.2020.03.001
98. Cevik, M., Bamford, C., & Ho, A. (2020). COVID-19 pandemic—A focused review for clinicians. *Clinical Microbiology and Infection*. https://doi.org/10.1016/j.cmi.2020.04.023

99. Li, X., Geng, M., Peng, Y., Meng, L. & Lu, S. (2020). Molecular immune pathogenesis and diagnosis of COVID-19. *Journal of Pharmaceutical Analysis*. https://doi.org/10.1016/j.jpha.2020.03.001
100. Abd El-Aziz, T. M., & Stockand, J. D. (2020). Recent progress and challenges in drug development against COVID-19 coronavirus (SARS-CoV-2)-an update on the status. *Infection, Genetics and Evolution*, 104327. https://doi.org/10.1016/j.meegid.2020.104327
101. Li, Y., & Xia, L. (2020). Coronavirus disease 2019 (COVID-19): Role of chest CT in diagnosis and management. *American Journal of Roentgenology, 214*(6), 1280–1286.
102. https://www1.nyc.gov/assets/doh/downloads/pdf/imm/covid-19-daily-data-summary-deaths-04152020-1.pdf
103. https://www.populationpyramid.net/
104. https://en.wikipedia.org/wiki/Demographics_of_India
105. Prem, K., Cook, A. R., & Jit, M. (2017). Projecting social contact matrices in 152 countries using contact surveys and demographic data. *PLoS computational biology, 13*(9), 1005697.
106. Kermack, W. O., & McKendrick, A. G. (1927). A contribution to the mathematical theory of epidemics. *Proceedings of the Royal Society of London. Series A, Containing Papers of a Mathematical and Physical Character*, *115*(772), 700–721. Royal Society. https://doi.org/10.1098/rspa.1927.0118
107. Macdonald, G. (1957). *The epidemiology and control of malaria*. Oxford University Press.
108. GIThub home page https://github.com/CSSEGISandData/COVID-19. Accessed 20 April, 2020.
109. Forbes home page https://www.forbes.com/sites/brucelee/2020/05/05/how-long-does-it-take-to-recover-from-covid-19-coronavirus-and-return-to-work/#d99094c43476. Accessed 5 May, 2020.
110. WHO home page https://www.who.int/docs/default-source/coronaviruse/who-china-joint-mission-on-covid-19-final-report.pdf#:~:text=Using%20available%20preliminary%20data%2C,severe%20or%20critical%20disease, Accessed 4 May, 2020.
111. New Indian express home page https://www.newindianexpress.com/nation/2020/apr/29/17-districts-with-no-fresh-covid-19-cases-in-28-days-but-is-it-really-an-achievement-2137000.html. Accessed 29 April, 2020.

Improved Estimation in Logistic Regression Through Quadratic Bootstrap Approach: An Application in Indian Agricultural E-learning System During COVID-19 Pandemic

Pramit Pandit, Bishvajit Bakshi, and K. N. Krishnamurthy

1 Introduction

Regression analysis is one of the most preferred statistical techniques for investigating the relationships involving multiple variables. Its appeal stems from the conceptually logical process of utilising a functional form to describe the relationship between a response variable (i.e. the variable of interest) and a set of related explanatory variables. Regression analysis, mostly due to its elegant underlying mathematics and well-developed statistical foundation, has dominated divergent research domains in dealing with the real-world data. A model working satisfactorily for a particular situation may fail drastically in a slightly different set-up. Therefore, development of reliable models is warranted to obtain information well in advance under varied conditions. Theory of multiple linear regression (MLR) analysis conventionally deals with the quantitative response variable. Hence, to deal with qualitative response variable or more specifically binary response variable, alternative models are necessitated. Among the various statistical approaches useful for classification and prediction, models based on regression, stochastic frameworks and various multivariate techniques are in vogue. Each of these approaches, with respect to classification and prediction ability, has its own advantages and limitations. Johnson et al. [1] performed linear discriminant and logistic regression analyses to investigate the weather effect on potato late blight occurrence in South Central Washington. Gent

P. Pandit
Department of Agricultural Statistics, Bidhan Chandra Krishi Viswavidyalaya, Mohanpur, West Bengal 741252, India

B. Bakshi (✉)
Centre for Management of Health Services, Indian Institute of Management-Ahmedabad, Ahmedabad, Gujarat 380015, India

K. N. Krishnamurthy
Department of Agricultural Statistics, Applied Mathematics and Computer Science, University of Agricultural Sciences, Bengaluru, Karnataka 560065, India

M. Niranjanamurthy et al. (eds.), *Intelligent Data Analysis for COVID-19 Pandemic*, Algorithms for Intelligent Systems, https://doi.org/10.1007/978-981-16-1574-0_10

et al. [2] used logistic regression for classifying the geographical regions of origin of *Xanthomonas* strains. Mila et al. [3] utilised logistic regression to estimate the probability of *Sclerotinia* outbreak in soybean using tillage practice, soil texture and weather variables as inputs. Bhowmik et al. [4] employed logistic regression for classification purposes in the area of agricultural ergonomics. Ramosacaj et al. [5] employed logistic regression in investigating students' performance level. Shukla et al. [6] developed students' placement prediction model using logistic regression.

Even though discriminant analysis is a common choice for the researchers to deal with classification problems, it relies on the assumption of multivariate normality. However, if a mixture of categorical and continuous variables serves as a set of explanatory variables, the assumption of multivariate normality will not hold good. To overcome this lacuna, logistic regression analysis is mostly preferred as it is free from any stringent assumption regarding the distribution of the explanatory variables. Practical situations dealing with mixture of categorical and continuous explanatory variables and qualitative response variable are quite common phenomena in agriculture, medical science, etc. The binary logistic regression model, extensively used to deal with such binary (dichotomous) responses, was developed primarily by Cox [7] and Walker and Duncan [8]. Like discriminant function analysis, logistic regression modelling can be also utilised for the classification purposes by considering two distinct responses as two groups. Then, the distinct observations with pre-defined group memberships along with associated variables are analysed as well as separated and the new observations are allotted to these pre-defined groups. In spite of the vast potential of the logistic regression model, there is still scope for developing an improved estimation procedure, assessing the model adequacy thereof and validating the same for their utilisation for the classification purposes.

In agricultural education framework, classification techniques are much needed for effective learning. However, not much work has been done so far on the application of logistic regression in the field of agricultural education in India. Due to the COVID-19 pandemic, a major shift from offline to online mode has been observed in education systems around the world including India. Many reports from different sources have clearly emphasised that many students, especially from rural area, are not at ease with the online mode of learning due to several socio-economic constraints. Hence, there is a necessity to analyse the effect of this shift with utmost care. With this backdrop, logistic regression analysis has been performed in the current study as a classification technique by utilising data relating to discomfort of Indian agricultural students in e-learning during COVID-19 pandemic. An attempt has also been made to identify the most influential explanatory variable.

For estimating the parameters of logistic regression model, method of maximum likelihood estimation (MLE) is mostly used. Lately, however, methods based on bootstrap have found numerous applications in regression analysis, specifically in the domain of nonlinear modelling. In ordinary bootstrap methodology, from the original sample, several independent samples are drawn randomly with replacement with size of the original sample, and then, the parameter estimates of the population are computed on the basis of the estimates obtained from these resamples. Over time, a spate of modifications is observed in the bootstrap methodology. It is now a well-recognised fact that the bootstrap can be very computer-intensive, especially if any analytical method cannot be implemented and approximations based on simulation are necessitated. Plenty of research works have been conducted by using bootstrap; however, its use under logistic regression set-up is still very limited [9–11]. Utilising the underprintings from Claeskens and Aerts [12], Claeskens et al. [13] proposed a quadratic bootstrap method for improved estimation. They also moved another step further by constructing a bias-corrected estimator. In this study, we have also obtained the quadratic bootstrap estimates under logistic regression model based on a single explanatory variable (i.e. the most influential explanatory variable). Quadratic bootstrap and maximum likelihood estimators, based on the original sample, have been compared in terms of width of the confidence interval. Classificatory abilities of the fitted logistic regression models based on these estimators have also been assessed. Further, a bias-corrected estimator has also been obtained on the lines of Claeskens et al. [13], and its performance is compared with the usual maximum likelihood estimator in terms of efficiency through a simulation study.

Rest of the chapter is organised as follows. In the next section, we have elaborately discussed the logistic regression model and its parameter estimation procedures. Empirical results obtained from the real data are presented in Sect. 3, and finally, Sect. 4 concludes the chapter.

2 Logistic Regression Model

2.1 *Preliminaries*

Consider a simple linear regression model with binary response variable.

$$Y_i = \beta_0 + \beta_1 X_i + \varepsilon_i; \quad i = 1, 2, \ldots, n$$

where the outcome Y_i is binary, i.e. it can take value either 0 or 1, $\varepsilon_i \sim N(0, \sigma_\varepsilon^2)$, ε_i and ε_j $(i \neq j)$ are independent, and n is the number of observations.

Let π_i denote the probability that $Y_i = 1$ when $X_i = x$, which implies

$$\pi_i = P(Y_i = 1 | X_i = x) = P(Y_i = 1) \quad \text{and thus,} \quad P(Y_i = 0) = 1 - \pi_i$$

Based on the assumption $E(\varepsilon_i) = 0$, the expected value of the response variable can be expressed as

$$E(Y_i) = 1.(\pi_i) + 0.(1 - \pi_i) = \pi_i$$

Now, as the response variable is binary in nature, the error terms ε_i also can take two values such as

$$\varepsilon_i = 1 - \pi_i, \quad \text{when} \quad Y_i = 1$$
$$\varepsilon_i = -\pi_i, \quad \text{when} \quad Y_i = 0$$

This dichotomous nature of the error terms clearly indicates the violation of normality assumption. The error variance, moreover, is not a constant but a function of π_i in this case. Thus, the assumption of homoscedasticity also does not hold good.

$$V(\varepsilon_i) = \pi_i(1 - \pi_i)^2 + (1 - \pi_i)(-\pi_i)^2 = \pi_i(1 - \pi_i)$$

Under such condition of non-normality and heteroscedasticity, ordinary least square estimation procedure cannot be applied. One of the commonly used alternatives to deal with this kind of situations is weighted least square estimation procedure; however, this procedure also fails to ascertain that the fitted values will be constrained to the interval (0, 1) so that these can be interpreted as probabilities. Few error variance, moreover, may appear in negative. In one way, this problem can be simply solved if π is constrained to the unit interval, and simultaneously, the linear relation between π and the regressor X is retained within the interval. Thus,

$$\pi = \begin{cases} 0, & \beta_0 + \beta_1 X < 0 \\ \beta_0 + \beta_1 X, & 0 \leq \beta_0 + \beta_1 X \leq 1 \\ 1, & \beta_0 + \beta_1 X > 1 \end{cases}$$

However, this constrained model also suffers from certain unattractive features such as abrupt changes in slope at the extremes 0 and 1, whereas between π and X, a smoother relation is more sensible in general [55]. To overcome this lacuna, transformation of $(\beta_0 + \beta_1 X_i)$ to unit interval with the help of a positive monotone function is necessitated with a view to meet the requirement of any cumulative probability distribution function. The model is now respecified as $\pi_i = P(\beta_0 + \beta_1 X_i)$. Clearly, it would be advantageous in case of a strictly increasing P and one-to-one transformation as then rewriting the model as $P^{-1}(\pi_i) = (\beta_0 + \beta_1 X_i)$ will be possible. Thus, smooth and symmetric property of the nonlinear model for π can be ascertained, approaching $\pi = 0$ and $\pi = 1$ as asymptotes. Consequently, estimated procedure can now be carried out as per the maximum likelihood method. The graphical representation of logistic response function is typically an S-shaped curve, where the probability (π) shows an initial slow increase, followed by accelerated increase and stabilisation, respectively, with increase in X. However, it never goes beyond 1. For a single explanatory variable, the probabilities can be modelled as

$$\pi = P(Y = 1|X = x) = 1/\left(1 + \mathrm{e}^{-z}\right)$$

where $z = \beta_0 + \beta_1 x$, and e is the base of the natural logarithm. This can be extended further for more than one (say r) explanatory variables to obtain the usual form of logistic regression equation.

$$\pi = P(Y = 1|X_1 = x_1, X_2 = x_2, \ldots, X_r = x_r) = 1/(1 + e^{-z})$$

where $z = \beta_0 + \beta_1 x_1 + \beta_2 x_2 + \cdots + \beta_r x_r$. The widespread popularity of logistic regression model is mostly due to the fact that the combined effect of several explanatory variables on the probability of an event can be modelled in an appealing *S*-shape and its ability to provide estimates ranging between 0 and 1.

2.2 *Identification of the Most Influential Variable*

2.2.1 Standardised Logistic Regression Coefficients

Reasons behind considering the standardised coefficients in logistic regression set-up are necessarily same as the reasons of utilising standardised coefficients in ordinary least squares regression (OLS) [14]. First of all, for the variables without any natural metric, a scale-independent standardised coefficient makes more sense than an unstandardised one [15]. However, the unstandardised coefficient can directly indicate the impact of one-unit increase or decrease in the explanatory variable on the response variable. But if the unit itself does not have any specific meaning, one-unit change will also become meaningless. For variables measured in grams, metres or any other such natural metric, a unit possesses some intrinsic meaning, but in many cases, social sciences in particular, even if the assumption of interval scale is made, impact of a change of 0.1 unit will remain ambiguous with respect to the scale [16]. In OLS, utilisation of standardised coefficients transforms the explanatory variables into variables measured in terms of standard deviation units [15, 17].

According to the inequality theorem provided by Chebycheff, at least 96% cases will fall within ten standard deviations from the mean for any distribution, even for a very non-normal one. However, in case of normal distribution, the lower ceiling for the same is 99.999999713% [18]. Thus, a one standard deviation change, regardless of distribution, is reasonably substantial typically encompassing about 10% of the total range of an explanatory variable.

Consequently, a standardised coefficient of an explanatory variable without any natural metric can ensure the amount of change required in that explanatory variable to impact the response variable substantially, provided these variables are related [19]. Second reason to use standardised coefficients is to compare the relative influence of different explanatory variables within an OLS or logistic regression model, when units of measurement of different variables are not same [20, 21]. That is, it makes the influence of different explanatory variables directly comparable.

The usual standardisation procedure under logistic regression set-up, as suggested by Agresti [22] and mentioned by Menard [23], is to standardise only the explanatory variables, yielding in

$$b_A^* = (b)(s_x)$$

where b denotes the sample estimate of the unstandardised logistic regression coefficient, and s_x represents the sample standard deviation of the explanatory variable (X).

2.3 Estimation in Logistic Regression Model

The usual estimation procedure for estimating the parameters of logistic regression model is maximum likelihood estimation (MLE) method. However, in the literature, few alternative estimation procedures such as resampling-based estimations and exact logistic regression also exist [24–26]. In the subsequent sections, we employ a quadratic bootstrap method [13, 55] along with MLE for the purpose of comparative assessment.

2.3.1 Method of Maximum Likelihood Estimation

The maximum likelihood estimates, in simple terms, are those values of the estimated parameters, which maximise the log-likelihood function. Computer-intensive numerical search procedures are often necessitated to find out the maximum likelihood estimates in case of logistic regression model as there does not exist any closed-form solution for the values of the parameters.

Let X denote an explanatory variable with p levels, and all the p levels of the explanatory variable are considered as p different populations. Let $Y_{i1}, \ldots, Y_{\text{in}_i}$ be independent and identically distributed Bernoulli random variables with probability function $f_i(y) = \pi_i^{y_{ij}}(1-\pi_i)^{1-y_{ij}}$; $y = 0, 1$; $i = 1, 2, \ldots, p$; $j = 1, 2, \ldots, n_i$ where Y_{ij} indicates whether the jth outcome in ith population is a 'success' or not, and the probability of success is represented by π_i. Let n_i be the number of replications at x_i. The number of levels (p) is assumed to be fixed, whereas number of observations (n_i) of distinct populations become large when total number of observations tends to infinity $\left(n = \sum_{i=1}^{p} n_i \to \infty\right)$.

In case of logistic regression model, the probability of success is modelled as a function of covariates through model parameters, i.e. for r number of explanatory variables, $\beta = (\beta_0, \beta_1, \ldots, \beta_r)$. Now, the maximum likelihood estimates for associated populations are based on the score functions of $(r+1)$ dimension (including the intercept) as:

$$\psi_i\left(Y_{ij}, \hat{\beta}_n\right) = \left(\partial/\partial\hat{\beta}\right) \log f_i(y, \beta); \quad i = 1, 2, \ldots, p$$

Score vector for logistic regression model with single explanatory variable can be given as follows:

$$\psi_i\left(Y_{ij}, \hat{\beta}_n\right) = \left[\psi_{i1}\left(Y_{ij}, \hat{\beta}_n\right)\psi_{i2}\left(Y_{ij}, \hat{\beta}_n\right)\right]'$$

$$= \left[y_{ij} - \frac{1}{1+\exp\left\{-\left(\hat{\beta}_0+\hat{\beta}_1 x_i\right)\right\}} y_{ij} - \frac{x_i}{1+\exp\left\{-\left(\hat{\beta}_0+\hat{\beta}_1 x_i\right)\right\}} \right]'$$

Now, the maximum likelihood estimator $\hat{\beta}_n$ for β can be obtained by solving the system of equations, $\sum_{i=1}^{p}\sum_{j=1}^{n_i}\psi_i\left(Y_{ij},\beta\right)=0$.

2.3.2 Method of Quadratic Bootstrap-Based Estimation and Bias-Corrected Estimator

As the key concern of any statistical analysis is to extract information as much as possible from the data under study, computer-intensive resampling techniques are of prime importance [27–29]. Among the resampling methods, bootstrap has gained immense popularity because of its robustness, compelling simplicity and computational demands [30–32]. The bootstrap approach was originally developed by Efron [33]. Davison and Hinkley [34] and Wu [35] made further developments in the context of regression analysis.

The fundamental principle behind the bootstrap technique is that the relationship between population and the original sample should closely resemble the relation between original sample and resample. Bootstrap provides one solution by taking several new samples from the original samples, assuming that that there is a sample of a given size for which more reliable estimates in terms of bias and standard errors are required. The statistic, thereafter, is computed each time along with the average and standard error from the empirical distribution of the bootstrap samples. Considering the average as estimate and the estimate obtained from the original sample as true value of the parameter, bias is calculated with a view to obtain a bias-corrected estimate. Bootstrapping approach is particularly useful in obtaining reliable estimates of the standard errors in situations where there is no standard procedure available or where the available methods are only approximate techniques because they are based on large sample or asymptotic theory.

The quadratic bootstrap approach is generally utilised to improve estimates by reducing bias and mean squared error, which consequently leads to the construction of a bias-corrected estimator. In logistic regression, the quadratic bootstrap method of estimation is employed for finite sample bias correction as follows [13, 55].

Let a large number (say B) of resamples are taken, which in turn results in a set of B quadratic bootstrap estimators $\left(\hat{\beta}_n^{*1}, \hat{\beta}_n^{*2}, \ldots, \hat{\beta}_n^{*B}\right)$. From this set of quadratic bootstrap estimators, a bias-corrected estimator can be obtained as

$$\hat{\beta}_n^{bc} = 2\hat{\beta}_n - \frac{1}{B}\sum_{u=1}^{B}\hat{\beta}_n^{*u}$$

The quadratic bootstrap estimator $\hat{\beta}_n^{*u}$ is here defined as

$$\hat{\beta}_n^{*u} = \hat{\beta}_n + U_n^* - \frac{1}{2}\left(\sum_{i=1}^{p}\sum_{j=1}^{n_i}\widetilde{\psi}_{ij}^*\left(\hat{\beta}_n\right)\right)^{-1}\left(\sum_{k=0}^{r}\sum_{l=0}^{r}\sum_{i=1}^{p}\sum_{j=1}^{n_i}\widetilde{\widetilde{\psi}}_{ij}^*\left(\hat{\beta}_n\right)_{k,l}U_{nk}^*U_{nl}^*\right)$$

for all $i = 1, 2, \ldots, p;\quad j = 1, 2, \ldots, n_i$ and $u = 1, 2, \ldots, B$ with

$$U_n^* = -\left(\sum_{i=1}^{p}\sum_{j=1}^{n_i}\widetilde{\psi}_{ij}^*\left(\hat{\beta}_n\right)\right)^{-1}\left(\sum_{i=1}^{p}\sum_{j=1}^{n_i}\psi_{ij}^*\left(\hat{\beta}_n\right)\right)$$

The quadratic bootstrap estimators are based on the values of $\left(\psi_{ij}^*\left(\hat{\beta}_n\right), \dot{\psi}_{ij}^*\left(\hat{\beta}_n\right), \widetilde{\widetilde{\psi}}_{ij}^*\left(\hat{\beta}_n\right)\right)$, $j = 1, 2, \ldots, n_i$ and $i = 1, 2, \ldots, p$ taken with replacement from the set

$$\left\{\begin{array}{l}\left(\psi_i\left(Y_{ij}, \hat{\beta}_n\right), (\partial/\partial\beta)\psi_i\left(Y_{ij}, \hat{\beta}_n\right), (\partial^2/\partial\beta\partial\beta^T)\psi_i\left(Y_{ij}, \hat{\beta}_n\right)\right);\\ j = 1, 2, \ldots, n_i;\quad i = 1, 2, \ldots, p\end{array}\right\}$$

It is expected that the representation of the random variation about estimator $\hat{\beta}_n^{*u}$ would be improved through the last term at the right hand side of its defining equation. Now, $\psi_i\left(Y_{ij}, \hat{\beta}_n\right)$ is a 2×1 vector, and the first derivatives of the score function can be expressed in a 2×2 matrix as follows:

$$(\partial/\partial\beta)\psi_i\left(Y_{ij}, \hat{\beta}_n\right) = \begin{bmatrix}(\partial/\partial\beta_0)\psi_{i1}\left(Y_{ij}, \hat{\beta}_n\right) & (\partial/\partial\beta_1)\psi_{i1}\left(Y_{ij}, \hat{\beta}_n\right)\\ (\partial/\partial\beta_0)\psi_{i2}\left(Y_{ij}, \hat{\beta}_n\right) & (\partial/\partial\beta_1)\psi_{i2}\left(Y_{ij}, \hat{\beta}_n\right)\end{bmatrix}_{\beta_0=\hat{\beta}_0\beta_1=\hat{\beta}_1}$$

$$= \begin{bmatrix}\frac{-\exp\left\{-\left(\hat{\beta}_0+\hat{\beta}_1x_i\right)\right\}}{\left(1+\exp\left\{-\left(\hat{\beta}_0+\hat{\beta}_1x_i\right)\right\}\right)^2} & \frac{-x_i\exp\{-(\hat{n}_0+\hat{n}_1x_i)\}}{(1+\exp\{-(\hat{n}_0+\hat{n}_1x_i)\})^2}\\ \frac{-x_i\exp\left\{-\left(\hat{\beta}_0+\hat{\beta}_1x_i\right)\right\}}{\left(1+\exp\left\{-\left(\hat{\beta}_0+\hat{\beta}_1x_i\right)\right\}\right)^2} & \frac{-x_i^2\exp\{-(\hat{n}_0+\hat{n}_1x_i)\}}{(1+\exp\{-(\hat{n}_0+\hat{n}_1x_i)\})^2}\end{bmatrix}$$

With respect to (k, l)th components of β, the second partial derivatives of $\psi_i\left(Y_{ij}, \hat{\beta}_n\right)$ are taken; where $k, l = 0, 1$. The corresponding vectors with dimensionality of (2×1) are given as follows.

The second partial derivative of $\psi_i\left(Y_{ij}, \hat{\beta}_n\right)$ with respect to $(0, 0)$th component is

$$\begin{bmatrix}(\partial^2/\partial\beta_0^2)\psi_{i1}\left(Y_{ij}, \hat{\beta}_n\right)\\ (\partial^2/\partial\beta_0^2)\psi_{i2}\left(Y_{ij}, \hat{\beta}_n\right)\end{bmatrix}_{\beta_0=\hat{\beta}_0, \beta_1=\hat{\beta}_1}$$

$$= \begin{bmatrix} \dfrac{\exp\left\{-\left(\hat{\beta}_0+\hat{\beta}_1 x_i\right)\right\}-\exp\left\{-2\hat{\beta}_0-2\hat{\beta}_1 x_i\right\}}{\left(1+\exp\left\{-\left(\hat{\beta}_0+\hat{\beta}_1 x_i\right)\right\}\right)^3} \\ \dfrac{x_i \exp\left\{-\left(\hat{\beta}_0+\hat{\beta}_1 x_i\right)\right\}-x_i \exp\left\{-2\hat{\beta}_0-2\hat{\beta}_1 x_i\right\}}{\left(1+\exp\left\{-\left(\hat{\beta}_0+\hat{\beta}_1 x_i\right)\right\}\right)^3} \end{bmatrix}$$

The second partial derivative of $\psi_i\left(Y_{ij}, \hat{\beta}_n\right)$ with respect to (0, 1)th component is

$$\begin{bmatrix} \left(\partial^2/\partial\beta_0\partial\beta_1\right)\psi_{i1}\left(Y_{ij},\hat{\beta}_n\right) \\ \left(\partial^2/\partial\beta_0\partial\beta_1\right)\psi_{i2}\left(Y_{ij},\hat{\beta}_n\right) \end{bmatrix}_{\beta_0=\hat{\beta}_0,\beta_1=\hat{\beta}_1}$$

$$= \begin{bmatrix} \dfrac{x_i\exp\left\{-\left(\hat{\beta}_0+\hat{\beta}_1 x_i\right)\right\}-x_i\exp\left\{-2\hat{\beta}_0-2\hat{\beta}_1 x_i\right\}}{\left(1+\exp\left\{-\left(\hat{\beta}_0+\hat{\beta}_1 x_i\right)\right\}\right)^3} \\ \dfrac{x_i^2\exp\left\{-\left(\hat{\beta}_0+\hat{\beta}_1 x_i\right)\right\}-x_i^2\exp\left\{-2\hat{\beta}_0-2\hat{\beta}_1 x_i\right\}}{\left(1+\exp\left\{-\left(\hat{\beta}_0+\hat{\beta}_1 x_i\right)\right\}\right)^3} \end{bmatrix}$$

The second partial derivative of $\psi_i\left(Y_{ij}, \hat{\beta}_n\right)$ with respect to (1, 0)th component is

$$\begin{bmatrix} \left(\partial^2/\partial\beta_1\partial\beta_0\right)\psi_{i1}\left(Y_{ij},\hat{\beta}_n\right) \\ \left(\partial^2/\partial\beta_1\partial\beta_0\right)\psi_{i2}\left(Y_{ij},\hat{\beta}_n\right) \end{bmatrix}_{\beta_0=\hat{\beta}_0,\beta_1=\hat{\beta}_1}$$

$$= \begin{bmatrix} \dfrac{x_i \exp\left\{-\left(\hat{\beta}_0+\hat{\beta}_1 x_i\right)\right\}-x_i \exp\left\{-2\hat{\beta}_0-2\hat{\beta}_1 x_i\right\}}{\left(1+\exp\left\{-\left(\hat{\beta}_0+\hat{\beta}_1 x_i\right)\right\}\right)^3} \\ \dfrac{x_i^2 \exp\left\{-\left(\hat{\beta}_0+\hat{\beta}_1 x_i\right)\right\}-x_i^2 \exp\left\{-2\hat{\beta}_0-2\hat{\beta}_1 x_i\right\}}{\left(1+\exp\left\{-\left(\hat{\beta}_0+\hat{\beta}_1 x_i\right)\right\}\right)^3} \end{bmatrix}$$

The second partial derivative of $\psi_i\left(Y_{ij}, \hat{\beta}_n\right)$ with respect to (1, 1)th component is

$$\begin{bmatrix} \left(\partial^2/\partial\beta_1^2\right)\psi_{i1}\left(Y_{ij},\hat{\beta}_n\right) \\ \left(\partial^2/\partial\beta_1^2\right)\psi_{i2}\left(Y_{ij},\hat{\beta}_n\right) \end{bmatrix}_{\beta_0=\hat{\beta}_0,\beta_1=\hat{\beta}_1}$$

$$= \begin{bmatrix} \dfrac{x_i^2 \exp\left\{-\left(\hat{\beta}_0+\hat{\beta}_1 x_i\right)\right\}-x_i^2 \exp\left\{-2\hat{\beta}_0-2\hat{\beta}_1 x_i\right\}}{\left(1+\exp\left\{-\left(\hat{\beta}_0+\hat{\beta}_1 x_i\right)\right\}\right)^3} \\ \dfrac{x_i^3 \exp\left\{-\left(\hat{\beta}_0+\hat{\beta}_1 x_i\right)\right\}-x_i^3 \exp\left\{-2\hat{\beta}_0-2\hat{\beta}_1 x_i\right\}}{\left(1+\exp\left\{-\left(\hat{\beta}_0+\hat{\beta}_1 x_i\right)\right\}\right)^3} \end{bmatrix}$$

The estimated bias of the quadratic bootstrap estimator is calculated as $\frac{1}{B}\sum_{u=1}^{B}\hat{\beta}_n^{*u} - \hat{\beta}_n$.

For the current study, first of all, from the original sample, we have obtained a good number of quadratic bootstrap samples. Then, the quadratic bootstrap estimates of the model parameters with single explanatory variable along with the maximum likelihood estimates of the original sample are obtained. The width of the confidence intervals for both the estimates of model parameters has been computed as well as compared through the original sample. Further, from the original sample, a large number of simulated samples have also been generated in order to obtain both maximum likelihood and bias-corrected estimates for each of the simulated sample. Finally, in terms of mean square error (MSE) and efficiency, comparative assessment of two approaches of estimation is carried out. For maximum likelihood and bias-corrected estimators, the mean square errors are computed as

$$\mathrm{MSE}\left(\hat{\beta}_n^{\mathrm{MLE}}\right) = \mathrm{variance}\left(\hat{\beta}_n^{\mathrm{MLE}}\right) + \left[\mathrm{bias}\left(\hat{\beta}_n^{\mathrm{MLE}}\right)\right]^2$$

$$\mathrm{MSE}\left(\hat{\beta}_n^{bc}\right) = \mathrm{variance}\left(\hat{\beta}_n^{bc}\right) + \left[\mathrm{bias}\left(\hat{\beta}_n^{bc}\right)\right]^2$$

2.4 Goodness of Fit

Hosmer–Lemeshow test is extensively used to check the goodness of fit of logistic regression models [36–38]. To employ this test for a binary logistic regression model, the observations are first arranged according to the increasing order of their estimated event probability [39]. In the next step, on the basis of the estimated probabilities, the observations are split into approximately ten groups [40, 41]. Subsequently, observed and expected frequency for each group are compared. If there exists less than ten patterns of explanatory variables, number of groups can be reduced; however, not less than 3.

For a $(2 \times g)$ table of observed and expected frequencies, where g indicates the number of groups, the Hosmer–Lemeshow goodness of fit statistic is obtained by calculating the Pearson chi-square statistic as follows:

$$\chi^2_{HL} = \sum_{i=1}^{g} \frac{\left(O_i - N_i \overline{\widehat{\pi}_i}\right)^2}{N_i \overline{\widehat{\pi}_i}\left(1 - \overline{\widehat{\pi}_i}\right)} \sim \chi^2_{g-2}$$

where O_i and N_i are the observed number of events and the number of subjects, respectively, in the ith group, and $\overline{\widehat{\pi}_i}$ denotes the average estimated probability of an event in the ith group.

2.5 Predictive Ability

After measuring the goodness of fit of the fitted models, predictive ability is judged in terms of Somers' D and Gamma statistic. Both these measures are conceptualised on the basis of concordance and discordance. The pair of subjects can be classified as concordant or discordant on the basis of ordering of two subjects on each of two variables. If the subject ranking is higher on both the variables, the pair is concordant. Otherwise, i.e. if the subject ranking is higher on only one of these variables and consequently, lower on another, the pair is considered to be discordant. However, if on both of the variables, the subjects have the same prediction, and the situation is considered as a tie. The Gamma statistic, ranging from -1 to 1, is defined as

$$\frac{N_s - N_d}{N_s + N_d}$$

where N_s and N_d denote the number of same and different pairs, respectively. Gamma statistic, being simplest among the predictive ability measures, ignores all tied pairs of cases. Consequently, there is a chance of exaggeration of the actual strength of association. However, Somers' D, unlike Gamma, takes tied pairs into account in one way or another. It can be considered as a simple modification of Gamma statistic, which is expressed as

$$\frac{N_s - N_d}{N_s + N_d + T_y}$$

where T_y represents the number of tied pairs. Like Gamma, Somers' D also ranges between -1 and 1.

2.6 Comparison Measures

Comparison measures rely on 2×2 classification tables. In columns, the observed values of the dependent variable are provided, whereas the predicted values are presented in rows. In a perfect model, i.e. when the overall percent correct is 100, all cases will be on the diagonal. The key words associated with the classification table are as follows.

2.6.1 Sensitivity

Sensitivity indicates the correct predictions in the reference class (usually 1) of the dependent variable in terms of percentage. Likewise, it also implies the model's capability to classify an event correctly.

2.6.2 Specificity

Specificity indicates the correct predictions in the given category (usually 0) of the dependent variable in terms of percentage. Likewise, it also implies the model's capability to classify a non-event correctly.

2.6.3 False Positive Rate

False positive rate is defined as the percentage of predicted event responses to the total actual non-event responses.

2.6.4 False Negative Rate

False negative rate is defined as the percentage of predicted non-event responses to the total actual event responses.

Higher the sensitivity as well as the specificity and lower the false positive rate as well as the false negative rate, better classificatory ability a model has.

3 Empirical Results

3.1 Data and Implementation

Responses from the agricultural students of all over India have been collected through Google form from 15 April 2020 to 15 May 2020. During that period, 1370 students from 43 agricultural institutions including different state agriculture universities and Indian Council of Agricultural Research (ICAR) - deemed to be universities have responded. Out of these 1370 responses available, 80%, i.e. 1096 responses have been selected randomly for the training purpose, and the remaining 20%, i.e. 274 responses have been retained as test data set. A pilot study has also been done prior to this with a view to obtain preliminary idea about the explanatory variables.

Presence ($Y = 1$) or absence ($Y = 0$) of discomfort of Indian agricultural students in e-learning has been considered as the response variable. As explanatory variables, Internet speed (X_1), gender (X_2), family income (X_3), proficiency in using Internet (X_4), pursuing degree programme (X_5), average family education (X_6) and lack of first-hand experience (X_7) have been taken, as indicated by the pilot study. Among the explanatory variables, Internet speed and family income are quantitative in nature. Rest of the explanatory variables are qualitative in nature each having two levels, as given in Table 1.

Evaluation of the responses received has revealed that male to female ratio among the respondents (i.e. students responded in this study) is nearly 1. Majority of the

Table 1 List of qualitative explanatory variables

Explanatory variable	Levels	
	0	1
Gender	Male	Female
Proficiency in using Internet	High	Low
Pursuing degree programme	Post-graduation	Graduation
Average family education	More or equal to 10th standard	Less than 10th standard
Lack of first-hand experience	Disagree	Agree

students (57%) are pursuing their graduation, while rest of them (43%) are pursuing their post-graduation. Average Internet speed experienced by the students has been found to be 71 Kilo Byte per second with a standard error of 61.5 Kilo Byte per second, which indicates the instable nature of the network strength. Per month family income has ranged from ₹5000.00 to ₹1,10,000.00 with an average of ₹18,300.00, whereas average family education of majority of the students (54%) is more than 10th standard. 86% students have found themselves proficient in using Internet, whereas 14% students have placed themselves below the proficiency level. Lack of first-hand experience has been felt by most of the students (93%); however, some of the students (7%) have not felt any such difference between offline and online mode of education.

In order to find out the best model under logistic regression set-up, stepdown method is employed [42, 43]. Stepdown logistic regression procedure starts with considering all the variables in the model, i.e. with a full model, and then, variable selection and model building are carried out simultaneously [44–48]. Table 2 reveals that the best model identified as per the stepdown logistic methodology consists of only three explanatory variables, viz. Internet speed, family income and lack of first-hand experience. Result of the Hosmer–Lemeshow test (p-value of chi-square statistic = 0.98) has also confirmed the goodness of fit of the model.

Values of Somers' D and Gamma statistics in Table 3 have clearly revealed that the selected model has the highest predictive ability among the fitted models. Outcomes of this study clearly indicate that emphasis should be given on high Internet speed, higher family income and strategies to provide first-hand experience to decrease the discomfort of Indian agricultural students with a view to increase the efficacy of e-learning process.

As there are only two continuous explanatory variables considered in the study, utilisation of various collinearity diagnostics such as pairwise correlation coefficients, variance inflation factors (VIF) or Belsley's variance decomposition proportion procedure will not be meaningful to compare the impacts of the explanatory variables. Hence, with a view to identify the most influential explanatory variable, standardised regression coefficients of the best fitted model are compared [49–53] and have found that Internet speed is the most influential among them.

Table 2 Results of stepdown regression analysis

Variables included in the model	$\widehat{\beta_0}$	$\widehat{\beta_1}$	$\widehat{\beta_2}$	$\widehat{\beta_3}$	$\widehat{\beta_4}$	$\widehat{\beta_5}$	$\widehat{\beta_6}$	$\widehat{\beta_7}$	p-value of H-M
$X_1, X_2, X_3, X_4, X_5, X_6, X_7$	−0.81	−0.97	0.88	−0.39	1.86	0.99	−0.04	0.39	0.87
	(0.17)	(0.07)	(0.76)	(0.11)	(0.44)	(0.46)	(0.02)	(0.12)	
$X_1, X_3, X_4, X_5, X_6, X_7$	−4.22	−1.45	–	−0.48	4.47	3.16	0.02	0.45	0.83
	(2.16)	(0.10)		(0.09)	(2.16)	(1.79)	(0.01)	(0.11)	
X_1, X_3, X_4, X_5, X_7	−6.83	−1.53	–	−0.64	6.54	4.31	–	0.21	0.9
	(3.84)	(0.09)		(0.1)	(3.84)	(3.55)		(0.08)	
X_1, X_3, X_4, X_7	−2.11	−1.85	–	−0.43	4.54	–	–	0.33	0.93
	(1.27)	(0.07)		(0.08)	(4.01)			(0.06)	
X_1, X_3, X_7	−3.07	−1.97	–	−0.51	–	–	–	5.82	0.98
	(1.34)	(0.06)		(0.07)				(1.18)	

Note Figures in brackets indicate standard errors, and p-value of H-M indicates p-value of chi-square statistic of Hosmer–Lemeshow test

Table 3 Predictive ability of the fitted models

Variables included in the model	Percent concordant	Percent discordant	Percent tied	Somers' D statistic	Gamma statistic
$X_1, X_2, X_3, X_4, X_5, X_6, X_7$	95.70	4.20	0.10	0.92	0.92
$X_1, X_3, X_4, X_5, X_6, X_7$	89.80	10.20	0.00	0.79	0.79
X_1, X_3, X_4, X_5, X_7	96.30	3.60	0.10	0.93	0.93
X_1, X_3, X_4, X_7	96.80	3.20	0.00	0.94	0.94
X_1, X_3, X_7	98.60	1.40	0.00	0.97	0.97

3.2 Comparative Assessment Between MLE and Quadratic Bootstrap Estimation

For the purpose of comparative assessment, 2500 quadratic bootstrap estimates have been obtained first by utilising the original sample of size 1096. Mean value of these 2500 estimates is obtained and taken as a single quadratic bootstrap estimate given by $\hat{\boldsymbol{\beta}}_0^* = -0.06$ and $\hat{\boldsymbol{\beta}}_1^* = -1.43$. Along with these, maximum likelihood estimates are also obtained as $\hat{\boldsymbol{\beta}}_0 = -0.04$ and $\hat{\boldsymbol{\beta}}_1 = -1.77$ from the original sample. Table 4 presents the 95% confidence interval for both the estimates. Smaller width of confidence interval is observed in case of quadratic bootstrap estimates as compared to maximum likelihood estimates. Quadratic bootstrap method, thus, efficiently reduces the confidence interval outperforming the maximum likelihood method. The 2500 quadratic bootstrap estimates are further classified in ten groups, and group frequencies are calculated accordingly in order to obtain an idea about the distribution pattern (specially, symmetry of the distribution) of the parameter estimates. The distribution of the intercept parameter is positively skewed, whereas negative skewness is observed for the slope parameter.

The fitted models based on quadratic bootstrap and maximum likelihood method of estimation are assessed for their classification abilities by utilising the test data set. Table 5 shows that both the models possess highly satisfactory classificatory power, however, quadratic bootstrap method performs slightly superior as compared to the maximum likelihood method in terms of different employed measures of comparison.

Table 4 95% confidence intervals for maximum likelihood and quadratic bootstrap estimates

Method of estimation	Estimates	95% confidence interval	Width of confidence interval
Maximum likelihood	$\hat{\beta}_0 = -0.04$	(−0.0498, −0.0302)	0.0196
	$\hat{\beta}_1 = -1.77$	(−1.7740, −1.7662)	0.0078
Quadratic bootstrap	$\hat{\beta}_0^* = -0.06$	(−0.0659, −0.0541)	0.0118
	$\hat{\beta}_1^* = -1.43$	(−1.4319, −1.4281)	0.0038

Table 5 Classificatory abilities of the fitted logistic regression models based on maximum likelihood and quadratic bootstrap method

Method of estimation	Sensitivity	Specificity	False positive rate	False negative rate
Maximum likelihood	94.10	90.00	10.00	5.90
Quadratic bootstrap	94.80	91.20	8.80	5.20

3.3 Outcomes of the Simulation Study

From the logistic regression model, 25,000 simulated samples each of size 1096 are also generated with a view to investigate further the properties of quadratic bootstrap estimation procedure. As the initial values of the model parameters, maximum likelihood estimates of the original sample are utilised. Thus, the logistic regression model fitted initially is

$$\hat{\pi}_1 = P(Y = 1) = \frac{1}{1 + e^{0.04+1.77X_1}}$$

Here, X_1 (Internet speed) is categorised into five groups such as 0–30 Kilo Byte per second, 30–60 Kilo Byte per second, 61–90 Kilo Byte per second, 91–120 Kilo Byte per second and more than 120 Kilo Byte per second. These five groups are considered as five populations. Now, if we put the value of X_1 in the initially fitted logistic regression model, probability that Y can take value 1 can be obtained corresponding to each value of X_1. By multiplying these probabilities with the size of corresponding population, the expected frequencies of occurrences of '1' in the respective populations can be computed, based on which 25,000 simulated samples each of size 1096 are generated. From each simulated data set, 2500 bootstrap resamples have been taken and used for obtaining quadratic bootstrap estimates. Each of these 2500 quadratic bootstrap estimates are utilised to obtain bias-corrected estimates $\left(\hat{\beta}_0^{bc}, \hat{\beta}_1^{bc}\right)$ for the corresponding simulated sample. Consequently, 25,000 such bias-corrected estimates can be obtained in total from the simulated samples. Maximum likelihood estimates ($\hat{\beta}_0^{\mathrm{MLE}}$, $\hat{\beta}_1^{\mathrm{MLE}}$) have also been obtained along with the bias-corrected estimates from each of the corresponding simulated samples resulting in a total of 25,000 maximum likelihood estimates. Table 6 shows the simulated means, standard deviation and mean square error values of maximum likelihood and bias-corrected estimates. The simulated standard deviation $\sigma\left(\hat{\beta}_0^{bc}\right)$ and $\sigma\left(\hat{\beta}_1^{bc}\right)$ of the bias-corrected estimates are found to be comparatively smaller than its maximum likelihood counterparts, $\sigma\left(\hat{\beta}_0^{\mathrm{MLE}}\right)$ and $\sigma\left(\hat{\beta}_1^{\mathrm{MLE}}\right)$ indicating the vital role of bias correction in decreasing variance. Moreover, MSEs for bias-corrected estimators are also much lesser as compared to corresponding maximum likelihood estimators. Consequently, substantially higher efficiency is evident in case of bias-corrected estimators, which is in consonance with the findings of Bhowmik et al. [54]. The

Table 6 Comparison between simulated mean, standard deviation and mean square error values of maximum likelihood and bias-corrected estimates

Estimates of intercept	Estimates of slope		
$E\left(\hat{\beta}_0^{\text{MLE}}\right)$	−0.051	$E(\hat{\beta}_1^{\text{MLE}})$	−1.789
$E(\hat{\beta}_0^{bc})$	−0.038	$E(\hat{\beta}_1^{bc})$	−1.831
$\sigma\left(\hat{\beta}_0^{\text{MLE}}\right)$	0.008	$\sigma(\hat{\beta}_1^{MLE})$	0.001
$\sigma(\hat{\beta}_0^{bc})$	0.002	$\sigma(\hat{\beta}_1^{bc})$	1.1×10^{-4}
$\text{MSE}(\hat{\beta}_0^{\text{MLE}})$	1.6×10^{-4}	$\text{MSE}(\hat{\beta}_1^{\text{MLE}})$	1.2×10^{-5}
$\text{MSE}(\hat{\beta}_0^{bc})$	1.9×10^{-5}	$\text{MSE}(\hat{\beta}_1^{bc})$	5.5×10^{-7}
$\frac{\text{MSE}(\hat{\beta}_0^{\text{MLE}})}{\text{MSE}(\hat{\beta}_0^{bc})}$	8.42	$\frac{\text{MSE}(\hat{\beta}_1^{\text{MLE}})}{\text{MSE}(\hat{\beta}_1^{bc})}$	21.82

efficiency factor of $\hat{\beta}_0^{bc}$ and $\hat{\beta}_1^{bc}$ with respect to $\hat{\beta}_0^{\text{MLE}}$ and $\hat{\beta}_1^{\text{MLE}}$ is 8.42 and 21.82, respectively.

4 Conclusion

In the current study, logistic regression model has been successfully used for classification of overall discomfort of Indian agricultural students in e-learning during COVID-19 pandemic. The best model identified as per the stepdown logistic methodology consists of only three explanatory variables, viz. Internet speed, family income and lack of first-hand experience. All the parameter estimates of the model have been found to be significant at 1% level. Findings emanated from this study clearly indicate that high-speed Internet as well as higher family income has direct impact on effective e-learning and there is a necessity to adopt alternative strategies to provide first-hand experience to the students. The present study would considerably help the policy makers and educationists to eradicate or at least to decrease the discomfort of Indian agricultural students in e-learning process. However, among the explanatory variables, Internet speed is identified as the most influential in causing discomfort in e-learning system.

Further, based on this variable, we have obtained the quadratic bootstrap estimates along with maximum likelihood estimates under logistic regression model for comparative study. From the estimation point of view, quadratic bootstrap outperforms MLE in terms of confidence intervals of the estimates based on the original sample as smaller width is observed in case of the former as compared to the later. Both the fitted models show satisfactory classificatory ability; however, marginal superiority is evident for the model fitted based on quadratic bootstrap estimators. A simulation study has also been conducted, which clearly shows the high relative efficiency of quadratic bootstrap-based bias-corrected estimators as compared to its maximum likelihood counterparts. The bias correction leads to a significant decrease in the variance. The present study, thus, validates the theoretical findings of the literature on the basis of real-world data in the field of agricultural education.

It is worth mentioning in the context of current study that efficient statistical models are always sought over the existing widely used models with a view to depict the various perspectives of the observed phenomena for improved classification and prediction. The extensively used usual logistic regression methodology may perform satisfactorily in some particular situations and, however, may fail in slightly different set-up. In such cases, the improved methodology, which are bias corrected and robust in nature, is warranted for more reliable modelling. In this era of high-speed statistical computing, such tasks do not remain herculean at all. These can be readily relegated to high-speed computers for model fitting and analysis. This improved methodology as employed in the current investigation is worth the efforts as it provides bias-corrected estimates besides being more efficient than the existing one.

References

1. Johnson, D. A., Alldredge, J. R., & Vakoch, D. L. (1996). Potato late blight forecasting models for the semiarid environment of south-central Washington. *Phytopathology, 86*(5), 480–484.
2. Gent, D. H., Schwartz, H. F., Ishimaru, C. A., Louws, F. J., Cramer, R. A., & Lawrence, C. B. (2004). Polyphasic characterization of Xanthomonas strains from onion. *Phytopathology, 94*(2), 184–195.
3. Mila, A. L., Carriquiry, A. L., & Yang, X. B. (2004). Logistic regression modeling of prevalence of soybean Sclerotinia stem rot in the north-central region of the United States. *Phytopathology, 94*(1), 102–110.
4. Bhowmik, A., Ramasubramanian, V., & Kumar, A. (2011). Logistic regression for classification in agricultural ergonomics. *Advances in Applied Research, 3*(2), 163–170.
5. Ramosacaj, M., Hasani, V., & Dumi, A. (2015). Application of logistic regression in the study of students' performance level (case study of Vlora University). *Journal of Educational and Social Research, 5*(3), 239.
6. Shukla, M. K., Rambade, P., Torasakar, J., Prabhu, R., & Maste, D. (2017). Students placement prediction model using logistic regression. *International Journal of Engineering Research and Technology, 5*(1), 1–4.
7. Cox, D. R. (1958). The regression analysis of binary sequences (with discussion). *Journal of the Royal Statistical Society Series B (Statistical Methodology), 20*, 215–242.
8. Walker, S. H., & Duncan, D. B. (1967). Estimation of the probability of an event as a function of several independent variables. *Biometrika, 54*, 167–178.
9. Aerts, M., & Claeskens, G. (2001). Bootstrap tests for misspecified models, with application to clustered binary data. *Computational Statistics & Data Analysis, 36*, 383–401.
10. Lee, K. W. (1990). Bootstrapping logistic regression models with random regressors. *Communications in Statistics-Theory and Methods, 19*, 2527–2539.
11. Swapnepoel, C. J., & Frangos, C. C. (1994). Bootstrap confidence intervals for slope parameter of a logistic model. *Communications in Statistics-Simulation and Computation, 23*(4), 1115–1126.
12. Claeskens, G., & Aerts, M. (2000). Bootstrapping local polynomial estimators in likelihood-based models. *Journal of Statistical Planning and Inference, 86*, 63–80.
13. Claeskens, G., Aerts, M., & Molenberghs, G. (2003). A quadratic bootstrap method and improved estimation in logistic regression. *Statistics & Probability Letters, 61*, 383–394.
14. Mayer, L. S., & Younger, M. S. (1976). Estimation of standardized regression coefficients. *Journal of American Statistical Association, 71*, 154–157.

15. Shamshirband, S., Hashemi, S., Salimi, H., Samadianfard, S., Asadi, E., Shadkani, S., Kargar, K., Mosavi, A., Nabipour, N., & Chau, K. (2020). Predicting standardized streamflow index for hydrological drought using machine learning models. *Engineering Applications of Computational Fluid Mechanics, 14*(1), 339–350.
16. Menard, S. (2004). Six approaches to calculating standardized logistic regression coefficients. *American Statistician, 58*(3), 218–223.
17. Aristya, V. E., Taryono, T., & Wulandari, R. A. (2016). Genetic variability, standardized multiple linear regression and principal component analysis to determine some important sesame yield components. *AGRIVITA, Journal of Agricultural Science, 39*(1), 83–90.
18. Bohrnstedt, G. W., & Knoke, D. (1988). *Statistics for social data analysis*. Peacock Publishers.
19. Kim, J., & Ferree, G. D. (1981). Standardization in causal analysis. *Sociological Methods & Research, 10*, 187–210.
20. Agresti, A., & Finlay, B. (1986). *Statistical methods for the social sciences*. Collier Macmillan.
21. Thompson, C. G., Kim, R. S., Aloe, A. M., & Becker, B. J. (2017). Extracting the variance inflation factor and other multicollinearity diagnostics from typical regression results. *Basic and Applied Social Psychology, 39*(2), 81–90.
22. Agresti, A. (1996). *An introduction to categorical data analysis*. Wiley.
23. Menard, S. (1995). *Applied logistic regression analysis*. Sage.
24. King, E. N., & Ryan, T. P. (2002). A preliminary investigation of maximum likelihood logistic regression versus exact logistic regression. *American Statistician, 56*(3), 163–170.
25. Shao, J., & Tu, D. (1995). *The jackknife and bootstrap*. Springer.
26. Simonoff, J. S., & Tsai, C. L. (1988). Jackknifing and bootstrapping quasi-likelihood estimators. *Journal of Statistical Computation and Simulation, 30*, 213–232.
27. Cheng, G., & Huang, J. Z. (2010). Bootstrap consistency for general semiparametric M-estimation. *Annals of Statistics, 38*(5), 2884–2915.
28. Maghyereh, A. I., & Awartani, B. (2012). Financial integration of GCC banking markets: A non-parametric bootstrap DEA estimation approach. *Research in International Business and Finance, 26*(2), 181–195.
29. Wright, D. B., London, K., & Field, A. P. (2011). Using bootstrap estimation and the plug-in principle for clinical psychology data. *Journal of Experimental Psychopathology, 2*(2), 252–270.
30. Freiman, M., Perez-Rossello, J. M., Callahan, M. J., Voss, S. D., Ecklund, K., Mulkern, R. V., & Warfield, S. K. (2013). Reliable estimation of incoherent motion parametric maps from diffusion-weighted MRI using fusion bootstrap moves. *Medical Image Analysis, 17*(3), 325–336.
31. Lee, S., Bolic, M., Groza, V. Z., Dajani, H. R., & Rajan, S. (2011). Confidence interval estimation for oscillometric blood pressure measurements using bootstrap approaches. *IEEE Transactions on Instrumentation and Measurement, 60*(10), 3405–3415.
32. Liu, H., & Verrall, R. J. (2010). Bootstrap estimation of the predictive distributions of reserves using paid and incurred claims. *Variance, 4*, 121–135.
33. Efron, B. (1979). Bootstrap methods: Another look at the jackknife. *Annals of Statistics, 9*(6), 1218–1228.
34. Davison, A. C., & Hinkley, D. V. (1997). *Bootstrap methods and their application*. Cambridge University Press.
35. Wu, C. F. J. (1986). Jackknife, bootstrap and other resampling methods in regression analysis. *Annals of Statistics, 14*, 1261–1295.
36. Bertolini, G., D'amico, R., Nardi, D., Tinazzi, A., & Apolone, G. (2000). One model, several results: The paradox of the Hosmer-Lemeshow goodness-of-fit test for the logistic regression model. *Journal of Epidemiology and Biostatistics, 5*(4), 251–253.
37. Fagerland, M. W., & Hosmer, D. W. (2012). A generalized Hosmer-Lemeshow goodness-of-fit test for multinomial logistic regression models. *The Stata Journal, 12*(3), 447–453.
38. Yu, W., Xu, W., & Zhu, L. (2017). A modified Hosmer-Lemeshow test for large data sets. *Communications in Statistics-Theory and Methods, 46*(23), 11813–11825.

39. Hosmer, D. W., Hosmer, T., Le, C. S., & Lemeshow, S. (1997). A comparison of goodness-of-fit tests for the logistic regression model. *Statistics in Medicine, 16*(9), 965–980.
40. Lai, X., & Liu, L. (2018). A simple test procedure in standardizing the power of Hosmer-Lemeshow test in large data sets. *Journal of Statistical Computation and Simulation, 88*(13), 2463–2472.
41. Paul, P., Pennell, M. L., & Lemeshow, S. (2013). Standardizing the power of the Hosmer-Lemeshow goodness of fit test in large data sets. *Statistics in Medicine, 32*(1), 67–80.
42. Furmańczyk, K. (2015). On some stepdown procedures with application to consistent variable selection in linear regression. *Statistics, 49*(3), 614–628.
43. Hegyi, G., & Garamszegi, L. Z. (2011). Using information theory as a substitute for stepwise regression in ecology and behavior. *Behavioral Ecology and Sociobiology, 65*(1), 69–76.
44. Abraham, S., Raisee, M., Ghorbaniasl, G., Contino, F., & Lacor, C. (2017). A robust and efficient stepwise regression method for building sparse polynomial chaos expansions. *Journal of Computational Physics, 332*, 461–474.
45. Bauweraerts, J. (2016). Predicting bankruptcy in private firms: Towards a stepwise regression procedure. *International Journal of Financial Research, 7*(2), 147–153.
46. Nazarpour, A., Paydar, G. R., & Carranza, E. J. M. (2016). Stepwise regression for recognition of geochemical anomalies: Case study in Takab area, NW Iran. *Journal of Geochemical Exploration, 168*, 150–162.
47. Wang, M., Wright, J., Brownlee, A., & Buswell, R. (2016). A comparison of approaches to stepwise regression on variables sensitivities in building simulation and analysis. *Energy and Buildings, 127*, 313–326.
48. Zhou, X., & Jiang, T. (2016). Metamodel selection based on stepwise regression. *Structural and Multidisciplinary Optimization, 54*(3), 641–657.
49. Cosenza, A., Mannina, G., Vanrolleghem, P. A., & Neumann, M. B. (2013). Global sensitivity analysis in wastewater applications: A comprehensive comparison of different methods. *Environmental Modelling & Software, 49*, 40–52.
50. Menberg, K., Heo, Y., & Choudhary, R. (2016). Sensitivity analysis methods for building energy models: Comparing computational costs and extractable information. *Energy and Buildings, 133*, 433–445.
51. Mohammed, M. A., Manktelow, B. N., & Hofer, T. P. (2016). Comparison of four methods for deriving hospital standardised mortality ratios from a single hierarchical logistic regression model. *Statistical Methods in Medical Research, 25*(2), 706–715.
52. Neumann, M. B. (2012). Comparison of sensitivity analysis methods for pollutant degradation modelling: A case study from drinking water treatment. *Science of the Total Environment, 433*, 530–537.
53. Rahman, A., Haddad, K., Zaman, M., Kuczera, G., & Weinmann, P. E. (2011). Design flood estimation in ungauged catchments: A comparison between the probabilistic rational method and quantile regression technique for NSW. *Australasian Journal of Water Resources, 14*(2), 127–139.
54. Bhowmik, A., Ramasubramanian, V., Rai, A., Kumar, A., & Kundu, M. G. (2016). Improved estimation in logistic regression through quadratic bootstrap approach: An application in agricultural ergonomics. *Journal of the Indian Society of Agricultural Statistics, 70*(3), 227–235.
55. Bhowmik, A. (2009). A study on logistic regression modeling for classification in agriculture (Unpublished master's thesis). Indian Agricultural Research Institute, New Delhi, India.

COVID-19 and Stock Markets: Deaths and Strict Policies

Ali Altiner, Eda Bozkurt, and Yılmaz Toktaş

1 Introduction

In the literature of economics, there are numerous publications starting with the phrase "under the effect of globalization" and emphasizing the effect of globalization on the subject discussed in the paper. Globalization has accelerated the free movement of people, capital, money, knowledge, production factors, and commodities, and there are numerous opinions as to its consequences. One such consequence is COVID-19 from which everybody suffers. Known as the coronavirus, it first appeared in Wuhan, China, then spread across Asia before reaching Europe, the Americas, and the Middle East. The World Health Organization (WHO) announced a global pandemic on March 11, 2020. On the first days, it was thought that the virus has been transmitted to humans by bats or other animals. Moreover, it was widely expressed that this virus has been developed in a laboratory and released accidentally and that it was a biological weapon.

COVID-19 has led to catastrophic worldwide death and illness rates. Beyond these medical outcomes, COVID-19 has had a significant economic impact. That is, it also seems to be economically infectious [1]. To combat the spread, concepts like social distancing and isolation have come into our lives. Governments have shut down schools, converting face-to-face education into distance learning. Social gathering places, such as shopping malls, cafes, restaurants, and sports arenas, have been closed. Limited and full curfews have been declared, and travel between countries has been largely banned.

A. Altiner (✉)
Recep Tayyip Erdoğan University, 53100 Rize, Turkey
e-mail: lncs@springer.com

E. Bozkurt
Atatürk University, 25240 Erzurum, Turkey

Y. Toktaş
Amasya University, 05200 Amasya, Turkey

M. Niranjanamurthy et al. (eds.), *Intelligent Data Analysis for COVID-19 Pandemic*, Algorithms for Intelligent Systems, https://doi.org/10.1007/978-981-16-1574-0_11

Along with these social changes, governments have adopted economic measures to reduce the negative effects in real and financial sectors. Substantial funds have been allocated to healthcare systems. Liquidity support that has been provided to banks, households and businesses has received cash and non-cash aid, and taxes have been deducted or deferred. Besides that, unemployment funds have been increased, and disemployment bans have been introduced [2]. These policies aim to protect the whole macroeconomic structure, including employment, inflation, investment, trade, and consumption. Barro et al. [3] report that 150 million people died in 43 countries during the 1918–1920 influenza pandemic, and GDP and consumption decreased by 6% and 8%, respectively; they regard these as the upper bounds of COVID-19. There will likely be fewer deaths caused by COVID-19 due to healthcare improvements. However, all economic indicators will be affected negatively on a global scale.

The crisis arisen by COVID-19 pandemic is a multidimensional crisis, in which the demand, supply, and finance shocks are experienced at the same time. Differing from the previous global crises, the current pandemic crisis has not been triggered by a single main source. The sources of COVID-19 crisis can be listed as the cease of operations in various industries due to limitation measures, the demand shrinkage arising from the loss of income, the supply shock arising from the damage in commodity chains and supply chain and the loss of employment, and the decline of financial assets' value due to the decrease in commodity prices and asset values in global and local financial markets [4].

Stock markets are important indicators during global crises. They reflect future expectations and provide information about stability and risk perception. Furthermore, if the household investment is intense, as in developed countries, much of society, including politicians, will be interested in stock market developments. This study differs by attempting to determine the reaction of G7 and E7 countries to the epidemic, and our motivations are fivefold. First, big events such as disasters, environmental changes, political developments, and sports activities have a substantial effect on stock market returns [5], and the current pandemic is one of the most significant incidents to affect the global economy. Second, stock markets respond to incidents more rapidly than other economic indicators as data are obtained on a daily basis. Third, the G7 and E7 countries include the 10 countries with the highest reported cases. Few studies have explored the relationship between previous epidemics, including severe acute respiratory syndrome (SARS), MERS, Ebola virus disease (EVD), and stock returns, indicating there is a gap in the literature. In conclusion, the studies examining the relationship between COVID-19 and stock exchange markets are gathered under the section of the literature review. The present paper is the first providing a summary of studies in literature and providing convenience for the readers.

2 COVID-19 and Its Macroeconomic Effects

Although the COVID-19 pandemic has created a shock wave, the world actually has experience with the coronavirus family. Coronaviruses are a large group of viruses that might cause disease among animals and humans. According to the data published by WHO, SARS has come first in February 2003 as a viral respiratory tract disease. Emerging first in China, SARS is known to be transmitted by cats and bats. SARS is a disease that is similar to catarrh and might be transmitted directly through droplets or even indirectly by contact with surfaces, which any virus-carrier has contacted with. SARS, which can be easily and rapidly transmitted in the twenty-first century, has affected the people aged between 25 and 70 years. Among the affected people, symptoms such as cough, fever, head-neck pain, sweating, and weakness are observed. The incubation period is 2–7 days and may last up to 10 days. 8098 cases and 774 deaths were reported in 26 countries in total and the filiation chain was broken on the July 5, 2003. The death rate among the cases was approx. 3%. For this disease, in which the treatment is supportive, no vaccine could be developed [6]. In 2012, however, MERS has been reported as a disease caused by a coronavirus. The virus has infected humans through contact with dromedaries. In MERS affecting people aged between 45 and 85 years, the incubation period was 2–14 days. Eighty percent of the cases were in Saudi Arabia. The symptoms of MERS include fever, cough, shortness of breath, shivering, and muscle pain. In the absence of protection, it might be transmitted by human to a human. According to the current statistics, 2519 MERS cases and 866 deaths have been reported in 27 countries in total. Thirty-five percent of the confirmed cases have died. The disease has no specific treatment or vaccine [7]. The pandemic before COVID-19 is known as the Ebola pandemic. Seen in West Africa between 2014 and 2016, the pandemic is thought to have originated from the wild animals. Transmitted to humans through the blood and body fluids of animals, the virus is also transmitted by the blood and body fluids of humans. Moreover, close contact with patients causes transmission. The incubation period was reported to vary between 2 and 21 days. The symptoms include fatigue, fever, headache, muscle pain, sore throat, diarrhea, vomiting, and rash. For this virus that has affected 18 countries, the number of confirmed cases was 28,616, whereas the number of deaths was 11,310. The average rate of death is approx. 50%. Although there is no widespread treatment method, early diagnosis increases the chance of survival [8]. The last known coronavirus pandemic (COVID-19) arose from China in late 2019. It is estimated that the disease has been transmitted through the animals sold in the wild animal market. The most known symptoms include fever, cough, and shortness of breath, and the incubation period is 2–14 days. Although it is thought that the virus is transmitted through droplets and surface contact, the researches on this subject continue. Spread over more than 200 countries, the virus affected 22 million people and 792,000 persons have died. Diagnosed with laboratory tests, COVID-19 has no specific treatment or vaccine [9].

Table 1 shows the summary of pandemics during 2000s. Comparing them, it can be seen that all the viruses (including COVID-19) in the coronavirus family

Table 1 Coronavirus-caused pandemics and their characteristics

Pandemic	SARS	MERS	Ebola	COVID-19
Date	2003	2012	2014	2019
First appeared in	China	Saudi Arabia	West Africa	China
Reason	Bats and cats	Dromedaries	Wild animals	Wild animals
Symptoms	Fever, sweating, headache, sore throat, weakness, cough	Fever, cough, shortness of breath, shivering, muscle pain	Fatigue, fever, headache, muscle pain, sore throat, diarrhea, vomiting, rash	Fever, cough, shortness of breath
Incubation period	2–7 days	2–14 days	2–21 days	2–14 days
Mode of transmission	Droplet, surface contact	No exact information, close contact	Blood and body fluids	Droplet, surface contact, researches continuing
Diagnosis-identification-treatment	History of contact and presence of symptoms, no specific treatment or vaccine	History of contact and presence of symptoms, no specific treatment or vaccine	Laboratory tests-no specific treatment or vaccine	Laboratory tests-no specific treatment or vaccine
Status of spread	26 countries	27 countries	18 countries	200+ countries
Number of cases	8098	2519	28,616	22,000,000
Number of deaths	774	866	11,310	792,000
Rate of death (%)	3	35	50	3

Source Compiled from WHO data

have an animal origin. It can be stated that the diseases, which have the same mode of transmission and incubation period, have similar symptoms. The characteristic of COVID-19 distinguishing it from the others is that it could reach a very wide area of impact in a very short period. In this pandemic, which has become a global one, the number of confirmed cases is hundreds times of those reported in previous pandemics.

Besides its effects on public health, COVID-19 also had significant effects on social, cultural, political, and economic lives. Increasing the severity of disease created a domino effect together with the economic dependence brought by globalization. Distance, hygiene, mask, and isolation protected the public health at a global scale by decelerating the transmission of disease but these measures also negatively affected the economic achievements of countries. COVID-19 pandemic has various effects ranging between the lifestyles and social lives of people and the economic activities of individuals and companies. The uncertainty about the end of pandemic causes a deepening of effects and an increase of severity. The pandemic has micro- and macroeffects.

Barua drew a general theoretical map of potential economic effects of COVID-19 pandemic in 2020 [10]. The potential effects of the pandemic are presented in Fig. 1.

Figure 1 presents the theoretical map of the potential effects of COVID-19 pandemic, besides the period of effect and progression line. While mapping the macroeconomic effects of the COVID-19 pandemic, it would be appropriate to examine a single country. Although the first effects begin with the first wave involving

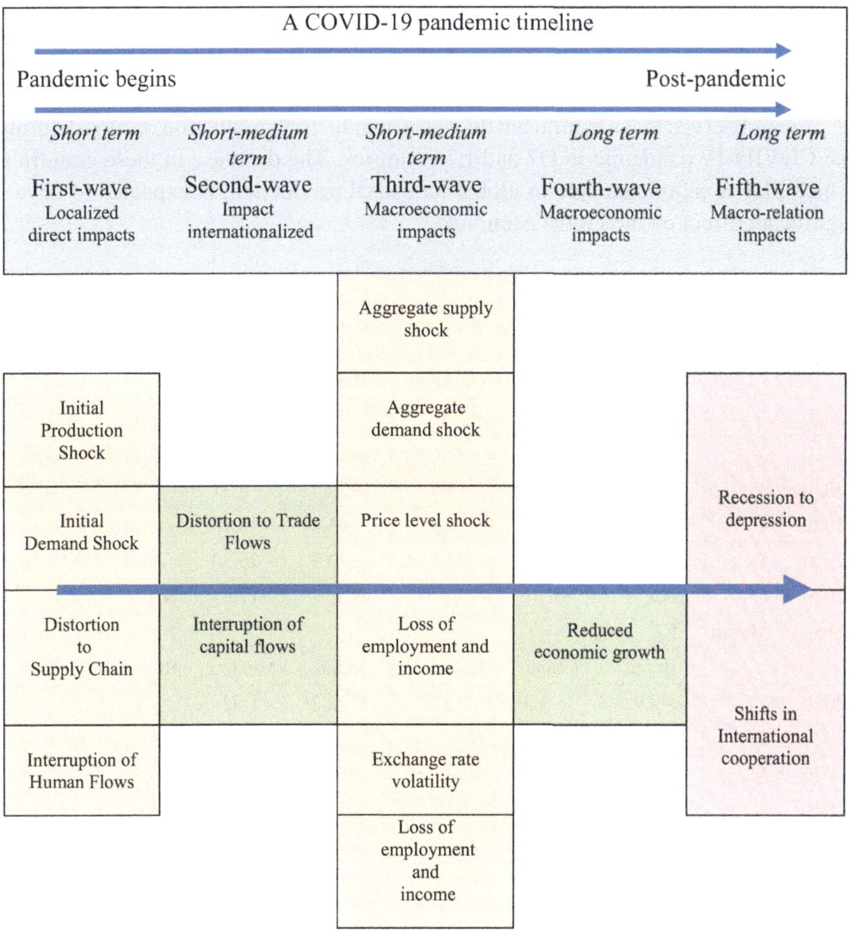

Fig. 1 A general map of the potential economic impacts of COVID-19 pandemic. *Source* [10]

the direct effects including temporary shutdowns of business places and factories, a process incorporating different waves begins in the course of time [10].

The first economic effect of the pandemic is the decrease in production because of social distance and lockdown.

As shown in Table 2, together with the COVID-19 pandemic, the National Institute of Statistics reported that the industrial production of China decreased by 13.5% in February 2020 and showed the worst performance of the last 30 years [11]. When compared to the previous year, the total industrial production in the USA decreased by 11% in April. This decrease is the highest monthly decrease in the history of 101 years of industrial production, and it reflects the effect of COVID-19 pandemic forcing many factories and companies to stop their operations following the government-led measures aiming to stop the spread of coronavirus [12]. Istat, the Italian statistics office, reported that industrial production rapidly decreased in March and the production of consumer goods, investment goods, intermediate goods, and energy products completely fell [13]. Among D7 countries, the highest decline in the production index in May was 26.6% in Japan, followed by France, Germany, Italy, UK, Canada, and the USA.

It was observed that a significant decrease in industrial production occurred during the COVID-19 pandemic in D7 and E7 countries. The decrease in these countries, which play a significant role in global industrial production, is expected to have a significant effect on the global economy.

Table 2 Industrial production, annual percent change

Year	Month	G7						
		Canada	France	Germany	Italy	Japan	UK	USA
2020	1	−0.15	−3.4	−3.5	−0.2	−2.4	−2.4	−0.85
2020	2	1.15	−1.5	−2.8	−2.3	−5.58	−3	−0.22
2020	3	−5.39	−17.6	−13.8	−29.4	−5.31	−7.7	−4.76
2020	4	−19.97	−35.6	−29.4	−43.4	−15.13	−23.4	−16.32
2020	5	−17.49	−24	−23.1	−20.3	−26.33	−19.9	−15.36
2020	6	NA	NA	NA	NA	−17.65	NA	−10.82
Year	Month	E7						
		Brazil	China	Indonesia	India	Mexico	Russia	Turkey
2020	1	−0.9	−3.3	−0.81	2.2	−1.82	1.1	7.7
2020	2	−0.4	−13.5	NA	5.2	−3.52	3.3	8.5
2020	3	−3.8	−1.1	NA	−18.3	−4.84	0.3	−1.7
2020	4	−27.2	3.9	NA	−57.6	−29.69	−6.6	−31.3
2020	5	−21.9	4.4	NA	−33.9	−29.69	−9.6	−19.9
2020	6	−9	4.8	NA	−16.6	NA	−9.4	NA

Source [14]

Stopping the production during the pandemic had a direct effect on the labor market. Differing from the global economic crises, the effects of COVID-19 on the employment were direct and without any delay. This is thought to be because of the lockdowns and the close of various businesses. At the beginning of April, approx. 81% of the global labor force was living in the regions implementing or recommending the lockdown measures. It is estimated that approx. 2.7 billion workers have been influenced by this [15].

In a research conducted by ILO, it is estimated that, in the second quartile of 2020, the working hours would decrease by 6.7% that equals to 195 million full-time workers. ILO estimates that 1.25 billion workers, which represent 38% of the global labor force, are employed in industries such as retail, hospitality, food services, and production that are under the risk of a significant decrease in production and increase in disemployment [15].

The effect of COVID-19 on the unemployment in D7 and E7 countries can be seen in Table 3.

Given the unemployment rates shown in Table 3, it can be seen that, among D7 countries, the USA and Canada are the countries affected by COVID-19 at most. In the USA, the rate of unemployment dramatically increased in April 2020 by 11.1% and March 2020 by 10.3%. In Canada, the rate of unemployment increased by 7.3 and 5.2% in the same period. However, in the UK, the rate of unemployment remained stable between January 2019 and June 2020 and was not affected by the pandemic. Moreover, it was also determined that Germany, France, and Japan have been affected by the first shock at a very low level. In Italy, the rate of unemployment decreased in April 2020 when compared to the previous year. It can be seen that, in comparison to the previous year, an improvement occurred in June 2020 due to the measures taken in the USA, Canada, and France and increases were observed in Germany, Italy, and Japan in April 2020. Moreover, the increase in unemployment rate between April and June 2020 was higher than in the other countries. In conclusion, it was found that the labor market in D7 countries (except for the UK) was directly affected by the lockdown decisions during the pandemic and the rate of unemployment increased in this period.

Although not as dramatic as in D7 countries, certain changes occurred in the unemployment rates in E7 countries during the COVID-19 period. Interestingly, when compared to the previous year, the unemployment rate in India increased by 16.1% in April 2020 and by 14.8% in March 2020. Then, since the lockdowns due to the coronavirus pandemic lasted for weeks but certain businesses continued their operations, this rate decreased to 11% in the June 2020. In China, Mexico, and Russia, the unemployment rate slightly increased by 1% in April 2020 due to the pandemic. Based on the available data, it can be seen that India was not affected by the pandemic. In Turkey, however, the rate of unemployment decreased in April 2020 in comparison to the same month of the previous year. In conclusion, the unemployment rates in E7 countries (except for Indonesia and Turkey) increased during the pandemic and the labor market was directly affected from the lockdown measures [14, 16, 17].

The exposure of production and employment to a shock crisis reflects on the growth performance of national economies. In Table 4, the values of D7 and E7

Table 3 Effects of COVID-19 on the unemployment

G7							
Date	Canada	France	Germany	Italy	Japan	UK	USA
2019M1	5.8	8.7	3.3	10.3	2.5	3.9	4
2019M2	5.8	8.7	3.2	10.4	2.3	3.9	3.8
2019M3	5.8	8.6	3.2	10.4	2.5	3.8	3.8
2019M4	5.7	8.5	3.1	10.3	2.4	3.8	3.6
2019M5	5.4	8.5	3.1	10.1	2.4	3.8	3.6
2019M6	5.5	8.5	3.0	9.6	2.3	3.9	3.7
2020M1	5.5	7.9	3.4	9.5	2.4	3.9	3.6
2020M2	5.6	7.6	3.6	9.2	2.4	4.0	3.6
2020M3	7.8	7.6	3.8	8.4	2.5	3.9	4.4
2020M4	13.0	8.8	3.9	6.8	2.6	3.9	14.7
2020M5	13.7	8.2	4.1	8.3	2.9	3.9	13.3
2020M6	12.3	7.7	4.2	8.8	2.8	3.9	11.1
E7							
Date	Brazil	China	Indonesia	India	Mexico	Russia	Turkey
2019M1	12.0	5.1	5.01	6.9	3.6	4.9	14.7
2019M2	12.4	5.3	5.01	7.2	3.3	4.9	14.7
2019M3	12.7	5.2	5.01	6.7	3.2	4.7	14.1
2019M4	12.5	5.0	5.01	7.4	3.5	4.7	13.0
2019M5	12.3	5.0	5.28	7.0	3.5	4.5	12.8
2019M6	12.0	5.1	5.28	7.9	3.6	4.4	13.0
2020M1	11.2	5.3	4.99	7.2	3.8	4.7	13.8
2020M2	11.6	6.2	4.99	7.8	3.6	4.6	13.6
2020M3	12.2	5.9	4.99	8.7	2.9	4.7	13.2
2020M4	12.6	6.0	4.99	23.5	4.7	5.8	12.8
2020M5	12.9	5.9		23.5	4.2	6.1	12.9
2020M6	13.3	5.7		11.0	5.5	6.2	

Source [14, 16, 17]

countries regarding the first two periods of 2020 can be seen. Having the second-largest economy of the world, China achieved a slight increase in the second quartile of 2020. When compared to the previous year, the economy grew by 3.2% in the April–June period and the decrease by 6.8% in the first quartile was reversed. Significant decreases were observed in the second quartile in Russia, Indonesia, and Mexico. Similar results were observed among the D7 countries in the second quartile and significant shrinkages were experienced.

Although significant economies of the world have shrunk, it is known that the pandemic crisis had different effects on different industries. Considering from the

Table 4 Economic growth

Period	G7 countries						
	Canada	France	Germany	Italy	Japan	UK	USA
2020Q1	−0.91	−5.73	−1.8	−5.49	−2.05	−1.7	0.3
2020Q2	NA	−18.96	−11.7	−17.26	NA	NA	-9.5
Period	E7 countries						
	Brazil	China	India	Indonesia	Mexico	Russia	Turkey
2020Q1	−0.25	−6.8	3.09	2.97	−1.37	1.6	4.54
2020Q2	NA	3.2	NA	−5.32	−18.9	−9.6	NA

Source [14, 16]

aspect of industries, it is thought that the tourism industry would be affected at most. In the scenario prepared by OECD, it is estimated that the tourism economy would shrink by 60–80% in 2020. Although more optimistic for 2020, UNWTO predicts an approx. 30–50 billion USD in the expenses of international visitors [18].

As seen in Fig. 2, the global tourism revenue in 2020 is expected to be 444.7 billion USD. According to the corrected estimations for 2020, the tourism revenues in 2020 are expected to be 34.7% lower than in 2019 and 37.1% lower than the original estimation. The most important reason for the decrease in tourism industry exactly is the close of borders to the foreign countries. The travel restrictions caused a significant decrease in the number of tourists. In Table 5, it can be seen that the revenue declines of airline transportation are due to the restrictions [19].

The global trade is another macroeconomic parameter indicating the devastating effect of the pandemic. From the aspect of exporting country, the pandemic is expected to decrease the export by decreasing the scale of production. The exports in countries and industries, which are less suitable for remote working, would decrease. From the aspect of importing country, however, the decreases in total demand would directly affect the foreign trade. The decrease in total demand might be because of the decreases in incomes of consumers or the decreases in the number of visits to the retail stores. The international trade of a country might also be affected by the COVID-19 load in a neighboring country. If the neighbor country has been affected by COVID-19 at a higher level, then an exporting opportunity may arise. However,

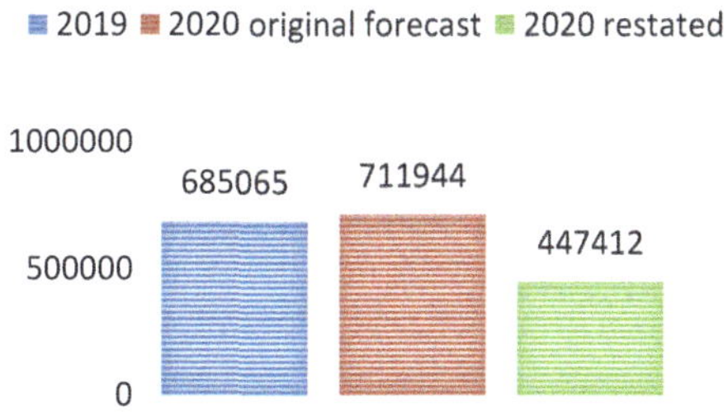

Fig. 2 Global change in travel and tourism revenue due to COVID-19 2019–2020 (in million U.S. dollars). *Source* [19]

Table 5 Revenue/loss distribution by the months (international and domestic flights) $

	Europe	Middle East	Africa	North America	Latin America/Caribbean
January	204,851,800	135,017,777	79,922,546	489,657,970	30,357,300
February	60,278,348	−34,754,010	35,875,428	679,410,234	48,840,567
March	−6,216,053,003	−1,868,062,693	−576,281,012	−5,633,659,947	−1,128,167,822
April	−12,666,176,732	−3,378,080,343	−1,221,584,964	−10,649,844,657	−2,507,490,647
May	−13,159,421,649	−2,999,010,205	−1,125,520,678	−10,737,562,876	−2,459,203,284
June	−13,608,648,646	−3,181,947,871	−1,230,903,925	−10,509,702,238	−2,424,588,239
Total	−45,385,169,882	−11,326,837,345	−4,038,492,605	−36,361,701,514	−8,440,252,125

Source [20]

Table 6 % Difference in trade value (USD) from the previous a long year

	January		February		March		April		May	
Partner	Import	Export	Import	Export	Import	Export	Import	Export	Import	Export
Canada	−0.07	0.00	−0.07	−0.03	0.09	−0.18	0.1	−0.35	−0.22	−0.43
Japan	0.01	0.07	−0.06	0.02	−0.05	−0.08	−0.28	−0.01	−0.31	−0.23
USA	−0.06	−0.03	−0.06	−0.04	0.06	0.12	0.03	0.05	−0.28	0.03
Germany	−0.02	0.02	−0.03	−0.05	−0.06	0.01	−0.23	−0.25	−0.29	−0.24
France	0.23	0.2	−0.16	−0.02	−0.15	−0.23	−0.35	−0.45	−0.32	−0.38
Italy	0.00	−0.03	0.00	0.02	−0.03	−0.1	−0.27	−0.31	−0.25	−0.36
UK	0.15	−0.09	−0.18	−0.2	0.38	−0.16	0.47	−0.41	−0.07	−0.41
India	0.02	0.04	0.07	−0.01	0.00	−0.34	−0.18	−0.86	−0.54	−0.87
Indonesia	−0.09	−0.13	−0.06	−0.01	0.02	0.00	0.15	−0.31	−0.06	−0.34
Russia	−0.09	−0.04	−0.02	−0.05	−0.16	−0.18	−0.17	−0.35	−0.40	−0.28
China	−0.04	−0.03	−0.37	0.00	−0.02	−0.09	0.11	−0.08	0.03	−0.07
Mexico	0.06	−0.05	0.07	−0.06	0.07	−0.05	−0.12	−0.22	−0.33	−0.55
Brazil	0.35	0.05	0.22	0.07	0.16	−0.05	−0.12	−0.19	−0.18	−0.22
Turkey	0.02	0.27	0.01	0.29	0.04	0.49	−0.32	−0.38	−0.19	−0.35

Source [22]

the negative production shocks in a country due to COVID-19 might decrease the production in other countries through the supply chain networks [21].

The changes in import and export values of D7 and E7 countries for the last 5 months can be seen in Table 6. As can be seen, the highest level of decrease was in Canada in May among the D7 countries and in India among the E7 countries.

Moreover, as can be seen in Table 7, the decreases in demand and supply during the pandemic caused price volatility. For this reason, even not in the short-term, significant increases may occur in the long-term inflation rates. In general, high inflation is considered as an economic problem for developing countries. However, given the first 6 months of 2020, it can be seen that the highest increase in the price level was in Germany among D7 countries and in Turkey among E6 countries.

3 COVID-19 and Stock Markets

As in the real industry, the finance industry was also influenced by the COVID-19 shock. Considering the expectation-based structure of financial markets, the crises cause rapid, momentary, and severe changes. The uncertainty can be easily observed by monitoring the daily data of stock exchange market indices. Moreover, the fluctuations in the stock exchange markets might also give hints about the future macroeconomic performances of the countries.

Table 7 Inflation, annual percent change in the CPI

G7								
Year	Month	Canada	France	Germany	Italy	Japan	UK	USA
2020	1	2.4	1.49	1.8	0.49	0.69	1.79	2.49
2020	2	2.16	1.43	1.8	0.29	0.49	1.69	2.33
2020	3	0.89	0.67	1.5	0.1	0.39	1.5	1.54
2020	4	−0.22	0.33	0.89	0	0.1	0.93	0.33
2020	5	−0.37	0.36	0.59	−0.19	0	0.65	0.12
2020	6	0.66	0.2	0.89	−0.19	0.1	0.83	0.65
E7								
Year	Month	Brazil	China	Indonesia	India	Mexico	Russia	Turkey
2020	1	4.19	5.16	1.79	7.59	3.24	2.36	12.15
2020	2	4.01	4.92	2.07	6.58	3.7	2.36	12.37
2020	3	3.3	4.05	2.05	5.27	3.25	2.67	11.86
2020	4	2.4	3.02	1.77	7.44	2.15	3.18	10.94
2020	5	1.88	2.19	1.25	6.97	2.84	3.18	11.39
2020	6	2.13	2.18	1.02	6.51	3.33	3.39	12.62

Source [14, 16, 17]

Due to the beginning of COVID-19 in early 2020, the positive trend in global stock exchange markets declined and a negative appearance emerged. Some authorities consider the COVID-19 pandemic as a new black swan creating shock in global stock exchange markets [23].

Black swan theory was developed by Taleb [24]. Black swan is considered as the rare and non-predictable events having destructive effects [25]. Taleb [24] narrated the story of the black swan theory as follows:

> Historically, before the discovery of Australia, humans have believed that all the swans were white. Until the first black swan has been seen, the empirical proofs have resulted in a completely confirmed finding. The appearance of the first black swan was a complete surprise for the ornithologists. Then, the interest in coloring the other birds has increased. In fact, the important point there was not that the swans might be black. That was not the point. The point there was that the fragility of information we gathered from our observations of experiences placed significant limitations. A general statement arising from the thousands of years of observation of millions of white swans can be invalidated by a single observation. The only thing needed is the presence of an ugly but black swan. [24]

According to Taleb [24], the "black swan" event, which has been considered impossible based on the common situation, has three characteristics. First of all, it is an outlier as it exceeds beyond the realm of regular expectations because nothing in the past has convincingly drawn attention to its possibility. Second, it also has an extreme impact. Third and last, in spite of its outlier status, our human nature makes us concoct explanations for its occurrence after the fact, making it explainable and predictable.

Anything such as natural disasters, terrorist attacks, and financial crises can be considered as a "black swan" case. The point to consider here is that the event must be impossible in reality and its effect must be significant due to the lack of preparation. For instance, the 9/11 attacks are considered as a "black swan" event. Although they have several conflicting effects on the stock exchange markets, the black swan events may decrease the possibility of profit or loss. In the financial markets that cannot be explained using rational analyses, the events create interesting and important effects and significantly influence the investment performances [25].

In Table 8, some of the important dates regarding the effects of COVID-19 pandemic on the stock exchange markets are summarized.

On December 31, 2019, China reported the disease to WHO and the first death due to this disease occurred on January 11, 2020. On March 11, WHO declared COVID-19 as a pandemic. In the tables, there are the dates, on which the first case in the relevant country has been seen. It can also be seen that remarkable changes arose in the stock exchange markets on the date, on which COVID-19 has been declared as a pandemic. For instance, the value of the stock exchange market in Brazil decreased from 90,000 to 70,000. The index values decreased from 14,000 to 12,000 in Canada and from 10,000 to 9000 in Germany. In fact, the factor playing role in the decrease in index values was not the disease itself but the measures taken by the governments to minimize the transmission of disease, as well as the transformation of these measures into economic contraction. For instance, under the conditions created by the travel restrictions, it seems not possible for the travel companies to gain value in the stock exchange market. Similarly, in the period of games without spectators, the sport clubs' return on equity declined. On the other hand, the increase in demand for food and retail sectors turned the pandemic into an opportunity for the companies in these sectors. In sum, the unnamed effect of the COVID-19 pandemic influenced the stock exchange markets too.

The authors such as Antipova [26], Ngwakwe (2020), Yarovaya [27] emphasized that, given the effects on the global community, numbers of deaths and cases, and the effects on stock exchange markets, COVID-19 might be considered as a black swan event. According to Taleb, however, the COVID-19 pandemic should not be considered as a black swan event because the black swan is unpredictable but white and gray ones are inevitable and worrying events. The most important lesson to learn from the pandemic is that avoiding the disease requires minimizing the permeability of world and having right to import additional controls in airports and borders of the countries, where the disease spread. The tests must be used for avoiding the supertransmitters before they enter the country. Thus, in case of a respiratory disease in the future, society would not need to learn something new. The societies should have better knowledge about their vulnerable aspects. In COVID-19, everybody understood that there are security vulnerabilities from the financial aspect [28].

In the entire world, it is discussed that China's reaction to disease, the measures taken in China, and the information provided to the international society were not sufficient at all. The case was not taken into consideration seriously until the cases started being seen in Europe and America. Especially the European countries failed in developing a shared strategy for struggling with the disease. Besides that, can the

Table 8 Outcomes of COVID-19 in stock exchange markets in G7 and E7 countries

	D7					
Date	March 11, 2020 (Declaration of pandemic)			The first case in relevant country		
Value of stock exchange market	Before	On the day of event	After	On the day of event	After	On the day of event
Canada (TSX60)	14,948.1	14,270.1	12,508.5	17,565.3	17,442.5 (26th January)	17,500.8
France (FCHI)	4636.6	4610.2	4044.2	6024.2	5863.0 (25th January)	5921.9
Germany (GDAXI)	10,475.5	10,438.7	9161.1	13,204.7	13,323.6 (28th January)	13,345.0
Italy (FTSE MIB)	17,870.2	17,928.6	14,894.4	49,515.8	48,383.0 (31st January)	48,847.3
Japan (Nikkei N225)	19,867.1	19,416.1	18,559.6	24,025.1	23,916.5 (15th January)	23,933.1
UK (FTSE100)	5960.2	5876.5	5237.4	7286.0	7326.3 (1st February)	7439.8
US (GSPC)	2882.2	2741.3	2480.6	3329.6	3320.7 (21st January)	3321.7
	E7					
Brazil (BVSP)	92,214.4	85,171.1	72,582.5	113,681.4	105,718.2 (26th February)	102,983.5
China (000,001.SS)	2996.7	2968.5	2923.4	3040.0	3050.1 (31st December)	3085.2
India (BSESN)	1010.6	1009.6	936.3	41,198.6	40,913.8 (30th January)	40,753.1
Indonesia (JKSE)	5220.8	5154.1	4895.7	5452.7	5361.2 (2nd March)	5518.6
Mexico (MXX)	39,565.4	38,678.5	36,636.7	41,324.3	42,167.2 (29th February)	42,472.2
Russia (IMOEX.ME)	3062.4	3097.5	3122.2	3076.6	3070.8 (1st February)	3097.6
Turkey (BIST100)	1010.6	1009.1	936.3	1009.1	936.3 (12th March)	956.0

failing medical services and not taking the warnings and reports of WHO, which are based on the previous diseases, be considered being at the end of rope against a known situation? While black swan discussions continue, it can be exactly seen that COVID-19 has effects on the stock exchange markets.

Together with the COVID-19 pandemic, the epidemics became a subject, economic effects of which are more comprehensively analyzed, such as terror, crises, and geographical disasters. At this point, all the policymakers conduct various researches on examining the effects of epidemics on region, country, and world. Even though the effect of pandemic became more popular, there also are studies examining the effects of previous epidemics on the share markets. In the studies such as those carried out by Nippani and Washer [29], Chen et al. [30, 31], Wang et al. [32], Yeung and Aman [33], Chen et al. [34], Ichev and Marinc [35], and Funck and Gutierrez [36], the relationship between pandemics such as SARS, MERS, and Ebola and the stock exchange markets were analyzed. The findings suggested that the epidemics negatively affected the stock exchange markets. In this section, the summary of studies examining the relationship between global COVID-19 pandemic and stock exchange market activities is presented.

Ahmar and Val [37] examined the relationship between COVID-19 and the stock exchange market in Spain between February 12, 2020 and April 9, 2020 by using the SutteARIMA method. SutteARIMA is the most suitable estimation method for Spain.

Using panel data analysis, Al-Awadhi et al. [5] examined the effects of COVID-19 on the Chinese stock exchange market between 10th January and 16th March. They found that the increases in both confirmed cases and number of deaths caused by COVID-19 had negative effects on the return on equity in all the companies.

Ashraf [38] analyzed the effects of COVID-19 cases and deaths on the stock returns in 64 countries between 22nd January and 17th April. The results achieved using panel random effects suggested that the stock exchange markets rapidly reacted to COVID-19 pandemic and the stock returns decreased as the number of confirmed cases increased. Moreover, it was also reported that, when compared to the reaction to the increase in the number of deaths, the stock exchange markets' reactions to the increase in the number of cases was found to be more proactive.

Using multifractal detrended fluctuation analysis (MFDFA), Aslam et al. [39] determined for the period between January 1, 2020 and March 23, 2020 that eight European stock exchange markets had intraday multifractal properties against the pandemic. These results indicate that the Spanish stock exchange market has the highest efficiency, whereas the lowest one belongs to the Austrian stock exchange market.

In their study examining different periods, Banerjee et al. [40] reported the relationship between increase in the number of confirmed COVID-19 cases in India and stock exchange market and foreign exchange market by using vector auto-regressive (VAR) model. The results they achieved revealed a positive correlation between the increase in number of confirmed cases and the increase in exchange rates and a negative correlation between stock exchange market index.

Using panel quantile regression method, Cepoi [41] analyzed the relationship between the COVID-19 news and the stock returns in stock exchange markets in the USA, UK, Germany, France, Spain, and Italy between February 3, 2020 and April 17, 2020. The results suggested that the correlations in February were relatively low but there were increases since March.

Using fixed-effect Dynamic Spatial Durbin Model (DSDM), Eleftheriou and Patsoulis [42] analyzed the effects of governments' social distancing measures in COVID-19 pandemic on 45 large stock exchange markets between 1st January and 8th April. The results showed that there were negative relationships between stock returns and intensity of COVID-19 measures and that the increase especially in the non-medical interventions resulted in a decrease in stock returns. It also decreases the stock returns in the markets of countries having relationship with.

Using dynamic conditional correlation multivariate GARCH (DCC-MVGARCH) and DCC-MVFIGARCH models, Gunay [43] investigated the effects of COVID-19 on the stock exchange markets in the USA, UK, China, Italy, Spain, and Turkey for four different periods. It was found that the relationship between Chinese and Turkish stock exchange markets, which has degraded between 2005 and 2019, increased by 20% after the pandemic. The effect in other stock exchange market pairs was at the level of 10%.

In their questionnaire conducted on the households in the USA, Hanspal et al. [44] determined that the collapse in stock markets and the beliefs about the recovery shaped the individuals' expectations about their own wealth and future activities.

He et al. [45] compared the relationship between COVID-19 and daily return in Chinese, Italian, South Korean, French, Spanish, German, Japanese, and USA stock exchange markets. For the period between June 1, 2019 and March 16, 2020, the results obtained from *t*-test and Mann–Whitney test indicated that COVID-19 had a negative and short-term effect on the stock exchange markets. Moreover, in the same study, there was no finding indicating that COVID-19 has affected the stock exchange markets of the countries beyond the global average.

Kandil Göker et al. [46] investigating the relationship between COVID-19 and sector index returns in Borsa İstanbul (BIST)—Turkey. Using the event study method, the results of 26 sectors in BIST suggested that most sectors had negative cumulative abnormal returns (CAAR) and the CAAR values were positive in several sectors in certain periods. The highest levels of loss were observed in sports, tourism, and transportation industries.

Using pooled OLS, *t*-test, and Mann–Whitney tests and efficient market theory and intertemporal asset price theory, Khan et al. [47] analyzed the effects of COVID-19 on the stock returns in 16 countries between 17th February and 29th March. They reported that COVID-19 negatively affected the stock returns in these countries. It was determined that increase in the number of cases significantly decreased the return for the next week. Especially the declaration that this disease was transmitted by humans significantly negatively affected the stock returns.

Using event study analyses, Khanthavit [48] measured the reactions of stock exchange markets against COVID-19. Accordingly, the author reported that the stock returns in nine countries showed significant and negative reactions against COVID-19.

Liu et al. [49, 50] examined the stock exchange market indexes of 21 for the period between February 21, 2019 and March 18, 2020 by using event study method and panel data analysis and they reported that the stock exchange market indexes of the large countries and regions rapidly declined after the pandemic. Moreover, when compared to the other countries, the negative abnormal returns were achieved in Asian countries.

Using the event study method, Liu et al. [49, 50] examined the abnormal returns within 10 business days after the COVID-19 in the Chinese economy and Asian stock markets. They determined that the cumulative abnormal returns decreased in both Chinese and Asian stock markets. Moreover, the cumulative returns in industries such as pharmacology, software, and information and communication technologies were positive, whereas those in hospitality and food & beverage industries were negative.

Using the March 2020 data of 1500 companies listed by Standard and Poor's, Mazur et al. [51] investigated the performance of USA stock market performance. The results obtained from event study analysis suggested significant decreases in entertainment, hospitality, oil, and real estate industries, as well as high levels of returns in food, natural gas, medicine, and software industries.

Using spectral causality and Granger causality, Morales and Andreosso-O'Callaghan [23] examined 11 stock exchange markets for the period between December 1, 2019 and March 9, 2020 and they reported that the stock markets did not respond to the volatility levels of Shanghai stock market but the effect in Europe begun after the first case in Italy.

Okorie and Lin [52] examined the fractal contagion effect of COVID-19 on stock exchange markets 32 countries by using the data of periods between October 1, 2019 and December 31, 2019 and January 1, 2020 and March 31, 2020. Detrended Moving Cross-Correlation Analysis (DMCA) and Detrended Cross-Correlation Analysis results suggested the presence of fractal contagion effect of the pandemic on the stock markets.

Onali [53] examined the effect of COVID-19 cases and deaths on the stock markets of USA, Spain, Italy, China, France, Iran, and China for the period of April 8, 2020 to April 9, 2020 by using GARCH, VAR, and Markov-switching models. The results showed that, except for the cases reported for China, the changes in the numbers of cases and deaths in the USA and other countries did not have an effect on the stock returns in the USA stock market. The numbers of deaths in Italy and France were found to have a negative effect on the returns in Dow Jones and a positive effect on VIX.

Using the fixed effects model, Öztürk et al. [54] analyzed the effects of COVID-19 on subsector price indexes of Borsa İstanbul (BIST) for the period between January 2, 2020 and April 15, 2020. The results showed that the sectoral indexes were affected by the numbers reported for Turkey, rather than the cases reported from Europe and world. Moreover, the pandemic affected metal products and machinery, sports, banking, and insurance industries at the highest level and food and beverage, wholesale-retail, and real estate investment industries at the lowest level.

Using Google trend synthetic index, Papadamou et al. [55] examined the volatility in 13 stock markets in Europe, Asia, USA, and Australia. The panel VAR results covering the period between January 2, 2020 and April 9, 2020 showed that the increasing number of search results for COVID-19 did not have a direct effect on the volatility. However, the effect in Europe was stronger than in the rest of the world. These results suggested that the Google-based concerns regarding the contagiousness of COVID-19 led to avoidance from high risk levels in the stock markets.

Using OLS and Bayesian model, Pavlyshenko [56] compared the effect of COVID-19 on the stock market with the effect of the 2008 Crisis. The results showed that the crises arising for different reasons had different effects and the uncertainty that COVID-19 brought had more negative effects on the stock markets.

Using PMG, MG, and ARDL methods, Rabhi [57] examined the relationship between Asian stock market and COVID-19 for the period between January 2, 2020 and April 1, 2020. The results showed that the news about the COVID-19 cases and deaths negatively affected the parameters such as performance of Asian stock markets, oil and gold prices, and exchange rates. Moreover, it was determined that the USA stock markets had also determinant effect on the Asian stock markets.

Sansa [58] analyzed the effect of COVID-19 on the financial markets for China and the USA by using the regression analysis for the period between March 1, 2020 and March 25, 2020. A significant positive relationship was found between confirmed COVID-19 cases and stock markets.

Sharif et al. [27] analyzed the relationships between COVID-19, oil prices, stock market, geopolitical risk, and political uncertainty in the USA by using the coherence wavelet method and the wavelet-based Granger causality tests. The study covered the period between January 21, 2020 and March 30, 2020. The results obtained showed that the USA stock market and geopolitical risk were sensitive to the COVID-19 and oil price volatility shocks at an unprecedented scale.

Using Morgan Stanley Capital International (MSCI) World, European, Emerging Market, and D7 countries' Fourier Cointegration test, Şenol and Zeren [59] examined the effects of global pandemic for the period between January 21, 2020 and April 7, 2020. They determined that there was a long-term relationship between stock prices and COVID-19.

Using the panel estimation method, Topcu and Gulal [60] examined the effect of COVID-19 on the stock markets in 26 emerging economies for the period between March 10, 2020 and April 30, 2020. The analysis results showed that the pandemic had negative effects on the emerging stock markets but the effect declined as of the mid of April. Moreover, the effect of the pandemic was at the highest level in emerging economies of Asia and the lowest level in Europe. On the other hand, the reaction times and stimulus package sizes of governments played a significant role in balancing the effects of the pandemic.

Using the structural vector autoregression (SVAR) model, Yilmazkuday [61] examined the effect of COVID-19 on the S&P 500 Index for the period between December 31, 2019 and March 12, 2020. The results showed that the S&P 500 index cumulatively decreased by 0.02% 1 day after the COVID-19 deaths, by 0.06% after a week, and 0.08% after a month.

Using panel data analysis for 67 countries, Zaremba et al. [21] tested if the governmental interventions aiming to prevent the spread of COVID-19 affected the volatility in the stock market. For the period between January 1, 2020 and April 3, 2020, the results showed that non-medical interventions increased the volatility.

Using Maki (2012) cointegration test, Zeren and Hızarcı [62] examined the effect of daily total numbers of COVID-19 cases and deaths on 6 stock markets for the period between January 23, 2020 and March 13, 2020. The results showed that all the stock markets acted synchronously in case of death and that the total number of cases was cointegrated with SSE, KOSPI, and IBEX35 and not cointegrated with FTSE MIB, CAC40, and DAX30.

In the literature review, the studies carried out using time series or panel data analyses employed different periods and different independent variables such as the number of confirmed cases and deaths and measures taken by the governments. The studies reported that COVID-19 had a destructive effect on the stock market concepts such as stock returns or volatility.

4 Data and Econometric Model

The effect of COVID-19 on stock markets (STOCK) was analyzed using daily data obtained between March 2, 2020 and May 12, 2020 in G7[1] countries and March 19, 2020 and May 12, 2020 in E7[2] countries—when deaths were first seen in all these countries. The rate of increase in death rates (DEATH) and measures taken by countries to prevent spread (STRING) are the independent variables. The STOCK variable was obtained from the Yahoo Finance and Investing website. The DEATH variable was obtained from CSSE (2020) database and the STRING variable was obtained from Thomas, Webster, Petheric, Phillips and Kira [63] database. The stringency index is computed using the average values of seven policy indicators, namely closing of schools and workplaces, restricting domestic and international travel, closing public transportation, canceling public events, and public information campaigns.

The model is as follows:

$$\text{STOCK}_{\text{it}} = \alpha_i + \alpha_1 \text{ DEATH}_{\text{it}} + \alpha_2 \text{ STRING}_{\text{it}} + u_{\text{it}}$$

First, the cross-sectional dependence of the variables used in the model was analyzed by using Breusch and Pagan's [64] Langrange multiplier CDLM_1 test and Pesaran's [65] CDLM_2 test. Next, the stationarity of the series was investigated using the Pesaran's [66] cross-sectional Augmented Dickey–Fuller (CADF) panel unit root

[1]G7 (Group of Seven) countries: Canada, France, Germany, Italy, Japan, UK, and USA.

[2]E7 (Emerging 7) countries: Brazil, China, India, Indonesia, Mexico, Russia, and Turkey.

test. As the series are stationary at their level values, diagnostic tests were conducted and coefficients were estimated using a fixed effects model for G7 countries and random effects model for E7 countries.

4.1 Diagnostic Statistics and Correlation Analysis

The descriptive statistics of variables used for examining the period 03.02.2020–05.12.2020 for D7 countries and the period 03.19.2020–05.12.2020 for E7 countries are presented in Table 9.

According to Table 9, for the STOCK prices indexed by taking the values of 11th March, when the pandemic has been declared by WHO, as 100, the mean values in D7 countries were higher than in E7 countries. Accordingly, the index values are 98.20 for D7 countries and 92.07 for E7 countries. Moreover, for the examined period, the highest index value was observed in D7 countries, whereas the lowest one was observed in E7 countries. The minimum index value was observed on March 23, 2020 in India, whereas the highest value was reached on March 4, 2020 in Italy. Considering the daily change in the numbers of deaths (DEATH), it can be seen that the mean value of D7 countries was higher than that of E7 countries. Besides that, although there were days with no death in both country groups, whereas the number of death had increased in comparison to the previous day by 550% in UK (D7 countries) on March 16, 2020 and by 825% in Turkey (E7 countries) on March 23, 2020. Considering the restrictive measures (STRING), it can be seen that the mean index value of E7 countries is higher than that of D7 countries. Moreover, whereas the minimum contraction levels were the same in both country groups, the maximum level of contraction was higher in E7 countries. The most contractionary measures in D7 countries were taken in Italy between April 13, 2020 and May 1, 2020 (index value of 94.29). In E7 countries, however, the most contractionary measures were taken in India between March 25, 2020 and April 17, 2020 (index value of 97.14).

Table 9 Diagnostics statistics

Variables	Obs	Mean	Std. dev.	Min	Max
G7					
STOCK	364	98.20	7.78	78.68	122.408
DEATH	364	23.21	49.43	0.00	550.00
STRING	364	67.28	22.19	2.86	94.29
E7					
STOCK	273	92.07	6.73	72.78	108.38
DEATH	273	21.83	56.99	0.00	825.00
STRING	273	77.48	14.87	2.86	97.14

Table 10 Correlation analysis

	STOCK	DEATH	STRING
G7			
STOCK	1.000		
DEATH	−0.294*** (0.000)	1.000	
STRING	0.003 (0.949)	−0.302*** (0.000)	1.000
E7			
STOCK	1.000		
DEATH	−0.207*** (0.001)	1.000	
STRING	0.171*** (0.005)	−0.005 (0.936)	1.000

Note The values in parentheses are probability values. *** indicate significance levels of 1%

The correlation matrix for the variables used in the present study is presented in Table 10. For both D7 and E7 countries, a statistically significant and negative relationship was found between STOCK and DEATH variables. However, no significant relationship was found between STRING and STOCK parameters for D7 countries but there was a positive and significant relationship in E7 countries. Moreover, even though a statistically significant and negative relationship was found between STRING and DEATH variables in D7 countries, no significant relationship could be found in E7 countries.

4.2 *Analysis Results*

The results of the cross-sectional dependence test are given in Table 11.

After determining there is cross-sectional dependence in the variables and models of all countries, a CADF unit root test was performed. A CIPS statistic specific to the whole panel was obtained by averaging the CADF statistics for each cross section. When the absolute value of the CIPS statistic is larger than the critical values, then the null hypothesis can be rejected, indicating there is no unit root for the panel. These results are presented in Table 12.

Next, static panel data analysis techniques were used for the regression analysis and tests were conducted to decide which of the classical models, fixed effects or random effects, will be used.

In the models established for the G7 and E7 countries, the effects of unit and/or time were investigated. The results of the F and LR tests for the fixed and random effects models, respectively, are given in Table 13.

Table 11 Results of cross-sectional dependence test

	G7		E7	
	$CDLM_1$	$CDLM_2$	$CDLM_1$	$CDLM_2$
STOCK	793.263*** (0.000)	119.163*** (0.000)	413.433*** (0.000)	60.554*** (0.009)
DEATH	470.186*** (0.000)	69.311*** (0.000)	203.709*** (0.000)	28.193*** (0.000)
STRING	463.252*** (0.000)	68.241*** (0.000)	338.360*** (0.000)	48.970*** (0.000)
Model	657.274*** (0.000)	98.179*** (0.000)	232.448*** (0.000)	32.627*** (0.000)

Note *** indicate cross-sectional dependence at significance levels of 1%

Table 12 Results of CADF panel unit root test

	G7	E7
Variables	Level	Level
STOCK	−4.309**	−2.321*
DEATH	−4.531***	−4.731***
STRING	−3.285***	−2.954***
Critical CIPS table values	(1%)	(5%) (10%)
	−2.55	−2.33 −2.21

Note ***, ** and * indicate cross-sectional dependence at significance levels of 1%, 5%, and 10%, respectively

Table 13 Results of unit and time effect test

	G7		E7	
	F-test	LR test	F-test	LR test
Unit effect	3.19*** (0.005)	3.70** (0.027)	80.08*** (0.000)	246.27*** (0.000)
Time effect	40.70*** (0.000)	400.78*** (0.000)	11.16*** (0.000)	2.39*** (0.061)

Note *** and ** indicates that there are unit/time effects with a significance level of 1% and 5%, respectively

As the existence of unit/time effects was proven, the Hausman (1978) specification test was used to investigate whether these effects were fixed or random; the results are given in Table 14.

Table 14 Results of Hausman test

	χ^2	*p*-value
G7	14.47	0.000
E7	0.20	0.904

Table 15 Results of diagnostic test

		G7	E7
Heteroscedasticity	Modified Wald test	92.29 (0.000)	–
	Breusch–Pagan LM test	–	2095.90 (0.000)
Autocorrelation	DW test	0.426	0.460
	LBI test	0.497	0.545

Since the probability value of χ^2 for the G7 countries is smaller than 0.05, H_0 was rejected, so the fixed effects model was used. For the E7 countries, the random effects model was chosen because the probability value of χ^2 was greater than 0.05. Before estimating the coefficient, the econometric model was examined to prevent issues such as heteroscedasticity and autocorrelation. The results of diagnostic test are presented in Table 15.

Based on the results of the modified Wald test of heteroscedasticity in the model generated for G7 countries, H0 was rejected; it was determined that the variance varies from unit to unit. According to the results of the Breusch–Pagan LM test of the model generated for E7 countries, the probability value of χ^2 was smaller than 0.10; a heteroscedasticity problem was observed. According to the results of the Durbin–Watson (DW) and locally best invariant (LBI) tests of autocorrelation in the model established for G7 and E7 countries, the statistics were below 2, the threshold value. Consequently, an autocorrelation problem was detected in both models. The results of the coefficient estimations made with robust estimators for G7 and E7 countries are given in Table 16.

The results of the estimation show that DEATH does not have any effect on stock prices in either country set, but STRING adversely affects stock prices. A 1 unit increase in the STRING index in E7 countries decreases the stock price index by –0.031 units and in G7 countries by −0.060 units. It was observed that the power of the effect is greater in G7 countries.

Table 16 Results of coefficient estimation

	G7			E7		
	Coefficient	Robust std. err	*p*-value	Coefficient	Robust std. err	*p*-value
DEATH	−0.001	0.002	0.743	−0.001	0.001	0.728
STRING	−0.060***	0.018	0.001	−0.031*	0.017	0.071
C	103.851***	2.002	0.000	86.082***	0.949	0.000

Note *** and * indicate significance levels of 1% and 10%, respectively

5 Conclusion

Due to increased financial liberalization, markets have become increasingly dependent on each other. Increased liberalization has made stock markets more sensitive to economic, political, or social incidents. The COVID-19 pandemic has caused almost all economic activities to stop worldwide. Indeed, some believe this pandemic is the most critical event since World War II, and it has led to hard times for international markets. This study investigated the effect of developments arising from the COVID-19 epidemic on stock markets. The results of the empirical analysis of G7 and E7 countries revealed that the changes in the death rate caused by COVID-19 have not affected stock prices but measures taken by governments to reduce the spread of the coronavirus have affected stock markets negatively. Since the pandemic spread over the countries that are in commercial and financial partnerships, investment diversification should be preferred for avoiding the financial risk. Besides that, the direct protective instruments such as Automated Session Stop in Turkey should be put into practice. Although the results provide significant insight into the movements of stock markets, which can help in making predictions, the study has some limitations due to many the uncertainties surrounding the epidemic, including the actual increase in cases and deaths and time-consuming issues like the development of a vaccine or effective treatment methods.

References

1. Baldwin, R., & Di Mauro, B. W. (2020). Introduction. In R. Baldwin & B. W. Di Mauro (Eds.), *Economics in the time of COVID-19.*CEPR Press.
2. Elgin, C., Basbug, G., & Yalaman, A. (2020). Economic policy responses to a pandemic: Developing the Covid-19 economic stimulus index. In C. Wyplosz (Ed.), *COVID economics: Vetted and real-time papers.*CEPR Press.
3. Barro, R. J., Ursua, J. F., & Weng, J. (2020). *The coronavirus and the great influenza pandemic: Lessons from The "Spanish Flu" for the coronavirus's potential effects on mortality and economic activity*, NBER Working Paper Series, No. 26866 (pp. 1–27).
4. Voyvoda, E., & Yeldan, A. E. (2020). *A general equilibrium analysis of the impact of the COVID-19 outbreak on Turkey's economy and a policy alternative to protect labor incomes.* Political Economy Research Institute, Working Paper, No. 518 (pp. 1–12).
5. Al-Awadhi, A. M., Alsaifi, K., Al-Awadhi, A., & Alhammadi, S. (2020). Death and contagious infectious diseases: Impact of the COVID-19 virus on stock market returns. *Journal of Behavioral and Experimental Finance, 27*(100326), 1–5
6. World Health Organization (WHO). (2004). *WHO guidelines for the global surveillance of severe acute respiratory syndrome (SARS).* Department of Communicable Disease Surveillance and Response Updated Recommendations.
7. World Health Organization. (WHO). Public health measures for scaling up national preparedness Middle East Respiratory Syndrome (MERS).
8. World Health Organization (WHO). (2020). *Guidelines for the management of pregnant and breastfeeding women in the context of Ebola virus disease.* World Health Organization.
9. World Health Organization. (WHO). https://www.who.int/emergencies/diseases/novel-coronavirus-2019/events-as-they-happen

10. Barua, S. Understanding coronanomics: The economic implications of the coronavirus (COVID-19) pandemic. *SSRN Electronic Journal*. https://doi.org/10.2139/ssrn.3557504
11. Agencie EFE. *Covid-19 causes China's biggest 30-year industrial production low*. Retrieved on July 21, 2020, from https://www.efe.com/efe/english/portada/covid-19-causes-china-s-biggest-30-year-industrial-production-low/50000260-4197088
12. Alexander, J. *COVID-19 pandemic drives largest drop in U.S. factory production on record*. Retrieved on July 29, 2020, from https://realeconomy.rsmus.com/covid-19-pandemic-drives-largest-drop-in-u-s-factory-production-on-record
13. Chapman, B. *Coronavirus Italy's industrial production collapses by 28% as economy shuts down to deal with pandemic*. Retrieved on July 27, 2020, from https://www.independent.co.uk/news/business/news/italy-economy-coronavirus-impact-industrial-production-data-lockdown-a9508691.html
14. Tradingeconomics. Retrieved on July 28, 2020, from https://www.tradineconomics.com
15. ILO Statistics and Databases. Retrieved on July 29, 2020, from https://www.ilo.org/global/statistics-and-databases/lang--en/index.htm
16. OECD Database. Retrieved on July 28, 2020, from https://data.oecd.org/
17. Globaleconomy. Retrieved on July 21, 2020, from https://www.globaleconomy.com
18. UNWTO. *International tourism numbers*. Retrieved on August 8, 2020, from https://www.unwto.org/news/covid-19-international-tourist-numbers-could-fall-60-80-in-2020
19. Kazunobu, H., & Hinoshi, M. (2020). *Impacts of COVID-19 on international trade: Evidence from the first quarter of 2020*. IDE Discussion Paper (Vol. 791). https://hdl.handle.net/2344/00051734
20. IATA. Retrieved on July 29, 2020, from https://www.iata.org/
21. Zaremba, A., Kizys, R., Aharon, D. Y., & Demir, E. (2020). Infected markets: Novel coronavirus, government interventions, and stock return volatility around the globe. *Finance Research Letters, 35*, 101597
22. Comtrade Database. Retrieved on July 29, 2020, from https://comtrade.un.org/data/monitor
23. Morales, L., & Andreosso-O'Callaghan, B. (2020). Covid-19-global stock markets "Black Swan". *Critical Letters in Economics & Finance, 1*(1), 1–14.
24. Taleb, N. N. (2007). *The Black Swan: The impact of the highly improbable*. Random House.
25. Lin, W.-Y., & Tsai, I.-C. (2019). Black swans events in China's stock markets: Intraday price behaviours on days of volatility. *International Review of Economics and Finance, 59*, 395–411
26. Antipova, T. (2020). Coronavirus pandemic as Black Swan event. In: T. Antipova (Ed.), *ICIS 2020, LNNS 136*, (pp. 356–366). Springer Nature Switzerland AG 2021. https://doi.org/10.1007/978-3-030-49264-9_32
27. Sharif, A., Aloui, C., & Yarovaya, L. (2020). COVID-19 pandemic, oil prices, stock market, geopolitical risk and policy uncertainty nexus in the US economy. *Fresh Evidence from the Wavelet Based Approach, International Review of Financial Analysis, 70*, 101496, 1–9.
28. Sputniknews. Retrieved on July 21, 2020, from https://tr.sputniknews.com
29. Nippani, S., & Washer, K. M. (2004). SARS: A non-event for affected countries' stock markets? *Applied Financial Economics, 14*, 1105–1110
30. Chen, M.-H., Jang, S. C. S., & Kim, W. G. (2017). The impact of the SARS outbreak on Taiwanese hotel stock performance: An event-study approach. *International Journal of Hospitality Management, 26*(1), 200–212
31. Chen, C. D., Chen, C. C., Tang, W. W., & Huang, B. Y. (2009). The positive and negative impacts of the SARS outbreak: A case of the Taiwan industries. *The Journal of Developing Areas, 43*(1), 281–293.
32. Wang, T. H., Yang, F. J., & Chen, L. J. (2013). An investor's perspective on infectious diseases and their influence on market behaviour. *Journal of Business Economics and Management, 14*(1), 112–127
33. Yeung, W. H., & Aman, A. (2016). Sensitivity of stock indices to global events: The perspective for Pakistani Canadians. *Journal of Economic and Administrative Sciences, 32*(2), 102–119
34. Chen, M. P., Lee, C. C., Lin, Y. H., & Chen, W. Y. (2018). Did the SARS epidemic weaken the integration of Asian stock markets? *Evidence from Smooth Time-Varying Cointegration Analysis, Economic Research, 31*(1), 908–926

35. Ichev, R., & Marinc, M. (2018). Stock prices and geographic proximity of information. *Evidence from the Ebola Outbreak, International Review of Financial Analysis, 56*, 153–166
36. Funck, M., & Gutierrez, J. A. (2019). *Has Ebola infected the market: A contagious reaction to a (media) health care crisis?* (Working Paper), Sam Houston State University.
37. Ahmar, A. S., & del Val, E. B. (2020). SutteARIMA: Short-term forecasting method, a case: Covid-19 and stock market in Spain. *Science of the Total Environment, 729*, 138883, 1–6.
38. Ashraf, B. N. (2020). Stock markets' reaction to COVID-19: Cases or fatalities? *Research in International Business and Finance*. https://doi.org/10.1016/j.ribaf.2020.101249
39. Aslam, F., Mohti, W., & Ferreira, P. (2020). Evidence of intraday multifractality in European stock markets during the recent coronavirus (COVID-19) outbreak. *International Journal Financial Studies, 8*(31), 1–13
40. Banerjee, I., Kumar, A., & Bhattacharyya, R. (2020). Examining the effect of COVID-19 on foreign exchange rate and stock market—An applied insight into the variable effects of lockdown on Indian economy. arXiv:2006.14499
41. Cepoi, C. O. (2020). Asymmetric dependence between stock market returns and news during COVID-19 financial turmoil. *Finance Research Letters*. https://doi.org/10.1016/j.frl.2020.101658
42. Eleftheriou, K., & Patsoulis, P. (2020). *COVID-19 lockdown intensity and stock market returns: A spatial econometrics approach*. MPRA Paper No. 100662.
43. Gunay, S. (2020). A new form of financial contagion: COVID-19 and stock market responses. Available at SSRN: https://ssrn.com/abstract=3584243 or https://doi.org/10.2139/ssrn.3584243
44. Hanspal, T., Weber, A., & Wohlfart, H. (2020). *Exposure to the COVID-19 stock market crash and its effect on household expectations*. SAFE Working Paper No. 279.
45. He, Q., Junyi, L., Wang, S., & Jishuang, Y. (2020). The impact of COVID-19 on stock markets, economic and political studies. https://doi.org/10.1080/20954816.2020.1757570
46. Kandil Göker, İ. E., Eren, B. S., & Karaca, S. S. (2020). The impact of the COVID-19 (Coronavirus) on the Borsa Istanbul sector index returns: An event study. *Gaziantep University Journal of Social Sciences*, 2020 Special Issue, 14–41.
47. Khan, K., Zhao, H., Zhang, H., Yang, H., Shah, M. H., & Jahanger, A. (2020). The impact of COVID-19 pandemic on stock markets: An empirical analysis of world major stock indices. *Journal of Asian Finance, Economics and Business, 7*(7), 463–474
48. Khanthavit, A. (2020). World and national stock market reactions to COVID-19. *ABAC Journal, 40*(2), 1–20
49. Liu, H., Manzoor, A., Wang, C., Zhang, L., & Manzoor, Z. (2020). The COVID-19 outbreak and affected countries stock markets response. *International Journal of Environment Research Public Health, 17*(2800), 1–19
50. Liu, H., Wang, Y., He, D., & Wang, C. (2020). Short term response of Chinese stock markets to the outbreak of COVID-19. *Applied Economics*. https://doi.org/10.1080/00036846.2020.1776837
51. Mazur, M., Dang, M., & Vega, M. COVID-19 and the March 2020 stock market crash. Evidence from S&P1500. *Finance Research Letters*. https://doi.org/10.1016/j.frl.2020.101690
52. Okorie, D. I. & Lin, B. (2020). Stock markets and the COVID-19 fractal contagion effects. *Finance Research Letters*. https://doi.org/10.1016/j.frl.2020.101640
53. Onali, E. (2020). COVID-19 and stock market volatility. Project: Economic impacts of COVID-19. https://doi.org/10.2139/ssrn.3571453
54. Öztürk, Ö., Şişman, M. Y., Uslu, H., & Çıtak, F. (2020). Effects of Covid-19 outbreak on Turkish stock market: A sectoral-level analysis. *Hitit University Journal of Social Sciences Institute, 13*(1), 57–68
55. Papadamou, S., Fassas, A. P., Kenourgios, D., & Dimitriou, D. (2020). *Direct and indirect effects of covid-19 pandemic on implied stock market volatility: Evidence from panel data analysis*. MPRA Paper No. 100020. https://mpra.ub.uni-muenchen.de/100020/1/MPRA_paper_100020.pdf

56. Pavlyshenko, B. M. (2020). *Regression approach for modeling COVID-19 spread and its impact on stock market*. Available at https://arxiv.org/pdf/2004.01489.pdf
57. Rabhi, A. (2020). *Stock market vulnerability to the Covid-19 Pandemic: Evidence from emerging Asian stock markets*. MPRA Paper 101774, University Library of Munich.
58. Sansa, N. A. (2020). The impact of the COVID-19 on the financial markets: Evidence from China and USA. *Electronic Research Journal of Social Sciences and Humanities, 2*(2), 29–39
59. Şenol, Z., & Zeren, F. (2020). Coronavirus (Covid-19) and stock markets: The effects of the pandemic on the global economy. *Eurasian Journal of Researches in Social and Economics, 7*(4), 1–16
60. Topcu, M., & Gulal, O. S. The impact of COVID-19 on emerging stock markets. *Finance Research Letters*. https://doi.org/10.1016/j.frl.2020.101691
61. Yilmazkuday, H. (2020). COVID-19 effects on the S&P 500 index. SSRN: https://ssrn.com/abstract=3555433
62. Zeren, F., & Hızarci, A. E. (2020). The impact of COVID-19 coronavirus on stock markets: Evidence from selected countries. *Bulletin of Accounting and Finance Review, 3*(1), 78–84
63. Hale, T., Webster, S., Petherick, A., Phillips, T., Kira, B., & Angrist, N. (2020). Oxford COVID-19 government response tracker. Blavatnik School of Government. Available at: https://www.bsg.ox.ac.uk/research/research-projects/coronavirus-government-response-tracker2020
64. Breusch, T. S., & Pagan, A. (1980). The lagrange multiplier test and its applications to model specification in econometrics. *Review of Economic Studies, 47*(1), 239–253
65. Pesaran, M. H. (2004). *General diagnostic tests for cross section dependence in panels*. Cambridge Working Papers in Economics. No. 435 (pp. 1–39).
66. Pesaran, M. H. (2007). A simple panel unit root test in the presence of cross-section dependence. *Journal of Applied Econometrics, 22*(2), 265–312

Artificial Intelligence Techniques in Medical Imaging for Detection of Coronavirus (COVID-19/SARS-COV-2): A Brief Survey

Anindya Banerjee and Raj Krishan Ghosh

1 Introduction

In December 2019, a virus named severe acute respiratory syndrome coronavirus 2 (SARS-CoV-2) had begun to spread in Wuhan, China. It was declared as a pandemic by World Health Organization (WHO) on the March 11, 2020. It is considered as human to human spread deadly virus; however, all other causes remain unanswerable due to its least information discovered at present. Physical contact respiratory transmission [1] is also responsible for the rapid spread of the COVID-19 virus among humans.

Open-access databases such as Github [2] and Kaggle [3] help researchers around the globe to develop a novel deep convolutional neural network model (CNN) for earlier detection of COVID-19 by computer-aided diagnosis. In this study, it is also observed that chest X-ray images are the best choice for the detection of the COVID-19 disease.

Deep learning algorithms are broadly utilized for performing accuracy, sensitivity, specificity, pattern recognition, and in medical imaging. This review study evaluates the performance comparison of ResNet-50, Inception-ResNet-v2, InceptionV3, VGG-19, and MobileNet and determines other crucial factors such as F1-score and prevalence. A database of total 100 images used for testing yields 98% accuracy for ResNet-50 and Inception-ResNet-v2 yields 87% accuracy, while 1428 images used

Anindya Banerjee and Raj Krishan Ghosh—Both authors contributed equally to this work as first author.

A. Banerjee
Department of Electronics and Communication Engineering, Kalyani Government Engineering College, Kalyani, West Bengal, India

R. K. Ghosh (✉)
Centre of Excellence in Artificial Intelligence, Indian Institute of Technology Kharagpur, Kharagpur, West Bengal, India

M. Niranjanamurthy et al. (eds.), *Intelligent Data Analysis for COVID-19 Pandemic*, Algorithms for Intelligent Systems, https://doi.org/10.1007/978-981-16-1574-0_12

for testing in InceptionV3 which yields 97% accuracy, VGG-19 yields 98% accuracy, and MobileNet yields 97% accuracy.

2 Literature Survey

Zhang et al. [4] proposed a confidence-aware anomaly detection (CAAD) model on two chest X-ray databases, which can detect viral pneumonia on chest X-ray images, and achieved an area under the receiver operator curve (AUC) of 83.61% and 71.70% sensitivity rate over COVID-19 images. Adhikari's work [5] proposed a network, namely automatic diagnostic medical analysis for the COVID-19 detection system (ADMCDS) which is dedicated to finding diseased regions caused by COVID-19 in both X-ray images and CT scan images. This model is beneficial for the doctors for better accuracy in finding the infected regions in both X-ray and CT scan images. Punn et al. [6] have used baseline reset, Inception-v3, Inception-ResNet-v2, DenseNet169, and NASNetLarge for binary classification and multiclass classification of poster anterior chest X-ray images. NASNetLarge model exhibits better performance among all the said methods for binary classification of COVID-19 images. Jamil et al. [7] represented a deep CNN architecture for the classification of COVID-19 images and normal images of chest X-ray. More than 150 confirmed chest X-ray images of COVID-19 patients collected from Kaggle database were used in this study. The proposed method shows 93% accuracy. However, this model could not be used in the COVID-19 CT scan image database. Hemdan et al. [8] introduced a novel deep learning framework (CVOIDX-Net) for automatic detection of chest X-ray COVID-19 images on seven deep learning classifiers including ResNet-v2, VGG-19, DenseNet201, InceptionV3, MobileNetV2, etc. Furthermore, CVOIDX-Net performs best on VGG-19 and DenseNet201 models. This study was based on 50 chest X-ray images of COVID-19 due to its limited availability of database for public access. Khan et al. [9] proposed Xception architecture-based CNN model for automatic detection of COVID-19 from chest X-ray images. This model was trained using a publicly available dataset of COVID-19 images as well as chest pneumonia X-ray images. It achieves an accuracy of 89.6%. Farooq et al. [10] proposed a CNN framework called COVID-ResNet for differentiating between pneumonia cases and COVID-19 cases. The input images were resized into $128 \times 128 \times 3$, $224 \times 224 \times 3$ and $229 \times 229 \times 3$ pixels, and it also shows the importance of data augmentation for increasing the training set images and achieves 96.23% accuracy when used along with automatic learning rate. Alqudah et al. [11] utilized CNN using softmax classifier and support vector machine (SVM) and random forest (RF) algorithms for distinguishing between non-COVID-19 and COVID-19 X-ray images. Time consumption in softmax is comparatively less compared to other hybrid systems. Mohammadi et al. [12] used VGG-16, VGG-19, MobileNet, and Inception-ResNet-v2 models for the accurate detection of COVID-19 by using 348 chest X-ray images. MobileNet provided the highest accuracy of 99.1% among the other three models. It has also been observed that by increasing the no. of samples, the accuracy also increases.

Gozes et al. [13] developed an algorithm, which can detect and localize the infection caused by COVID-19 in chest CT scan images. This study was based on 270 slices of COVID-19 (120 COVID-19 infected slices and 150 normal slices). It also achieved 94% sensitivity and 98% specificity.

3 Artificial Intelligence

Artificial intelligence (AI) is defined by the imitation of human thinking and intelligence for machines programmed to think and decide like most humans and thus mimic their decisions. AI is identified by the automation for tasks that are associated with human thinking, including problem-solving, making of decisions, perception, learning, and reasoning [14]. The goal of AI is to rationalize and act to have the best probability of achieving a specified goal. AI is based upon the concept that the intelligence of a human can be defined in a sense that can be mimicked by machines to execute tasks, from the most simple to those that are immensely complex. As technology advances, newer benchmarks render the previous ones basic and trivial. As a result, AI is continuously evolving as an artificial thinking entity to benefit a massive number of vastly different industries [15] (Fig. 1).

Algorithms often play a tremendously significant role in the building of AI, where simple algorithms are used in simple applications, while complex ones develop strong

Fig. 1 Basic block diagram of an AI system

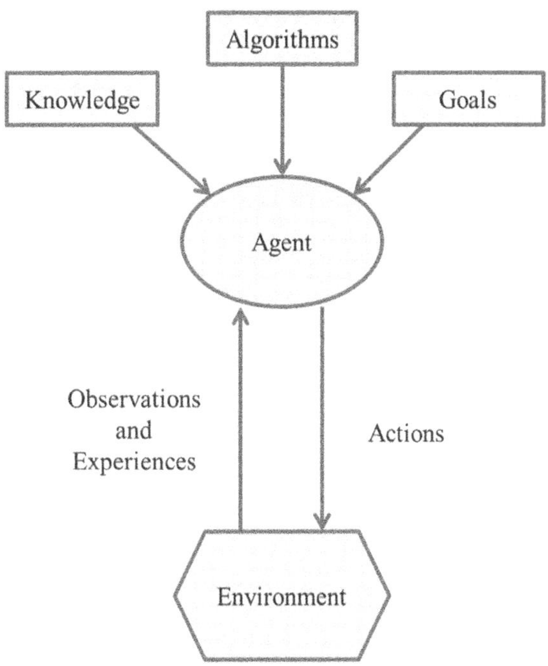

AI. Some of the most common algorithms associated with AI include fuzzy logic (FL), adaptive fuzzy logic (AFL), expert systems (ES), and genetic algorithms (GA).

Expert systems are an attempt to emulate the process of human thinking through representing knowledge and the mechanisms of inference. Within a closed domain for knowledge, the capability of ESs in making decisions is on a quality equivalent to human experts [16] (Fig. 2).

In FL, the representation of knowledge is more firmly connected to the method by which humans think. FL has the capabilities of strong inference of ESs in addition to natural (linguistic) representation of the knowledge. FL has been implemented fruitfully in control uses where the system model does not exist or the model is mathematically very complex as well as computationally intensive. AFL is a fuzzy logic-based model that holds the capabilities of optimization associated with GAs to enhance performance of intelligent systems using a priori knowledge [17–25] (Fig. 3).

GAs use human genetic evolution techniques to develop optimal resolutions. GAs are sometimes also known as a multi-dimensional optimization technique constructed upon a genetically random search engine [26] (Fig. 4).

Fig. 2 Block diagram of an expert system (ES)

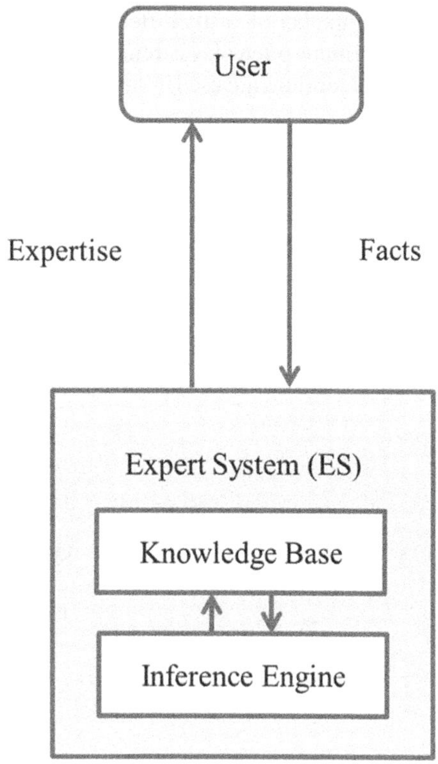

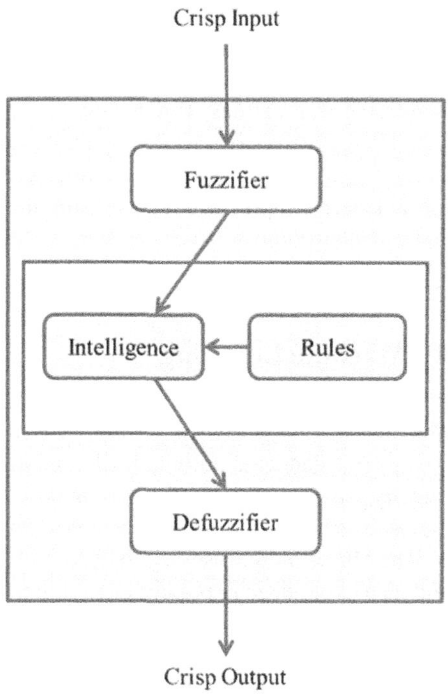

Fig. 3 Block diagram of a fuzzy logic system (FL)

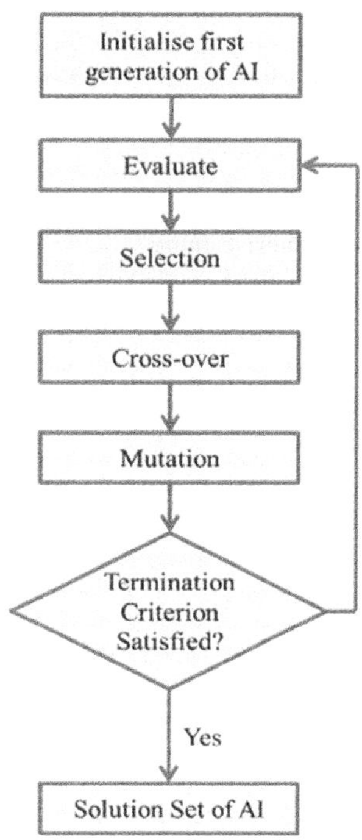

Fig. 4 Flowchart of a genetic algorithm (GA)

The applications for AI are seemingly endless. The technology can appeal in the healthcare industry to dose drugs, surgeries, and diagnosis; automotive industry including self-driving cars and wheelchairs, financial industry in detecting activity in unusual transactions, fraud prevention, and streamlined trading, just to name a few. These machines must decide the best course of action of any action they take, as each action will impact the result [27]. For example, self-driving cars must care for all external inputs and act to ensure the prevention of any collisions. Thus, AI is an ever-modifying and ever-evolving technology.

4 Machine Learning

Machine learning (ML) is a classification of artificial intelligence (AI) in which the systems can learn automatically and improve from circumstances without being directly programmed. ML focuses on the evolution of computer algorithms that learn themselves by accessing the available data [28] (Fig. 5).

The ML technique uses available data, known as training sets, to observe, analyze, and gain experience in prediction by looking for patterns. This is sometimes accompanied by reward functions and cost functions for artificial analysis in some of the training sets. The system iteratively corrects itself over the whole training set. The goal here is to enable the systems to learn automatically without human intervention [29–31]. After analyzing the training sets, the systems then predict the outcome or make decisions based on the data. The more training sets are available, the better the decision-making capability is. Algorithms of ML are often classified as supervised ML, semi-supervised ML, unsupervised ML, and reinforced ML [32].

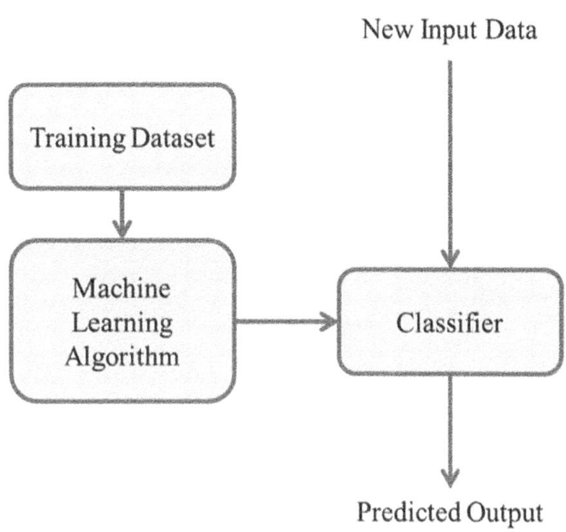

Fig. 5 Basic block diagram of machine learning

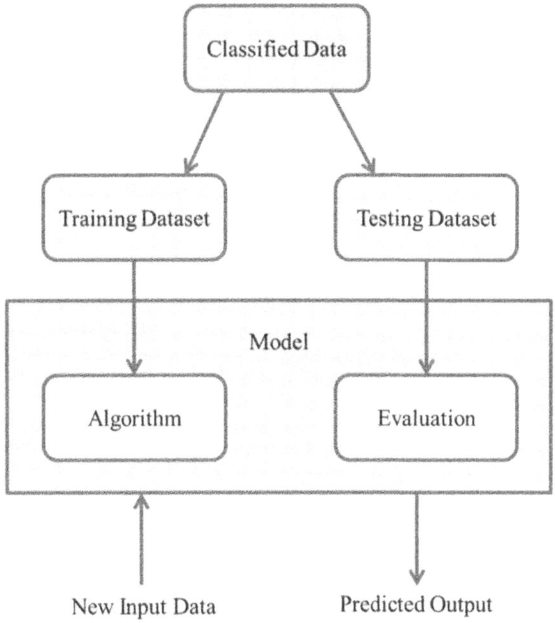

Fig. 6 Block diagram of supervised machine learning

Supervised ML algorithms can make a decision based on what has been learned from the training sets to new data to predict future events and take decisions. Beginning with the analysis of a known training set, the algorithm associates a function to make prognoses about the expected output values. Also, the algorithm can compare its output with the correct output to find parametric deviations to modify the model accordingly to minimize the cost function [33, 34] (Fig. 6).

Unsupervised ML algorithms are utilized when the data used in training the system are not classified. Machines using this type of learning technique study how to conclude a function for the description of a structure hidden in the training set. Unsupervised algorithms do not focus to infer a specific decision for output, but instead, try to find underlying patterns in the data. Thus, they often find new criteria and conditions for sorting and classifying data [35, 36] (Fig. 7).

Semi-supervised ML algorithms use the features of both supervised as well as unsupervised ML techniques for training and thus use classified as well as unclassified training datasets for learning. Typically, unclassified and unlabeled data are much more in volume compared to labeled or classified data. This type of learning has an advantage over both unsupervised and supervised learning as the learning accuracy is improved tremendously. These learning algorithms can also be used when the data in the training set are incomplete and have missing entries in the classification [37] (Fig. 8).

Reinforcement ML algorithms use a reinforcement signal, often treated as a reward or punishment corresponding to the decisions made by the machine. In principle, this is analogous to make a pet learn good and bad behaviors by offering rewards for

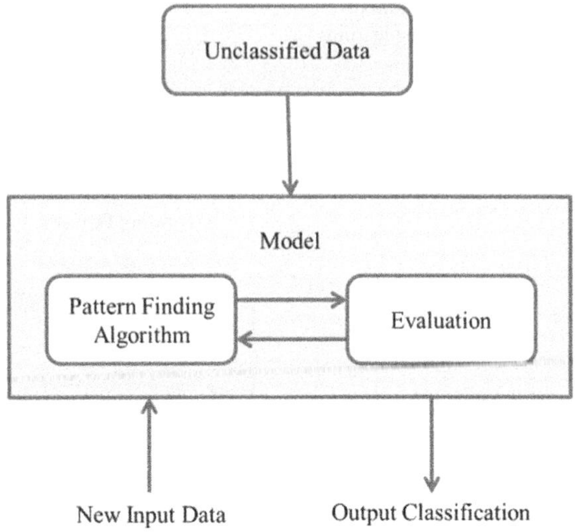

Fig. 7 Block diagram of unsupervised machine learning

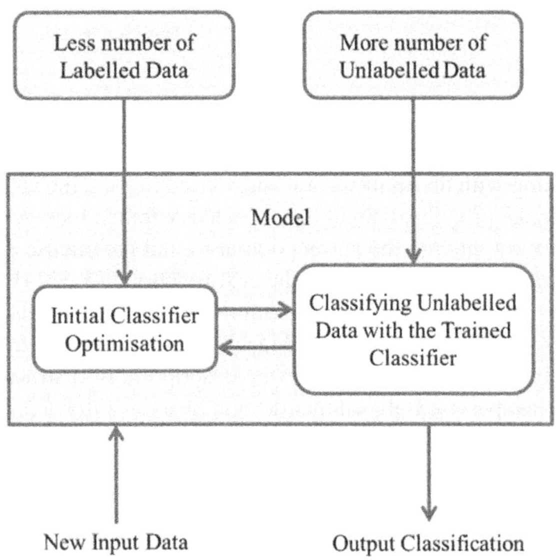

Fig. 8 Block diagram of semi-supervised machine learning

the good actions and punishments for the bad actions committed. Reward feedback ensures the correct identification of errors and helps the machine choose the best path for iterative learning. Thus, the system applies iterative changes to the parameters to maximize its performance based upon the reward or punishment received [38, 39] (Fig. 9).

Machine learning, while generally gives faster and accurate results, also requires additional time, data resources, and computational power for proper training. A

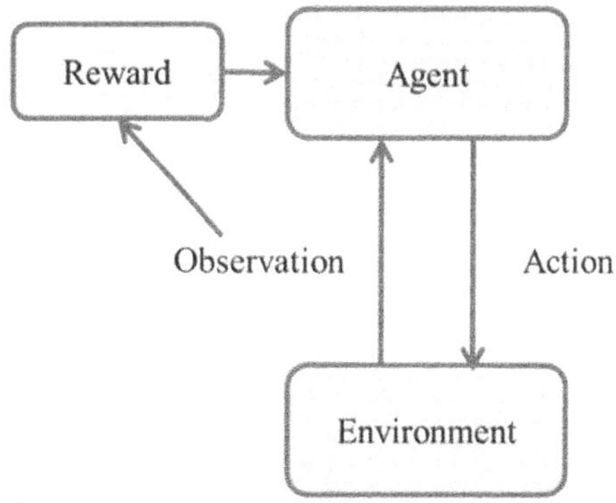

Fig. 9 Simplified block diagram of reinforced machine learning

lower number of training samples may drastically reduce the quality of machine learning. Also, incorporating machine learning in AI algorithms results in learning by processing massive volumes of data and finding patterns that are impossible to detect otherwise [40–43].

5 Neural Networks

A neural network (NN) is an algorithm that recognizes the underlying patterns and relationships in a data record through a process similar to the way the neurons and neural networks in a human brain does. Neural networks, in general, refer to the systems of neurons, which can be organic, or in our case, artificial. In this chapter, the use of the word "neural networks" corresponds to the discussion of artificial neural networks (ANNs) only.

In a neural network, the neuron is a basic building block defined by a mathematical function that classifies the information corresponding to a specific architecture. Neural networks have the power to adapt according to changing input values, and so the network constructs the optimal result without the need to continuously amend the criteria for output (Fig. 10).

A neural network contains layers of interconnected neurons. A neuron is often called a perceptron or node when defined for a neural network. Each neuron generally has a basic linear regression structure. The neuron feeds the signal from a multiple linear regression toward an activation function, which might be nonlinear. ANNs are effective in representing complicated (nonlinear) functions, and they acquire these functions with the help of examples.

In a multilayered perceptron (MLP), the neurons are sorted in interconnected layers, forming a web-like structure. The first layer, called the input layer, collects input data. The intermediate layers, called hidden layers, define the input-output mapping. The last layer, called the output layer, has classifications or output signals.

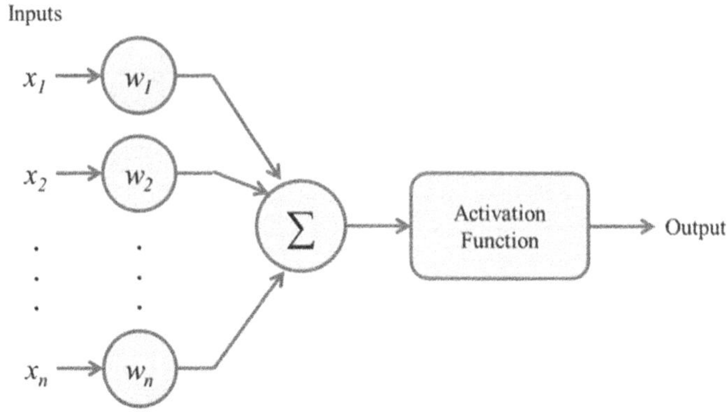

Fig. 10 Basic unit (Neuron) in an ANN

Hidden layers often iteratively adjust the input weightings until the error is minimized [44] (Fig. 11).

Neural networks have already been fruitfully used in many applications which may be grouped into two classes, namely optimization and associative retrieval or classification.

For optimization applications, the ANNs are used as state-space finding mechanisms. The synaptic weights are initially set before starting the search process. There is often no explicit learning procedure to determine the weights. Once the synaptic weights are set, the retrieving phase is performed. The gradient descent is used iteratively until convergence to an optimal state is achieved. The global optimal solution can be reached by using the Boltzmann machine. With a proper annealing schedule, the state of the Boltzmann machine will gradually move toward the global optimal solution [45].

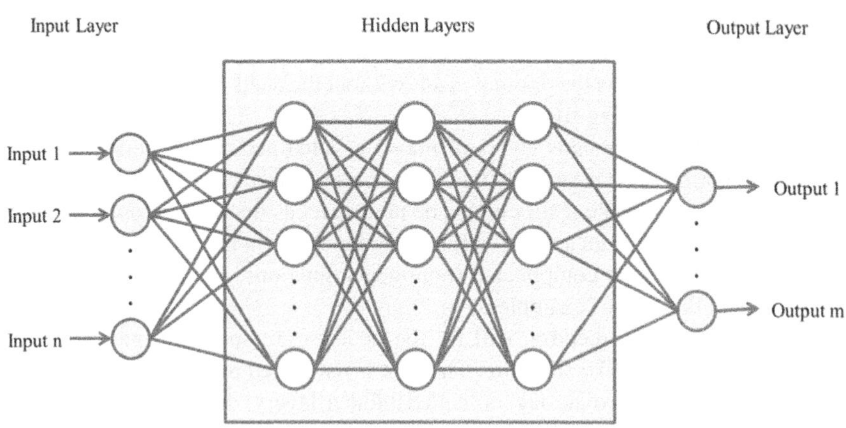

Fig. 11 ANN structure as a multilayered perceptron

Associative retrieval is defined either as the process of retrieving the complete pattern from given partial information about the desired pattern (auto-association) or retrieving a pattern in a subset, corresponding to the pattern given in another reference subset (pattern association). The associative classification is defined as identifying the corresponding category for a test pattern. For these types of applications, some learning schemes are sometimes used for training of the synaptic weights [46].

5.1 Deep Learning

Deep learning (DL) is a type of ML that can learn from unlabeled or unclassified data with the supervision or tweaking requirement by any human. It can handle a large amount of data that otherwise would take humans even decades to comprehend and process. As such, DL is used in the processing of bid data. The word "Deep" refers to the multiple layers of neural networks having multiple nodes in each layer typically processing big data—data that are very large in volume. It is based on the idea that neurons found in the human brain can understand abstract patterns and associations through multiple layers of neuron groups [47–49].

DL employs a hierarchical level with ANNs to implement the machine learning process. The ANNs are structured much like the brain of a human, in which neuron nodes are interconnected like a web structure. While traditional algorithms analyze the data linearly, the hierarchical structure of DL systems qualifies machines to operate on data in a nonlinear fashion [50–52].

5.2 Transfer Learning

Transfer learning (TL) is a part of ML that focuses upon storing the learned model while solving one set of data and then applying the model to a separate but correlated set of data. For example, an algorithm used to learn to detect liver tumors might be used to re-recognize brain tumors. Transferring or reusing information learned from previous models for the development of new models can greatly improve the speed and efficiency of a reinforcement learning agent [53–56] (Fig. 12).

5.3 Convolutional Neural Networks

A convolutional neural network (CNN or ConvNet) is a DL algorithm which takes a multi-dimensional array such as the pixel values in an image as a set input value, assigns weights (changeable parameter values) to various components in the array, and is capable of differentiating one from another. In primitive algorithms, filters are specifically defined manually, while CNNs can learn these filters/characteristics

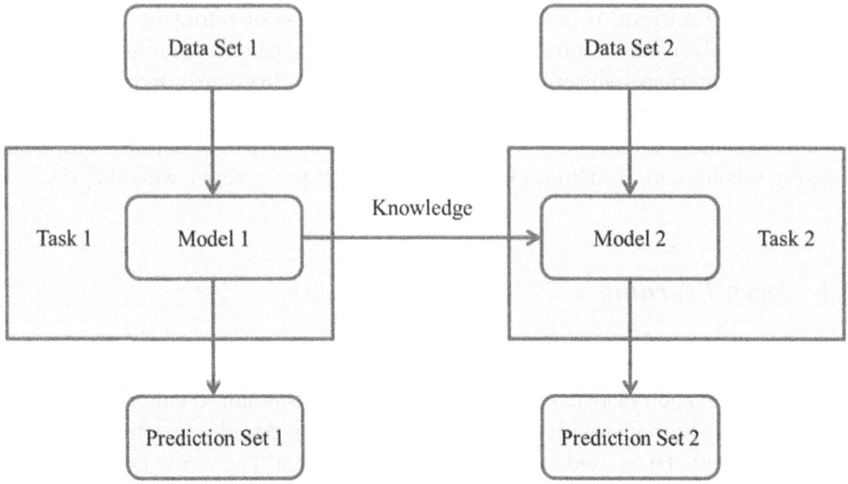

Fig. 12 Block diagram of machine learning

over a range of operation. The processing needed for CNN is much lower compared with other algorithms for classification [57–59].

A CNN generally can find and capture spatial and temporal dependencies successfully in an image with the use of corresponding necessary filters. The network can be trained to express the complexity of the image better, as the algorithm performs better fitting with the image dataset by reusability of weights and reduction in the number of involved parameters [60–65].

As the number of elements for the datasets increases in size for multiple dimensions, the computational load rises exponentially. The role of CNNs includes reducing the datasets so that they are easier to compute, without any loss in important critical characteristics to get a good prediction. The target is to design an architecture that excels at learning the features, as well as can be scaled for massive datasets. A typical CNN has two major components, a feature learning layer followed by a classification layer [66–71] (Fig. 13).

The feature learning layer (FLL) is accountable for the extraction of low-level as well as high-level features found in the array or image. The subset of the multi-dimensional dataset which is taken for calculation is called a Kernel. It can be one-dimensional as well as multi-dimensional itself, with multiple elements along each dimension, but less than the dataset which is being processed. The Kernel is the element that carries out convolution in the first section of a convolutional layer [71–93].

The Kernel first takes a specific dimension, and for the first element of the corresponding dimension, it moves along a different dimension each step until it parses it completely. Moving on, it takes the second element and repeats the process. For more than two dimensions, other dimensions are nested just like the second dimension is for the first one. This process is continued until the entire array, typically an image

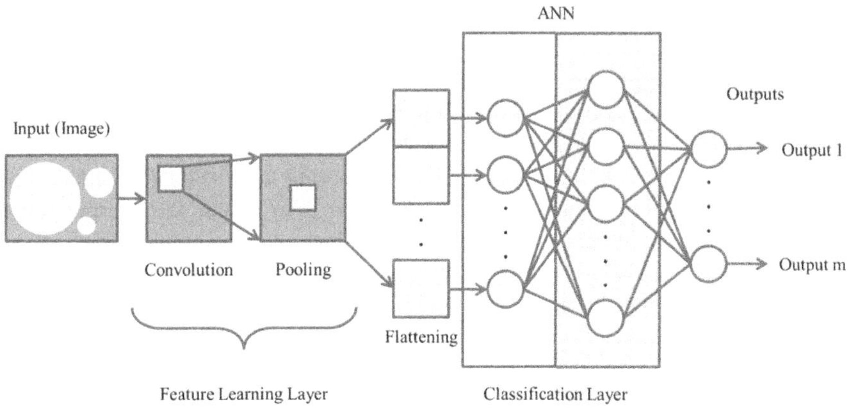

Fig. 13 Block diagram of a convolutional neural network (CNN)

is traversed. Finally, all results get summed with the bias and give us a compressed one-dimensional channel convoluted feature output [94–126] (Fig. 14).

The reason to use the convolution operation is for the extraction of the high-level features found from the input dataset, typically an image. CNN can have one or more than one convolutional layer. Generally, the first convolution layer captures the low-level features including edges and colors. By adding multiple layers, this architecture starts adapting to capture high-level features as well. Thus, the architecture now has an understanding of the dataset as a whole, similar to how humans perceive an image. The convolution operation can produce two types of results, namely, valid padding and same padding [127–139].

In valid padding, the convoluted output has a reduced number of elements in one or multiple dimensions of the array compared to the input. For example, if a valid

Fig. 14 Example of a Kernel producing convoluted output

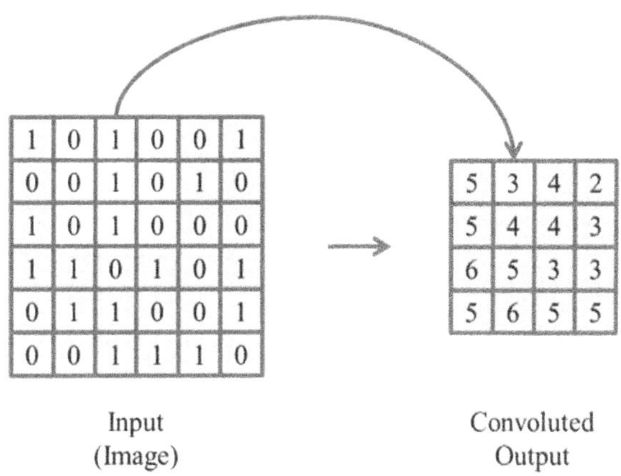

padding is done on a (5 × 5 × 2) array input, the result may be an array of size (3 × 3 × 1).

In the same padding, the dimensionality remains the same, hence the name. For example, if the same padding is done on a (5 × 5 × 2) array input, the result turns out to be an array of size (5 × 5 × 2) as well [66, 140–147].

Similar to the convolutional layer (CL), the pooling layer (PL) also reduces the spatial size for the convoluted output. The reason is to reduce the computational power that is required to process the data by the reduction in the number of elements. In addition to that, it is also useful for extracting dominant features. Thus, it maintains the process of training the model efficiently. Pooling can be of two types, namely average pooling and max pooling [148–155].

Average pooling returns the average of all values from a portion of the image covered by the Kernel. Average pooling uses spatial reduction also as a noise suppressing process.

Max pooling returns the maximum value from the portion of the image covered by the Kernel. It also acts as a noise suppressant and discards the noisy activations altogether while also performing de-noising. Hence, max pooling's performance is a lot better with respect to average pooling (Fig. 15).

The CL and PL together form a feature learning layer. Depending on the complexity of the problem, the feature learning layer may have multiple convolutional–pooling pairs. With more complexity, the number of pairs increases, and as a result, computational load also increases.

After the feature learning stage is completed, the resulting dataset is fed into the classification stage consisting of a regular ANN after proper flattening to a single dimension. The ANN then takes care of the classification process [102, 156–163].

Fig. 15 Average pooling versus max pooling

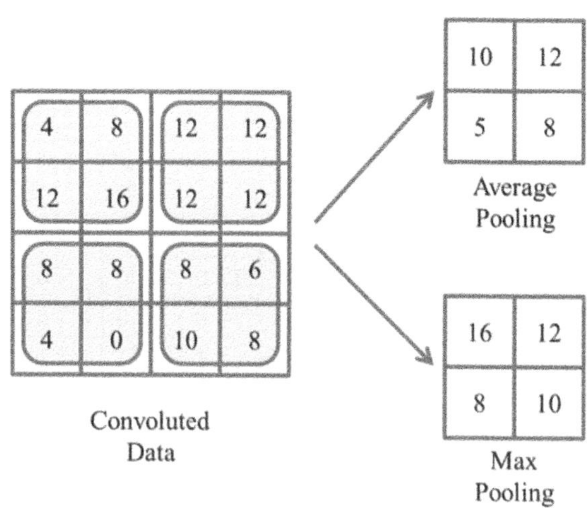

6 CNN Algorithms and Methods Used in the Survey

6.1 Inception V3

Inception convolution neural network has been widely accepted for its ability and performance accuracy for image classification and object detection. Inception networks were a 22-layer network; while the next versions are termed as Inception VN network(where n refers to version no: Inception V1, V2, V3). Inception V3 has 48 layers. Each block in the network consists of fully connected layers, average pooling, max pooling, convolutions, etc. [164]. The basic architecture of Inception V3 is shown below (Fig. 16).

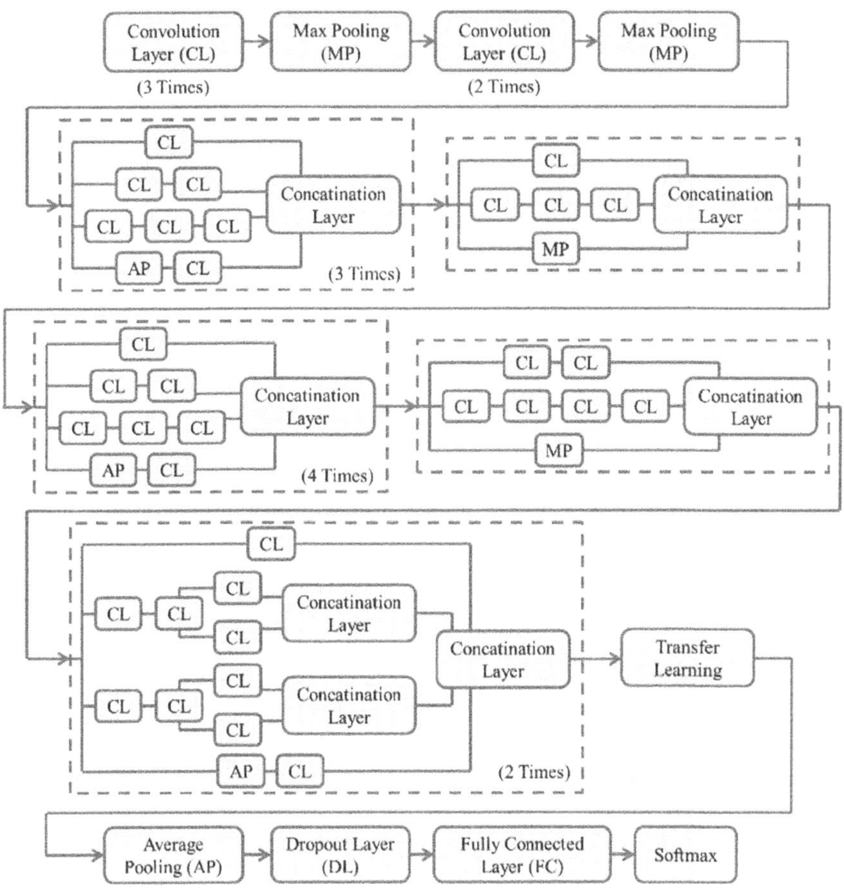

Fig. 16 Inception V3 architecture

6.2 ResNet-50

Residual networks or ResNet are extremely useful to solve complex computer vision problems. ResNets are widely accepted and popular for their functional form, allowing data to transfer directly over the network allowing the computations constant and stable [165]. ResNet utilizes the concept of skip connections. But skip connections are only applicable when both input and output size are the same. The illustrations of the skip connection are shown below (Fig. 17).

Here each block in the networks is learning the output $Y(x)$ unlike conventional networks where residual blocks tend to learn $F(x)$, thus it alleviates the difficulty of vanishing gradient.

Residual networks can be of different types such as ResNet-18, ResNet-152, and ResNet-50. Each model has 18, 152, and 50 layers,, respectively, including the first

Fig. 17 Sample diagram of ResNet residual block

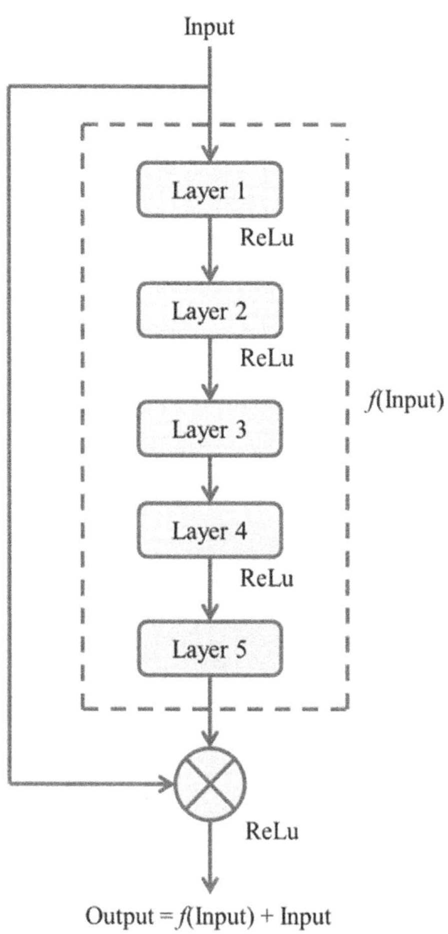

convolution layer and final convolution layer. It is also feasible to create a novel residual network according to our needs by manipulating the no of residual blocks and channels.

In this study, the performance accuracy of ResNet-50 has been analyzed. The architecture of ResNet-50 is represented below (Fig. 18).

6.3 *Inception-ResNet-v2*

In Inception-ResNet-v2, multiple dimensions of convolution blocks are interconnected by residual units. Residual units play a significant role in minimizing the training time [166]. It consists of max pooling, convolution blocks, etc. [167]. Figure 19 is the basic architecture of Inception-ResNet-v2.

6.4 *VGG-19*

Visual geometry group network (VGG) [168] CNN comprises of six main blocks. The input dimension is 224*224*3 and the filter dimension is 3*3, smaller than AlexNet (11*11) filter. The number of layers can be varied between 16 and 19 depending upon the requirement and architecture design. VGG-19 demonstrates higher accuracy for image recognition [169] and image classification applications. VGG-19 architecture design is shown below (Fig. 20).

The first two layers of blocks 1, 2, and 3 and the first four layers of block 4 and 5 are convolution layers having a 3*3 filter. Each block starting from block 1 to 4 has 64, 128, 256, and 512 filters, respectively. Max pooling is utilized to reduce the height and width of the initial data. Fully connected layers with 4096 channels followed by a string of convolution layers and the final layer are softmax with 1000 classes. The architecture of a fully connected layer remains the same in all networks.

6.5 *MobileNet*

MobileNet is particularly based upon depthwise convolution and pointwise convolution. Depthwise convolution is useful for filtering input without the need to create new features. It is also beneficial to abate the number of parameters than the normal convolution network. Pointwise convolution is useful for generating new features, and the computational time is also very less compared to the Inception-v3 network model [170]. Batch normalization (BN) and rectified linear unit(ReLU) are applied after each convolution [171]. MobileNet architecture also consists of a global average pooling layer, reshape layer, fully connected layer(FC) softmax, and dropout layer. Figure 21 is the basic representation of MobileNet architecture.

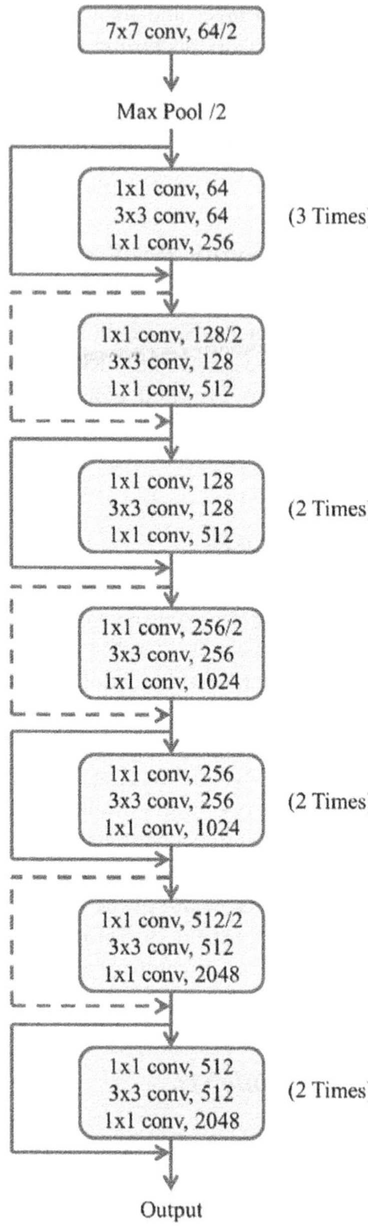

Fig. 18 ResNet-50 architecture

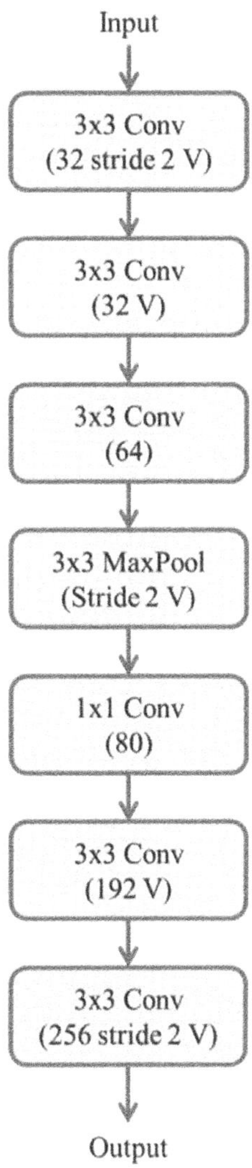

Fig. 19 Inception-ResNet-v2 architecture

7 Materials and Methods

7.1 Dataset

Three sets of different databases have been used in this survey. Due to the limitation of accessibility of real-time COVID-19 infected chest X-ray images, all the images (Figs. 1 and 2) shown below have been obtained from open-source Github

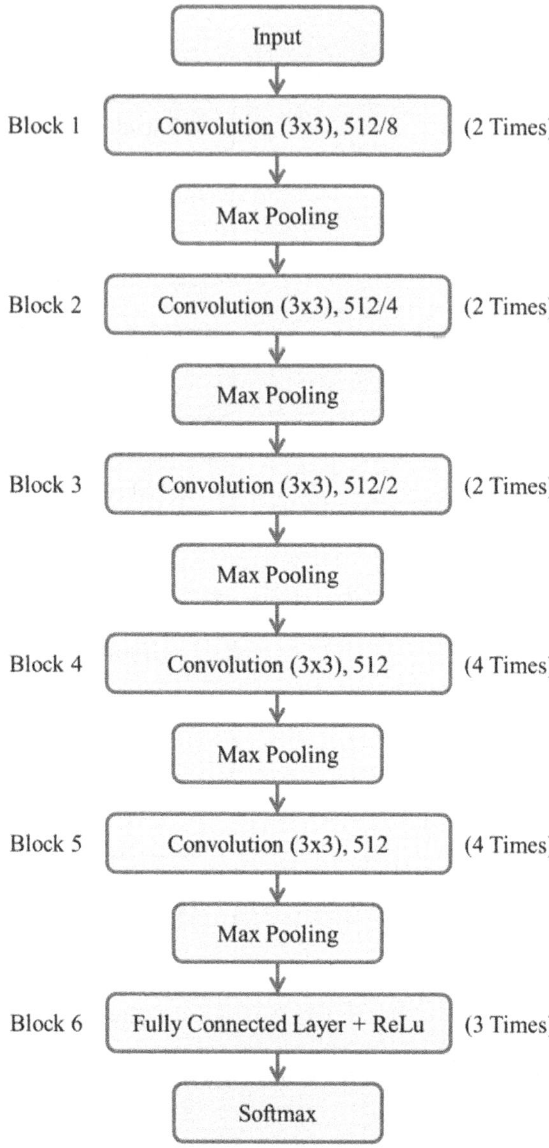

Fig. 20 VGG-19 architecture

repository [2] and Kaggle repository, namely "chest X-ray images (Pneumonia)" [3] for analyzing the performance of convolution neural network models ResNet-50, Inception-ResNet-v2, and Inception-v3; while for VGG-19, only Github repository [2] has been used. All the above-mentioned databases are being updated regularly by hospitals and/or respective authorities.

The performance analysis is being based on total 100 normal chest X-ray images and COVID-19 infected images [2, 3] for Resnet-50, Inception-ResNet-v2, and

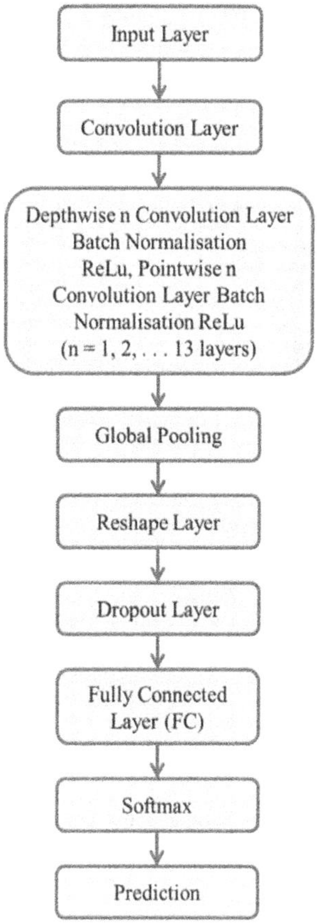

Fig. 21 MobileNet architecture

Inception-v3. For VGG-19 [172] and MobileNet [173], a dataset including 224 confirmed COVID-19 images, 700 images of pneumonia, and 504 normal chest X-ray images [2, 174, 175] has been used, respectively [176] (Figs. 22 and 23).

7.2 Performance Analysis Parameters

Basic parameters such as true positive (TP) are correctly identified as COVID-19 infected, false positive (FP) is normal chest X-ray image incorrectly identified as COVID-19 infected, true negative (TN) is normal chest X-ray identified correctly, and false negative (FN) is COVID-19 infected images detected as normal. A total of 12 performance parameters have been used for analyzing the performance of deep neural network models ResNet-50, Inception-ResNet-v2, VGG-19, MobileNet, and Inception-v3. Those are described briefly below.

$$\text{Accuracy} = (\text{TP} + \text{TN})/(\text{TP} + \text{TN} + \text{FP} + \text{FN}) \tag{1}$$

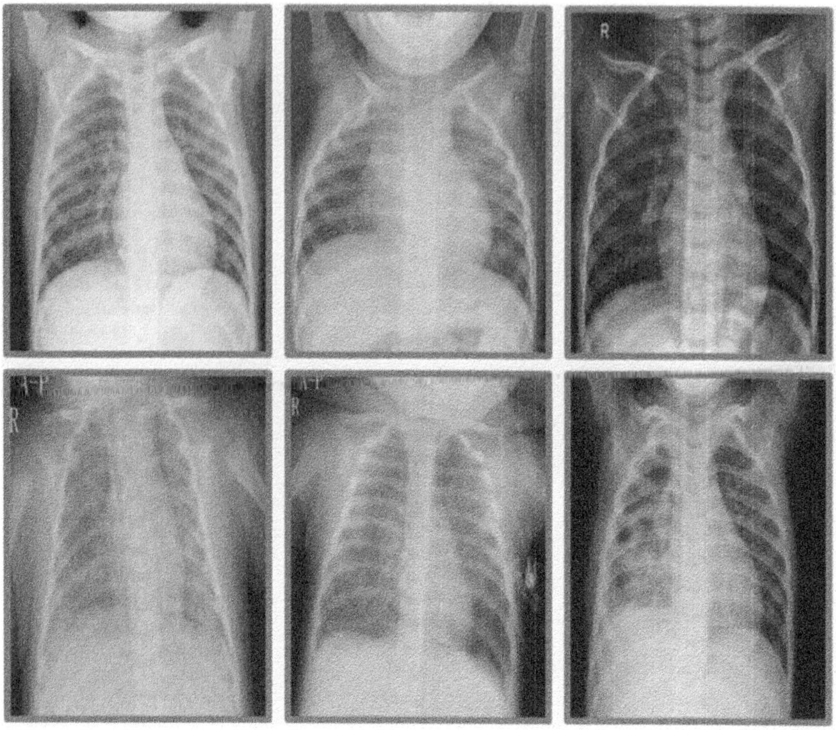

Fig. 22 Sample chest X-ray images from Github COVID-chest X-ray dataset [2]

$$\text{Sensitivity} = \text{TP}/(\text{TP} + \text{FN}) \tag{2}$$

$$\text{Negative Predictive Value} = \text{TN}/(\text{FN} + \text{TN}) \tag{3}$$

$$\text{Positive Predictive Value} = \text{TP}/(\text{TP} + \text{FP}) \tag{4}$$

$$\text{Specificity} = \text{TN}/(\text{TN} + \text{FP}) \tag{5}$$

$$\text{F1-Score} = 2\text{TP}/(2\text{TP} + \text{FP} + \text{FN}) \tag{6}$$

$$\text{False Discovery Rate} = \text{FP}/(\text{TP} + \text{FP}) \tag{7}$$

$$\text{False Omission Rate} = \text{FN}/(\text{FN} + \text{TN}) \tag{8}$$

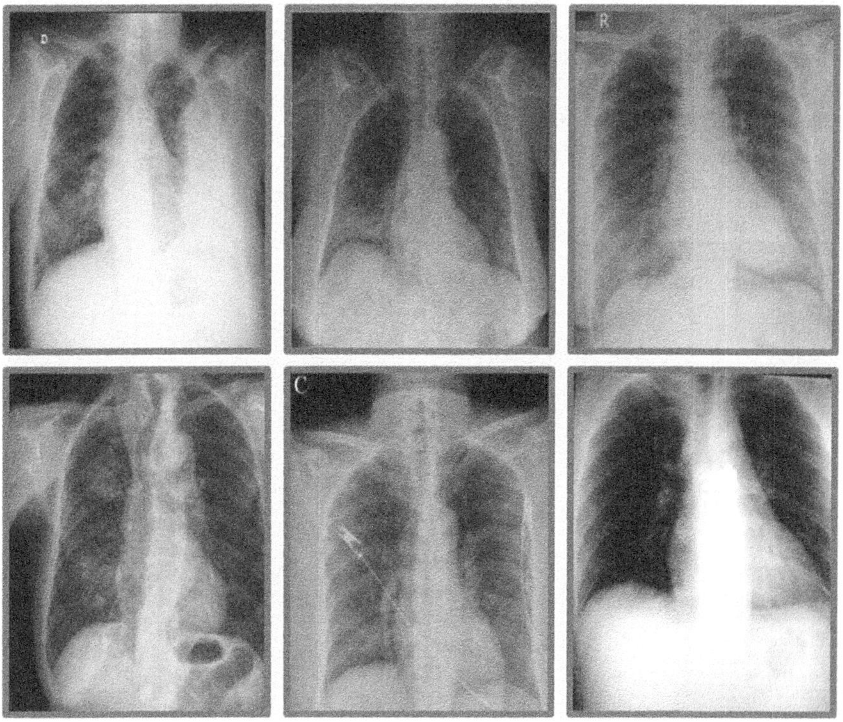

Fig. 23 Selected chest X-ray images from Kaggle database [3]

$$\text{False Positive Rate} = \text{FP}/(\text{FP} + \text{TN}) \quad (9)$$

$$\text{False Negative Rate (FNR)} = \text{FN}/(\text{TP} + \text{FN}) \quad (10)$$

$$\text{Negative Likelihood Ratio} = \text{FNR / Specificity} \quad (11)$$

$$\text{Prevalence} = (\text{TP} + \text{FN})/(\text{TP} + \text{TN} + \text{FP} + \text{FN}) \quad (12)$$

8 Results and Discussions

Table 2 is another performance attribute of all five models using test data and values obtained from Table 1. It is noted that the highest specificity of 100% has been observed in Inception-v3 and ResNet-50 models.

Table 1 Basic parameters

Parameters	Inception-v3 [2, 3, 176]	ResNet-50 [2, 3, 176]	Inception-ResNet-v2 [2, 3, 176]	VGG-19 [2, 3, 177]	MobileNet [2, 3, 177]
Dataset	100	100	100	1428	1428
True positive (TP)	47	48	42	208	222
False positive (FP)	0	0	5	15	35
False negative (FN)	3	2	8	16	2
True negative (TN)	50	50	45	1189	1169

Table 2 Calculated performance parameters

Parameters	Inception-v3	ResNet-50	Inception-ResNet-v2	VGG-19	MobileNet
Accuracy	0.97	0.98	0.87	0.98	0.97
Sensitivity	0.94	0.96	0.84	0.93	0.99
Negative predictive value	0.94	0.96	0.85	0.99	1.00
Positive predictive value	1.00	1.00	0.89	0.93	0.86
Specificity	1.00	1.00	0.90	0.99	0.97
F1-score	0.97	0.98	0.86	0.93	0.92
False discovery rate	0.00	0.00	0.11	0.07	0.14
False omission rate	0.06	0.04	0.15	0.01	0.00
False positive rate	0.00	0.00	0.10	0.01	0.03
False negative rate	0.06	0.04	0.16	0.07	0.01
Negative likelihood ratio	0.06	0.04	0.18	0.07	0.01
Prevalence	0.50	0.50	0.50	0.16	0.16

MobileNet model is having the highest sensitivity among the other five models of 99.10% ResNet-50 having the highest accuracy and F1-score.

In this comparative study, chest X-ray images collected from open-source databases [2, 3] are trained and tested in CNN models, namely ResNet-50, Inception-ResNet-v2, Inception-v3, VGG-19, and MobileNet. Accuracy, sensitivity, and negative predictive value of these five models are represented in Fig. 24; F1-score, specificity, and positive predictive value are represented in Fig. 25.

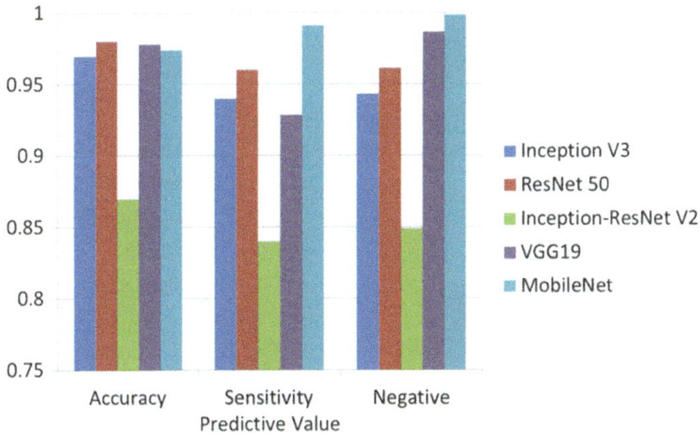

Fig. 24 Accuracy, sensitivity, and negative predictive value for different CNN models

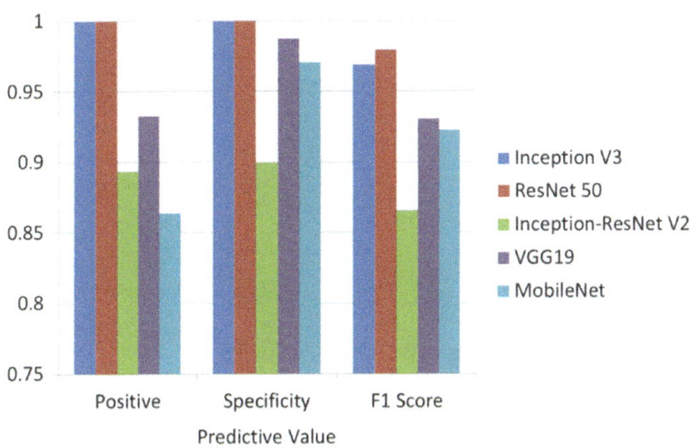

Fig. 25 Positive predictive value, specificity, and F1-score for different CNN models

False discovery rate, false omission rate, and false positive rate are represented as a bar chart in Fig. 26. Inception-ResNet-v2 having the highest false omission rate among the five models. Figure 27 represents the false negative rate, negative likelihood ratio, and prevalence as a bar graph.

9 Conclusion and Future Challenges

This study discusses the significance of different artificial intelligence techniques, algorithms for faster, and legitimate detection of COVID-19. Among the five methods, ResNet-50 and VGG-19 have the highest accuracy of 98%, MobileNet has

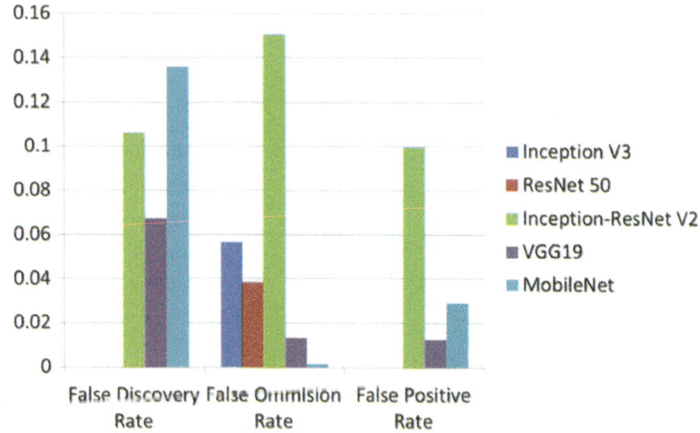

Fig. 26 False discovery rate, false omission rate, and false positive rate for different CNN models

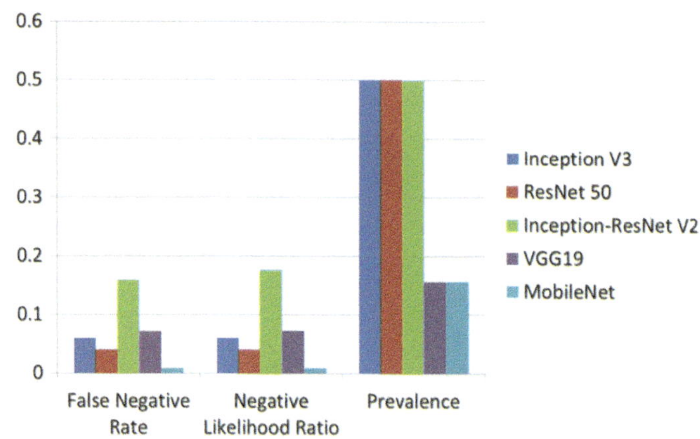

Fig. 27 False negative rate, negative likelihood ratio and prevalence for different CNN models

the highest sensitivity of 99%, Inception-v3 and ResNet-50 have the highest specificity of 100%, and ResNet-50 has the highest F1-score of 0.98. It is also important to finally summarize the result after carefully considering both clinical manifestations and computational results. This study also gives an overview of the importance of early prediction of COVID-19 patients with low cost and minimal time consumption.

In future studies, several other different CNN models are required with a larger patient database and should also be able to differentiate COVID-19 cases with respect to other viral fevers such as pneumonia and SARS.

References

1. Ilyas, M., Ilyas, M., Rehman, H., & Naït-Ali, A. (2020). *Detection of Covid-19 from chest x-ray images using artificial intelligence: An early review*. arXiv preprint arXiv:2004.05436.
2. Open database of COVID-19 cases with chest X-ray or CT images. https://github.com/iee e8023/covid-chestxray-dataset. Last accessed August 11, 2020.
3. Chest X-Ray Images (Pneumonia). https://www.kaggle.com/paultimothymooney/chest-xray-pneumonia. Last accessed August 11, 2020.
4. Zhang, J., Xie, Y., Liao, Z., Pang, G., Verjans, J., Li, W., Sun, Z., He, J., & Yi Li, C. S. (2020). *Viral pneumonia screening on chest X-ray images using confidence-aware anomaly detection*. arXiv preprint arXiv:2003.12338.
5. Adhikari, N. C. D. (2020). Infection severity detection of CoVID19 from X-Rays and CT scans using artificial intelligence. *International Journal of Computer (IJC), 38*(1), 73–92.
6. Punn, N. S., & Agarwal, S. (2020). *Automated diagnosis of COVID-19 with limited posteroanterior chest X-ray images using fine-tuned deep neural networks*. arXiv preprint arXiv:2004. 11676.
7. Jamil, M., & Hussain, I. (2020). *Automatic detection of COVID-19 Infection from chest X-ray using deep learning*. medRxiv. https://www.medrxiv.org/content/10.1101/2020.05.10.200970 63v1.
8. Hemdan, E. E. D., Shouman, M. A., & Karar, M. E. (2020). *Covidx-net: A framework of deep learning classifiers to diagnose covid-19 in x-ray images*. arXiv preprint arXiv:2003.11055.
9. Khan, A. I., Shah, J. L., & Bhat, M. M. (2020). Coronet: A deep neural network for detection and diagnosis of COVID-19 from chest x-ray images. *Computer Methods and Programs in Biomedicine, 196*, 105581.
10. Farooq, M., & Hafeez, A. (2020). *Covid-resnet: A deep learning framework for screening of covid19 from radiographs*. arXiv preprint arXiv:2003.14395.
11. Alqudah, A. M., Qazan, S., Alquran, H., Qasmieh, I. A., & Alqudah, A. *Covid-2019 detection using x-ray images and artificial intelligence hybrid systems*.
12. Mohammadi, R., Salehi, M., Ghaffari, H., Rohani, A. A., & Reiazi, R. (2020). Transfer learning-based automatic detection of coronavirus disease 2019 (COVID-19) from chest X-ray Images. *Journal of Biomedical Physics & Engineering, 10*(5), 559.
13. Gozes, O., Frid-Adar, M., Sagie, N., Zhang, H., Ji, W., & Greenspan, H. (2020). *Coronavirus detection and analysis on chest ct with deep learning*. arXiv preprint arXiv:2004.02640.
14. Ibrahim, W. A., & Morcos, M. M. (2002). Artificial intelligence and advanced mathematical tools for power quality applications: a survey. *IEEE Transactions on Power Delivery, 17*(2), 668–673.
15. Ramos, C., Augusto, J. C., & Shapiro, D. (2008). Ambient intelligence—the next step for artificial intelligence. *IEEE Intelligent Systems, 23*(2), 15–18.
16. Kozma, J. (1998). Intelligent agents. *IEEE Potentials, 17*(2), 16–19. https://doi.org/10.1109/ 45.666640.
17. Lee, C. C. (1990). Fuzzy logic in control systems: fuzzy logic controller. I. *IEEE Transactions on Systems, Man, and Cybernetics, 20*(2), 404–418.
18. Mendel, J. M. (1995). Fuzzy logic systems for engineering: A tutorial. *Proceedings of the IEEE, 83*(3), 345–377.
19. Jang, J. S. (1993). ANFIS: Adaptive-network-based fuzzy inference system. *IEEE Transactions on Systems, Man, and Cybernetics, 23*(3), 665–685.
20. Jang, J. S., & Sun, C. T. (1995). Neuro-fuzzy modeling and control. *Proceedings of the IEEE, 83*(3), 378–406.
21. Jang, J. S. R., Sun, C. T., & Mizutani, E. (1997). Neuro-fuzzy and soft computing-a computational approach to learning and machine intelligence [Book Review]. *IEEE Transactions on Automatic Control, 42*(10), 1482–1484.
22. Lin, C.-T., & Lee, C. S. G. (1991). Neural-network-based fuzzy logic control and decision system. *IEEE Transactions on Computers, 40*, 1320–1336.

23. Jang, J. S. R. (1992). Self-learning fuzzy controllers based on temporal backpropagation. *IEEE Transactions on Neural Networks, 3*(5), 714–723.
24. Horikawa, S. I., Furuhashi, T., & Uchikawa, Y. (1992). On fuzzy modeling using fuzzy neural networks with the back-propagation algorithm. *IEEE Transactions on Neural Networks, 3*(5), 801–806.
25. Belarbi, K., & Titel, F. (2000). Genetic algorithm for the design of a class of fuzzy controllers: an alternative approach. *IEEE Transactions on Fuzzy Systems, 8*(4), 398–405.
26. Wu, X. (2004, September). Data mining: Artificial intelligence in data analysis. In *Proceedings. IEEE/WIC/ACM International Conference on Intelligent Agent Technology, 2004. (IAT 2004)* (p. 7). IEEE.
27. Sodhro, A. H., Pirbhulal, S., & de Albuquerque, V. H. C. (2019). Artificial intelligence-driven mechanism for edge computing-based industrial applications. *IEEE Transactions on Industrial Informatics, 15*(7), 4235–4243.
28. Joo, E. M., & Zhou, Y. (Eds.) (2009). *Theory and novel applications of machine learning*. BoD–Books on Demand.
29. Alpaydin, E. (2020). *Introduction to machine learning*. MIT press.
30. Zurada, J. M., Mazurowski, M. A., Ragade, R., Abdullin, A., Wojtudiak, J., & Gentle, J. (2009). Building virtual community in computational intelligence and machine learning [research frontier]. *IEEE Computational Intelligence Magazine, 4*(1), 43–54.
31. Yen, G. G. (2009). Learning and Intelligence [Editor's remarks]. *IEEE Computational Intelligence Magazine, 4*(2), 2–2.
32. Mjolsness, E., & DeCoste, D. (2001). Machine learning for science: state of the art and future prospects. *Science, 293*(5537), 2051–2055.
33. Chang, C. C., & Lin, C. J. (2011). LIBSVM: A library for support vector machines. *ACM Transactions on Intelligent Systems and Technology (TIST), 2*(3), 1–27.
34. Fan, R. E., Chang, K. W., Hsieh, C. J., Wang, X. R., & Lin, C. J. (2008). LIBLINEAR: A library for large linear classification. *Journal of Machine Learning Research, 9,* 1871–1874.
35. Donoho, D. L., & Elad, M. (2003). Optimally sparse representation in general (nonorthogonal) dictionaries via $\ell 1$ minimization. *Proceedings of the National Academy of Sciences, 100*(5), 2197–2202.
36. Koh, K., Kim, S. J., & Boyd, S. (2007). An interior-point method for large-scale l1-regularized logistic regression. *Journal of Machine learning research, 8,* 1519–1555.
37. Murphy, K. P. (2012). *Machine learning: a probabilistic perspective*. MIT press.
38. Wu, M., Schölkopf, B., & Bakır, G. (2006). A direct method for building sparse kernel learning algorithms. *Journal of Machine Learning Research, 7,* 603–624.
39. Wang, G., Kalra, M., & Orton, C. G. (2017). Machine learning will transform radiology significantly within the next 5 years. *Medical Physics, 44*(6), 2041–2044.
40. Rudin, C., Waltz, D., Anderson, R. N., Boulanger, A., Salleb-Aouissi, A., Chow, M., et al. (2011). Machine learning for the New York City power grid. *IEEE Transactions on Pattern Analysis and Machine Intelligence, 34*(2), 328–345.
41. Zhang, J., Zhan, Z. H., Lin, Y., Chen, N., Gong, Y. J., Zhong, J. H., et al. (2011). Evolutionary computation meets machine learning: A survey. *IEEE Computational Intelligence Magazine, 6*(4), 68–75.
42. Ozay, M., Esnaola, I., Vural, F. T. Y., Kulkarni, S. R., & Poor, H. V. (2015). Machine learning methods for attack detection in the smart grid. *IEEE Transactions on neural Networks and Learning Systems, 27*(8), 1773–1786.
43. Wang, G., Ye, J. C., Mueller, K., & Fessler, J. A. (2018). Image reconstruction is a new frontier of machine learning. *IEEE Transactions on Medical Imaging, 37*(6), 1289–1296.
44. Pathak, B. K., Srivastava, S., & Srivastava, K. (2008). *Neural network embedded multi-objective genetic algorithm to solve non-linear time-cost tradeoff problems of project scheduling*.
45. Lee, C., Gen, M., & Kuo, W. (2001). Reliability optimization design using a hybridized genetic algorithm with a neural-network technique. *IEICE Transactions on Fundamentals of Electronics, Communications and Computer Sciences, 84*(2), 627–637.

46. Jin, Y., & Sendhoff, B. (2004, June). Reducing fitness evaluations using clustering techniques and neural network ensembles. In *Genetic and Evolutionary Computation Conference* (pp. 688–699). Springer.
47. Cheng, G., Yang, C., Yao, X., Guo, L., & Han, J. (2018). When deep learning meets metric learning: Remote sensing image scene classification via learning discriminative CNNs. *IEEE Transactions on Geoscience and Remote Sensing, 56*(5), 2811–2821.
48. Yin, C., Zhu, Y., Fei, J., & He, X. (2017). A deep learning approach for intrusion detection using recurrent neural networks. *Ieee Access, 5,* 21954–21961.
49. Mikołajczyk, A., & Grochowski, M. (2018, May). Data augmentation for improving deep learning in image classification problem. In *2018 International Interdisciplinary Ph.D. Workshop (IIPhDW)* (pp. 117–122). IEEE.
50. Chen, X. W., & Lin, X. (2014). Big data deep learning: challenges and perspectives. *IEEE access, 2,* 514–525.
51. Chen, Y., Lin, Z., Zhao, X., Wang, G., & Gu, Y. (2014). Deep learning-based classification of hyperspectral data. *IEEE Journal of Selected Topics in Applied Earth Observations and Remote Sensing, 7*(6), 2094–2107.
52. Zhou, Z., Liao, H., Gu, B., Huq, K. M. S., Mumtaz, S., & Rodriguez, J. (2018). Robust mobile crowd sensing: When deep learning meets edge computing. *IEEE Network, 32*(4), 54–60.
53. Jayaram, V., Alamgir, M., Altun, Y., Scholkopf, B., & Grosse-Wentrup, M. (2016). Transfer learning in brain-computer interfaces. *IEEE Computational Intelligence Magazine, 11*(1), 20–31.
54. Shao, L., Zhu, F., & Li, X. (2014). Transfer learning for visual categorization: A survey. *IEEE Transactions on Neural Networks and Learning Systems, 26*(5), 1019–1034.
55. Long, M., Wang, J., Ding, G., Pan, S. J., & Philip, S. Y. (2013). Adaptation regularization: A general framework for transfer learning. *IEEE Transactions on Knowledge and Data Engineering, 26*(5), 1076–1089.
56. Shao, S., McAleer, S., Yan, R., & Baldi, P. (2018). Highly accurate machine fault diagnosis using deep transfer learning. *IEEE Transactions on Industrial Informatics, 15*(4), 2446–2455.
57. Al-Saffar, A. A. M., Tao, H., & Talab, M. A. (2017, October). Review of deep convolution neural network in image classification. In *2017 International Conference on Radar, Antenna, Microwave, Electronics, and Telecommunications (ICRAMET)* (pp. 26–31). IEEE.
58. Lowe, D. G. (2004). Distinctive image features from scale-invariant keypoints. *International Journal of Computer Vision, 60*(2), 91–110.
59. Dalal, N., & Triggs, B. (2005, June). Histograms of oriented gradients for human detection. In *2005 IEEE Computer Society Conference on Computer Vision and Pattern Recognition (CVPR'05)* (Vol. 1, pp. 886–893). IEEE.
60. Hinton, G. E., & Salakhutdinov, R. R. (2006). Reducing the dimensionality of data with neural networks. *Science, 313*(5786), 504–507.
61. Tuerxun, T., & Dai, L. (2015). Deep neural network based uyghur large vocabulary continuous speech recognition. *Journal of Data Acquisition Processing, 30*(2), 365–371.
62. Fei-Fei, L., Fergus, R., & Perona, P. (2004, June). Learning generative visual models from few training examples: An incremental bayesian approach tested on 101 object categories. In *2004 Conference on Computer Vision and Pattern Recognition Workshop* (pp. 178–178). IEEE.
63. Deng, J., Dong, W., Socher, R., Li, L. J., Li, K., & Fei-Fei, L. I. (2009). A large-scale hierarchical image database. In *IEEE Conference on Computer Vision and Pattern Recognition, 2009. CVPR 2009* (pp. 248–255).
64. Ahonen, T., Hadid, A., & Pietikainen, M. (2006). Face description with local binary patterns: Application to face recognition. *IEEE Transactions on Pattern Analysis and Machine Intelligence, 28*(12), 2037–2041.
65. Russakovsky, O., Deng, J., Su, H., Krause, J., Satheesh, S., Ma, S., et al. (2015). Imagenet large scale visual recognition challenge. *International Journal of Computer Vision, 115*(3), 211–252.

66. Krizhevsky, A., Sutskever, I., & Hinton, G. E. (2017). Imagenet classification with deep convolutional neural networks. *Communications of the ACM, 60*(6), 84–90.
67. Zeiler, M. D., & Fergus, R. (2014, September). Visualizing and understanding convolutional networks. In *European Conference on Computer Vision* (pp. 818–833). Springer.
68. Szegedy, C., Liu, W., Jia, Y., Sermanet, P., Reed, S., Anguelov, D., Erhan, D., Vanhoucke, V. and Rabinovich, A. (2014). Going deeper with convolutions. In *2014 IEEE 12th International Conference on Computer Vision.*
69. He, K., Zhang, X., Ren, S., & Sun, J. (2015). Spatial pyramid pooling in deep convolutional networks for visual recognition. *IEEE Transactions on Pattern Analysis and Machine Intelligence, 37*(9), 1904–1916.
70. Jaderberg, M., Simonyan, K., & Zisserman, A. (2015). Spatial transformer networks. In *Advances in Neural Information Processing Systems* (pp. 2017–2025).
71. Girshick, R., Donahue, J., Darrell, T., Malik, J. (2014). Rich feature hierarchies for accurate object detection and semantic segmentation. In *Proceedings of the IEEE Conference on Computer Vision and Pattern Recognition* (pp. 580–587).
72. Ashraf, R., Habib, M. A., Akram, M., Latif, M. A., Malik, M. S. A., Awais, M., et al. (2020). Deep convolution neural network for big data medical image classification. *IEEE Access, 8,* 105659–105670.
73. Zhu, Q., Du, B., & Yan, P. (2019). Boundary-weighted domain adaptive neural network for prostate MR image segmentation. *IEEE Transactions on Medical Imaging, 39*(3), 753–763.
74. Zhu, Q., Du, B., Yan, P., Lu, H., & Zhang, L. (2018). Shape prior constrained PSO model for bladder wall MRI segmentation. *Neurocomputing, 294,* 19–28.
75. Zhu, Q., Du, B., Turkbey, B., Choyke, P., Yan, P. (2018). Exploiting interslice correlation for MRI prostate image segmentation, from recursive neural networks aspect. *Complexity, 2018.*
76. Kumar, K. K., & Gopal, T. V. (2014, March). A novel approach to self order feature reweighting in CBIR to reduce semantic gap using Relevance Feedback. In *2014 International Conference on Circuits, Power and Computing Technologies [ICCPCT-2014]* (pp. 1437–1442). IEEE.
77. Ashraf, R., Bajwa, K. B., & Mahmood, T. (2016). Content-based image retrieval by exploring bandletized regions through support vector machines. *Journal of Information Science and Engineering, 32*(2), 245–269.
78. Wan, J., Wang, D., Hoi, S. C. H., Wu, P., Zhu, J., Zhang, Y., Li, J. (2014, November). Deep learning for content-based image retrieval: A comprehensive study. In *Proceedings of the 22nd ACM International Conference on Multimedia* (pp. 157–166).
79. Shaukat, F., Raja, G., Ashraf, R., Khalid, S., Ahmad, M., & Ali, A. (2019). Artificial neural network based classification of lung nodules in CT images using intensity, shape and texture features. *Journal of Ambient Intelligence and Humanized Computing, 10*(10), 4135–4149.
80. Karpathy, A., Toderici, G., Shetty, S., Leung, T., Sukthankar, R., Fei-Fei, L. (2014). Large-scale video classification with convolutional neural networks. In *Proceedings of the IEEE conference on Computer Vision and Pattern Recognition* (pp. 1725–1732).
81. Wu, G., Lu, W., Gao, G., Zhao, C., & Liu, J. (2016). Regional deep learning model for visual tracking. *Neurocomputing, 175,* 310–323.
82. Hinton, G., Deng, L., Yu, D., Dahl, G. E., Mohamed, A. R., Jaitly, N., et al. (2012). Deep neural networks for acoustic modeling in speech recognition: The shared views of four research groups. *IEEE Signal Processing Magazine, 29*(6), 82–97.
83. Zhou, S., Chen, Q., & Wang, X. (2013). Active deep learning method for semi-supervised sentiment classification. *Neurocomputing, 120,* 536–546.
84. Shi, H. Y., Xie, J., & Miao, F. (2015). Pancreatic carcinosarcoma: First literature report on computed tomography imaging. *World Journal of Gastroenterology: WJG, 21*(4), 1357.
85. Zare, M. R., Mueen, A., & Seng, W. C. (2013). Automatic classification of medical X-ray images using a bag of visual words. *IET Computer Vision, 7*(2), 105–114.
86. Khan, S., Yong, S. P., & Deng, J. D. (2015, November). Ensemble classification with modified sift descriptor for medical image modality. In *2015 International Conference on Image and Vision Computing New Zealand (IVCNZ)* (pp. 1–6). IEEE.

87. Cireşan, D. C., Giusti, A., Gambardella, L. M., & Schmidhuber, J. (2013, September). Mitosis detection in breast cancer histology images with deep neural networks. In *International Conference on Medical Image Computing and Computer-Assisted Intervention* (pp. 411–418). Springer.
88. Kanerva, P. (2009). Hyperdimensional computing: An introduction to computing in distributed representation with high-dimensional random vectors. *Cognitive Computation, 1*(2), 139–159.
89. Yilmaz, O. (2015). Machine learning using cellular automata based feature expansion and reservoir computing. *Journal of Cellular Automata, 10.*
90. Cheng, D., Meng, G., Cheng, G., & Pan, C. (2016). SeNet: Structured edge network for sea–land segmentation. *IEEE Geoscience and Remote Sensing Letters, 14*(2), 247–251.
91. Chen, P., Song, Y., Yuan, D., & Liu, Z. (2019). Feature fusion adversarial learning network for liver lesion classification. In *Proceedings of the ACM Multimedia Asia* (pp. 1–7).
92. Bengio, Y., Lamblin, P., Popovici, D., & Larochelle, H. (2006). Greedy layer-wise training of deep networks. *Advances in Neural Information Processing Systems, 19,* 153–160.
93. Litjens, G., Kooi, T., Bejnordi, B. E., Setio, A. A. A., Ciompi, F., Ghafoorian, M., et al. (2017). A survey on deep learning in medical image analysis. *Medical Image Analysis, 42,* 60–88.
94. Al-Hadhrami, S., Altuwaijri, S., Alkharashi, N., & Ouni, R. (2019, May). Deep classification technique for density counting. In *2019 2nd International Conference on Computer Applications & Information Security (ICCAIS)* (pp. 1–6). IEEE.
95. Ashraf, R., Ahmed, M., Ahmad, U., Habib, M. A., Jabbar, S., & Naseer, K. (2020). MDCBIR-MF: multimedia data for content-based image retrieval by using multiple features. *Multimedia Tools and Applications, 79*(13), 8553–8579.
96. Szegedy, C., Liu, W., Jia, Y., Sermanet, P., Reed, S., Anguelov, D., Erhan, D., Vanhoucke, V., Rabinovich, A. (2015). Going deeper with convolutions. In *Proceedings of the IEEE Conference on Computer Vision and Pattern Recognition* (pp. 1–9).
97. He, K., Zhang, X., Ren, S., Sun, J. (2016). Deep residual learning for image recognition. In *Proceedings of the IEEE Conference on Computer Vision and Pattern Recognition* (pp. 770–778).
98. Ashraf, R., Ahmed, M., Jabbar, S., Khalid, S., Ahmad, A., Din, S., et al. (2018). Content based image retrieval by using color descriptor and discrete wavelet transform. *Journal of Medical Systems, 42*(3), 44.
99. Liu, Y., Gadepalli, K., Norouzi, M., Dahl, G. E., Kohlberger, T., Boyko, A., Venugopalan, S., Timofeev, A., Nelson, P. Q., Corrado, G. S., & Hipp, J. D. (2017). *Detecting cancer metastases on gigapixel pathology images.* arXiv preprint arXiv:1703.02442.
100. Esteva, A., Kuprel, B., Novoa, R. A., Ko, J., Swetter, S. M., Blau, H. M., et al. (2017). Dermatologist-level classification of skin cancer with deep neural networks. *Nature, 542*(7639), 115–118.
101. Kamnitsas, K., Ledig, C., Newcombe, V. F., Simpson, J. P., Kane, A. D., Menon, D. K., et al. (2017). Efficient multi-scale 3D CNN with fully connected CRF for accurate brain lesion segmentation. *Medical Image Analysis, 36,* 61–78.
102. Ashraf, R., Bashir, K., Irtaza, A., & Mahmood, M. T. (2015). Content based image retrieval using embedded neural networks with bandletized regions. *Entropy, 17*(6), 3552–3580.
103. Moeskops, P., Viergever, M. A., Mendrik, A. M., De Vries, L. S., Benders, M. J., & Išgum, I. (2016). Automatic segmentation of MR brain images with convolutional neural network. *IEEE Transactions on Medical Imaging, 35*(5), 1252–1261.
104. Prasoon, A., Petersen, K., Igel, C., Lauze, F., Dam, E., & Nielsen, M. (2013, September). Deep feature learning for knee cartilage segmentation using a triplanar convolutional neural network. In *International Conference on Medical Image Computing and Computer-Assisted Intervention* (pp. 246–253). Springer.
105. Antony, J., McGuinness, K., O'Connor, N. E., & Moran, K. (2016, December). Quantifying radiographic knee osteoarthritis severity using deep convolutional neural networks. In *2016 23rd International Conference on Pattern Recognition (ICPR)* (pp. 1195–1200). IEEE.
106. Brosch, T., Tam, R., & Alzheimer's Disease Neuroimaging Initiative. (2013, September). Manifold learning of brain MRIs by deep learning. In *International Conference on Medical Image Computing and Computer-Assisted Intervention* (pp. 633–640). Springer.

107. Plis, S. M., Hjelm, D. R., Salakhutdinov, R., Allen, E. A., Bockholt, H. J., Long, J. D., et al. (2014). Deep learning for neuroimaging: a validation study. *Frontiers in neuroscience, 8,* 229.
108. Shin, H. C., Orton, M. R., Collins, D. J., Doran, S. J., & Leach, M. O. (2012). Stacked autoencoders for unsupervised feature learning and multiple organ detection in a pilot study using 4D patient data. *IEEE Transactions on Pattern Analysis and Machine Intelligence, 35*(8), 1930–1943.
109. Suk, H. I., Lee, S. W., Shen, D., & Alzheimer's Disease Neuroimaging Initiative. (2014). Hierarchical feature representation and multimodal fusion with deep learning for AD/MCI diagnosis. *NeuroImage, 101,* 569–582.
110. Menegola, A., Fornaciali, M., Pires, R., Avila, S., Valle, E. (2016). *Towards automated melanoma screening: Exploring transfer learning schemes.* arXiv preprint arXiv:1609.01228.
111. Hoffman, A. J., & Singleton, R. R. (1960). On Moore graphs with diameters 2 and 3. *IBM Journal of Research and Development, 4*(5), 497–504.
112. Payan, A., & Montana, G. (2015). *Predicting Alzheimer's disease: A neuroimaging study with 3D convolutional neural networks.* arXiv preprint arXiv:1502.02506.
113. Kawahara, J., Brown, C. J., Miller, S. P., Booth, B. G., Chau, V., Grunau, R. E., et al. (2017). BrainNetCNN: Convolutional neural networks for brain networks; towards predicting neurodevelopment. *NeuroImage, 146,* 1038–1049.
114. Wang, F., Jiang, M., Qian, C., Yang, S., Li, C., Zhang, H., Wang, X., & Tang, X. (2017). Residual attention network for image classification. In *Proceedings of the IEEE conference on computer vision and pattern recognition* (pp. 3156–3164).
115. Shen, W., Zhou, M., Yang, F., Yang, C. and Tian, J., 2015, June. Multi-scale convolutional neural networks for lung nodule classification. In *International Conference on Information Processing in Medical Imaging* (pp. 588–599). Springer, Cham.
116. Gao, X., Lin, S., & Wong, T. Y. (2015). Automatic feature learning to grade nuclear cataracts based on deep learning. *IEEE Transactions on Biomedical Engineering, 62*(11), 2693–2701.
117. Nie, D., Zhang, H., Adeli, E., Liu, L., & Shen, D. (2016, October). 3D deep learning for multi-modal imaging-guided survival time prediction of brain tumor patients. In *International Conference on Medical Image Computing and Computer-Assisted Intervention* (pp. 212–220). Springer, Cham.
118. van Tulder, G., & de Bruijne, M. (2016). Combining generative and discriminative representation learning for lung CT analysis with convolutional restricted Boltzmann machines. *IEEE Transactions on Medical Imaging, 35*(5), 1262–1272.
119. Zhang, Q., Xiao, Y., Dai, W., Suo, J., Wang, C., Shi, J., et al. (2016). Deep learning based classification of breast tumors with shear-wave elastography. *Ultrasonics, 72,* 150–157.
120. Kallenberg, M., Petersen, K., Nielsen, M., Ng, A. Y., Diao, P., Igel, C., et al. (2016). Unsupervised deep learning applied to breast density segmentation and mammographic risk scoring. *IEEE Transactions on Medical Imaging, 35*(5), 1322–1331.
121. Xu, Y., Mo, T., Feng, Q., Zhong, P., Lai, M., Eric, I., & Chang, C. (2014, May). Deep learning of feature representation with multiple instance learning for medical image analysis. In *2014 IEEE International Conference on Acoustics, Speech and Signal Processing (ICASSP)* (pp. 1626–1630). IEEE.
122. Lim, K. J., Choi, C. S., Yoon, D. Y., Chang, S. K., Kim, K. K., Han, H., et al. (2008). Computer-aided diagnosis for the differentiation of malignant from benign thyroid nodules on ultrasonography. *Academic radiology, 15*(7), 853–858.
123. Savelonas, M. A., Maroulis, D. E., Iakovidis, D. K., & Dimitropoulos, N. (2008, August). Computer-aided malignancy risk assessment of nodules in thyroid US images utilizing boundary descriptors. In *2008 Panhellenic Conference on Informatics* (pp. 157–160). IEEE.
124. Iakovidis, D. K., Keramidas, E. G., & Maroulis, D. (2010). Fusion of fuzzy statistical distributions for classification of thyroid ultrasound patterns. *Artificial Intelligence in Medicine, 50*(1), 33–41.
125. Legakis, I., Savelonas, M. A., Maroulis, D., & Iakovidis, D. K. (2011). Computer-based nodule malignancy risk assessment in thyroid ultrasound images. *International Journal of Computers and Applications, 33*(1), 29–35.

126. Acharya, U. R., Sree, S. V., Swapna, G., Gupta, S., Molinari, F., Garberoglio, R., et al. (2013). Effect of complex wavelet transform filter on thyroid tumor classification in three-dimensional ultrasound. *Proceedings of the Institution of Mechanical Engineers. Part H, Journal of Engineering in Medicine, 227*(3), 284–292.
127. Zhang, F., Cai, N., Wu, J., Cen, G., Wang, H., & Chen, X. (2018). Image denoising method based on a deep convolution neural network. *IET Image Processing, 12*(4), 485–493.
128. Osher, S., Burger, M., Goldfarb, D., Xu, J., & Yin, W. (2005). An iterative regularization method for total variation-based image restoration. *Multiscale Modeling & Simulation, 4*(2), 460–489.
129. Elad, M., & Aharon, M. (2006). Image denoising via sparse and redundant representations over learned dictionaries. *IEEE Transactions on Image Processing, 15*(12), 3736–3745.
130. Mairal, J., Bach, F., Ponce, J., Sapiro, G., Zisserman, A. (2009, September). Non-local sparse models for image restoration. In *2009 IEEE 12th International Conference on Computer Vision* (pp. 2272–2279). IEEE.
131. Dong, W., Zhang, L., Shi, G., & Li, X. (2012). Nonlocally centralized sparse representation for image restoration. *IEEE Transactions on Image Processing, 22*(4), 1620–1630.
132. Xu, J., Zhang, L., Zuo, W., Zhang, D., & Feng, X. (2015). Patch group based nonlocal self-similarity prior learning for image denoising. In *Proceedings of the IEEE International Conference on Computer Vision* (pp. 244–252).
133. Dabov, K., Foi, A., Katkovnik, V., & Egiazarian, K. (2007). Image denoising by sparse 3-D transform-domain collaborative filtering. *IEEE Transactions on Image Processing, 16*(8), 2080–2095.
134. Ji, H., Liu, C., Shen, Z., Xu, Y. (2010, June). Robust video denoising using low rank matrix completion. In *2010 IEEE Computer Society Conference on Computer Vision and Pattern Recognition* (pp. 1791–1798). IEEE.
135. Gu, S., Zhang, L., Zuo, W., & Feng, X. (2014). Weighted nuclear norm minimization with application to image denoising. In *Proceedings of the IEEE Conference on Computer Vision and Pattern Recognition* (pp. 2862–2869).
136. Luo, E., Chan, S. H., & Nguyen, T. Q. (2016). Adaptive image denoising by mixture adaptation. *IEEE Transactions on Image Processing, 25*(10), 4489–4503.
137. Chen, F., Zhang, L., & Yu, H. (2015). External patch prior guided internal clustering for image denoising. In *Proceedings of the IEEE International Conference on Computer Vision* (pp. 603–611).
138. Xie, Y., Gu, S., Liu, Y., Zuo, W., Zhang, W., & Zhang, L. (2016). Weighted Schatten $ p $-norm minimization for image denoising and background subtraction. *IEEE Transactions on Image Processing, 25*(10), 4842–4857.
139. Chen, Y., & Pock, T. (2016). Trainable nonlinear reaction diffusion: A flexible framework for fast and effective image restoration. *IEEE Transactions on Pattern Analysis and Machine Intelligence, 39*(6), 1256–1272.
140. Jain, V., & Seung, S. (2008). Natural image denoising with convolutional networks. *Advances in Neural Information Processing Systems, 21*, 769–776.
141. Burger, H. C., Schuler, C. J., & Harmeling, S. (2012, June). Image denoising: Can plain neural networks compete with BM3D?. In *2012 IEEE Conference on Computer Vision and Pattern Recognition* (pp. 2392–2399). IEEE.
142. Wang, X., Tao, Q., Wang, L., Li, D., & Zhang, M. (2015, October). Deep convolutional architecture for natural image denoising. In *2015 International Conference on Wireless Communications & Signal Processing (WCSP)* (pp. 1–4). IEEE.
143. Huang, D. A., Kang, L. W., Wang, Y. C. F., & Lin, C. W. (2013). Self-learning based image decomposition with applications to single image denoising. *IEEE Transactions on Multimedia, 16*(1), 83–93.
144. Szegedy, C., Ioffe, S., Vanhoucke, V.,& Alemi, A. (2016). *Inception-v4, inception-resnet and the impact of residual connections on learning*. arXiv preprint arXiv:1602.07261.
145. Jia, Y., Shelhamer, E., Donahue, J., Karayev, S., Long, J., Girshick, R., Guadarrama, S., & Darrell, T. (2014, November). Caffe: Convolutional architecture for fast feature embedding. In *Proceedings of the 22nd ACM International Conference on Multimedia* (pp. 675–678).

146. Simonyan, K., & Zisserman, A. (2014). *Very deep convolutional networks for large-scale image recognition*. arXiv preprint arXiv:1409.1556.
147. Yang, J., Wright, J., Huang, T. S., & Ma, Y. (2010). Image super-resolution via sparse representation. *IEEE Transactions on Image Processing, 19*(11), 2861–2873.
148. Kumar, G. R., Kumar, R. K., & Sanyal, G. (2017, July). Facial emotion analysis using deep convolution neural network. In *2017 International Conference on Signal Processing and Communication (ICSPC)* (pp. 369–374). IEEE.
149. Shan, C., Gong, S., & McOwan, P. W. (2009). Facial expression recognition based on local binary patterns: A comprehensive study. *Image and Vision Computing, 27*(6), 803–816.
150. Mian, A., Bennamoun, M., & Owens, R. (2007). An efficient multimodal 2D-3D hybrid approach to automatic face recognition. *IEEE Transactions on Pattern Analysis and Machine Intelligence, 29*(11), 1927–1943.
151. Sebe, N., Cohen, I., Gevers, T., & Huang, T. S. (2006, August). Emotion recognition based on joint visual and audio cues. In *18th International Conference on Pattern Recognition (ICPR'06)* (Vol. 1, pp. 1136–1139). IEEE.
152. Liu, M., Wang, R., Li, S., Shan, S., Huang, Z. and Chen, X., 2014, November. Combining multiple kernel methods on riemannian manifold for emotion recognition in the wild. In *Proceedings of the 16th International Conference on multimodal interaction* (pp. 494–501).
153. Viola, P., & Jones, M. J. (2004). Robust real-time face detection. *International Journal of Computer Vision, 57*(2), 137–154.
154. Viola, P., & Jones, M. (2001, December). Rapid object detection using a boosted cascade of simple features. In *Proceedings of the 2001 IEEE Computer Society Conference on Computer Vision and Pattern Recognition. CVPR 2001* (Vol. 1, pp. I–I). IEEE.
155. Lucey, P., Cohn, J. F., Kanade, T., Saragih, J., Ambadar, Z., & Matthews, I. (2010, June). The extended cohn-kanade dataset (ck +): A complete dataset for action unit and emotion-specified expression. In *2010 IEEE Computer Society Conference on Computer Vision and Pattern Recognition-Workshops* (pp. 94–101). IEEE.
156. Fu, R., Li, B., Gao, Y., & Wang, P. (2016, October). Content-based image retrieval based on CNN and SVM. In *2016 2nd IEEE International Conference on Computer and Communications (ICCC)* (pp. 638–642). IEEE.
157. Hu, K., Dong, Y., & Bai, H. (2016, November). Multi-level convolutional channel features for content-based image retrieval. In *2016 Visual Communications and Image Processing (VCIP)* (pp. 1–4). IEEE.
158. Varga, D., & Szirányi, T. (2016, October). Fast content-based image retrieval using convolutional neural network and hash function. In *2016 IEEE International Conference on Systems, Man, and Cybernetics (SMC)* (pp. 002636–002640). IEEE.
159. Liu, X., Tizhoosh, H. R., & Kofman, J. (2016, July). Generating binary tags for fast medical image retrieval based on convolutional nets and radon transform. In *2016 International Joint Conference on Neural Networks (IJCNN)* (pp. 2872–2878). IEEE.
160. Muneesawang, P., & Guan, L. (2001, October). A neural network approach for learning image similarity in adaptive CBIR. In *2001 IEEE Fourth Workshop on Multimedia Signal Processing (Cat. No. 01TH8564)* (pp. 257–262). IEEE.
161. Yap, K. H., & Wu, K. (2005, July). Fuzzy relevance feedback in content-based image retrieval systems using radial basis function network. In *2005 IEEE International Conference on Multimedia and Expo* (pp. 4). IEEE.
162. Li, J., & Wang, J. Z. (2003). Automatic linguistic indexing of pictures by a statistical modeling approach. *IEEE Transactions on Pattern Analysis and Machine Intelligence, 25*(9), 1075–1088.
163. Wang, J. Z., Li, J., & Wiederhold, G. (2001). SIMPLIcity: Semantics-sensitive integrated matching for picture libraries. *IEEE Transactions on Pattern Analysis and Machine Intelligence, 23*(9), 947–963.
164. Szegedy, C., Vanhoucke, V., Ioffe, S., Shlens, J., & Wojna, Z. (2016). Rethinking the inception architecture for computer vision. In *Proceedings of the IEEE Conference on Computer Vision and Pattern Recognition* (pp. 2818–2826).

165. He, K., Zhang, X., Ren, S., & Sun, J. (2016). Deep residual learning for image recognition. In *Proceedings of the IEEE Conference on Computer Vision and Pattern Recognition* (pp. 770–778).
166. Szegedy, C., Ioffe, S., Vanhoucke, V., & Alemi, A. (2016). *Inception-v4, inception-resnet and the impact of residual connections on learning*. arXiv preprint arXiv:1602.07261.
167. Nguyen, L. D., Lin, D., Lin, Z., & Cao, J. (2018, May). Deep CNNs for microscopic image classification by exploiting transfer learning and feature concatenation. In *2018 IEEE International Symposium on Circuits and Systems (ISCAS)* (pp. 1–5). IEEE.
168. Hemdan, E. E. D., Shouman, M. A., & Karar, M. E. (2020). *Covidx-net: A framework of deep learning classifiers to diagnose covid-19 in x-ray images*. arXiv preprint arXiv:2003.11055.
169. Xiao, J., Wang, J., Cao, S., & Li, B. (2020, April). Application of a novel and improved VGG-19 network in the detection of workers wearing masks. *Journal of Physics: Conference Series, 1518*(1), 012041. IOP Publishing.
170. Bhavani, R., Prakash, V., Kumaresh, R. V., & Sundra Srinivasan, R. (2019) Vision-based skin disease identification using deep learning. *International Journal of Engineering and Advanced Technology (IJEAT) 8*(6). https://doi.org/10.35940/ijeat.f9391.088619. ISSN: 2249 – 8958.
171. Sae-Lim, W., Wettayaprasit, W., & Aiyarak, P. (2019, July). Convolutional neural networks using MobileNet for skin lesion classification. In *2019 16th International Joint Conference on Computer Science and Software Engineering (JCSSE)* (pp. 242–247). IEEE.
172. Howard, A. G., Zhu, M., Chen, B., Kalenichenko, D., Wang, W., Weyand, T., Andreetto, M., & Mobilenets, H. A. (2017). *Efficient convolutional neural networks for mobile vision applications*. arXiv preprint arXiv:1704.04861.
173. Apostolopoulos, I. D., & Mpesiana, T. A. (2020). Covid-19: automatic detection from x-ray images utilizing transfer learning with convolutional neural networks. *Physical and Engineering Sciences in Medicine*, p. 1.
174. COVID-19 X rays (X rays and CT snapshots of CONVID-19 patients) https://www.kaggle.com/andrewmvd/convid19-x-rays. Last accessed August 11, 2020.
175. Kermany, D. S., Goldbaum, M., Cai, W., Valentim, C. C., Liang, H., Baxter, S. L., et al. (2018). Identifying medical diagnoses and treatable diseases by image-based deep learning. *Cell, 172*(5), 1122–1131.
176. Narin, A., Kaya, C., & Pamuk, Z. (2020). *Automatic detection of coronavirus disease (covid-19) using x-ray images and deep convolutional neural networks*. arXiv preprint arXiv:2003.10849.
177. Apostolopoulos, I. D., & Mpesiana, T. A. (2020). Covid-19: automatic detection from x-ray images utilizing transfer learning with convolutional neural networks. *Physical and Engineering Sciences in Medicine*, p. 1.

A Travelling Disinfection-Man Problem (TDP) for COVID-19: A Nonlinear Binary Constrained Gaining-Sharing Knowledge-Based Optimization Algorithm

Said Ali Hassan, Prachi Agrawal, Talari Ganesh, and Ali Wagdy Mohamed

A newly arrived problem which is call the travelling disinfection-man problem (TDP) in network is defined for a disinfection group who want to settle on the foremost effective route for disinfection of several candidate places. The group begins from a predetermined position and next wants to go to each infected place exactly once within the day working time. The target of the TDP is to maximize the utilization of daily available time calculated as the total active disinfection time minus the total wasted travelling time between places in the chosen route. This definition is somewhat resembling that the problem of travelling salesman (TSP) and its variations with some basic indicated differences.

The second section includes useful information about the new coronavirus (COVID-19). This information covers the COVID-19 outbreak world map, geographic risk assessment for COVID-19 transmission, the total cases and deaths of coronavirus worldwide, and the growth factor for every day new cases.

Section 3 is devoted to demonstrating the coronavirus decontamination planning process to increase the efficiency of purification and decontamination operation and minimizing any unneeded costs according to the latest WHO instructions to combat the coronavirus and limit its spreading.

S. A. Hassan
Department of Operations Research and Decision Support, Faculty of Computers and Artificial Intelligence, Cairo University, Giza, Egypt

P. Agrawal · T. Ganesh
Department of Mathematics and Scientific Computing, National Institute of Technology Hamirpur, Himachal Pradesh Hamirpur 177005, India

A. W. Mohamed (✉)
Operations Research Department, Faculty of Graduate Studies for Statistical Research, Cairo University, Giza 12613, Egypt

Wireless Intelligent Networks Center (WINC), School of Engineering and Applied Sciences, Nile University, Giza, Egypt

M. Niranjanamurthy et al. (eds.), *Intelligent Data Analysis for COVID-19 Pandemic*, Algorithms for Intelligent Systems, https://doi.org/10.1007/978-981-16-1574-0_13

Section 4 introduces the new coronavirus travelling disinfection-man problem (TDP). As universities are considered one of the important gathering places that must be cleaned and disinfected perfectly, a number of faculties will be chosen as a real application for the application of the TDP. The main differences between TDP and TSP are also revealed in this section.

Section 5 presents a concise review of the problem of travelling salesman and related variations like: the problem of travelling salesman with priority prizes, deliveries and collections, pickup and delivery, backhauls, multiple depots, specifications of salesmen number, and problems with time windows and that with fixed charges. It deals also with problems of multiple travelling salesman, generalized travelling salesman, generalized vehicle routing, and travelling repairman one.

The mathematical model of a travelling disinfection-man problem is designed in Sect. 6 including all needed formulations. The model proposed is a nonlinear binary one with a dimension that depends on the number of places to be disinfected, and the details of the solution procedure are also shown.

A real case study for Ain Shams University in Cairo is explained in Sect. 7; its complete mathematical model is formulated including the binary decision variables, constraints comprising positions, places, sequencing route positions and working hours/day, and the objective function.

In Sect. 8, a novel discrete binary version of a recently developed gaining-sharing knowledge-based technique (GSK) is presented for solving the TDP. GSK cannot solve the problem with discrete binary space; therefore, discrete binary-GSK optimization algorithm (DBGSK) is proposed with two new discrete binary junior and senior stages. These stages allow DBGSK to inspect the problem search space efficiently.

Section 9 represents the experimental results of TDP obtained by DBGSK, and Sects. 10 and 11 give the main conclusions and the proposed points for future researches, respectively.

1 Coronavirus (COVID-19): An Overview

Nowadays, the whole world is distressed with the COVID-19 epidemic which has affected millions of persons in almost all countries [1]. In December last year, Wuhan, in China, was the origin of a pneumonia of unknown cause. Cases of COVID-19 are not limited to this city, and by January in this year, assured cases were detected outside Wuhan [2].

Nowadays, the newly emerged COVID-19 put people in all countries in face of the huge hazard. To safeguard against the pandemic, centres of virus disinfection recommend various safe measures among them to stay at home except in case of severe necessity. The Centres for Diseases Control and Prevention (CDC) declares the main symptoms of coronavirus so that people can discover clearly these signs [3, 4].

The risk in these diseases is that there is no vaccine for treatment; yet, antibiotics will not help with them. The matter is further complicated by the fact that the incubation period of the virus is up to 14 days; therefore, officials of the examination at airports and other examination places will not be able to discover all the possible patients carrying the disease.

Figure 1 displays the number of confirmed infected cases with the new coronavirus as of 2 April 2020; from the map, it is clear that all countries suffer from the virus attack, taking into consideration that it is a vast evolving case, and new situation changes may not be represented at once [5]. The confirmed number in Egypt is moderate till now. Egypt reported 850 cases, 52 deaths and 179 recoveries on 2020–04-2, but numbers are expected to increase exponentially as new cases are discovered and since the daily increasing rate is about 12% [6].

The greatest risk also lies in travelling from one country to another, and the following map shows that the risks of travel recently include all countries of the world, including Egypt as of 2 April 2020, as shown in Fig. 2 [7]. Figure 3 shows the worldwide total cases and deaths of coronavirus indicated as of 3 April 2020, coronavirus cases: 1,016,310; deaths: 53,236 and recovered: 213,126 [8].

Figure 4 presents the growth factor of daily new cases as of 3 April 2020, which is the factor by which a value multiplies itself in the future periods. As an example, increasing with 9% every day has a growth factor of 1.09. A growth in the range 0 to 1 is an indication of decreasing, whereas a growth rate permanently bigger than 1 may indicate an exponentially growth, [9]. Nowadays, it is shown that the growth factor is above 1 indicating that daily new cases multiply itself over time. Figure 3

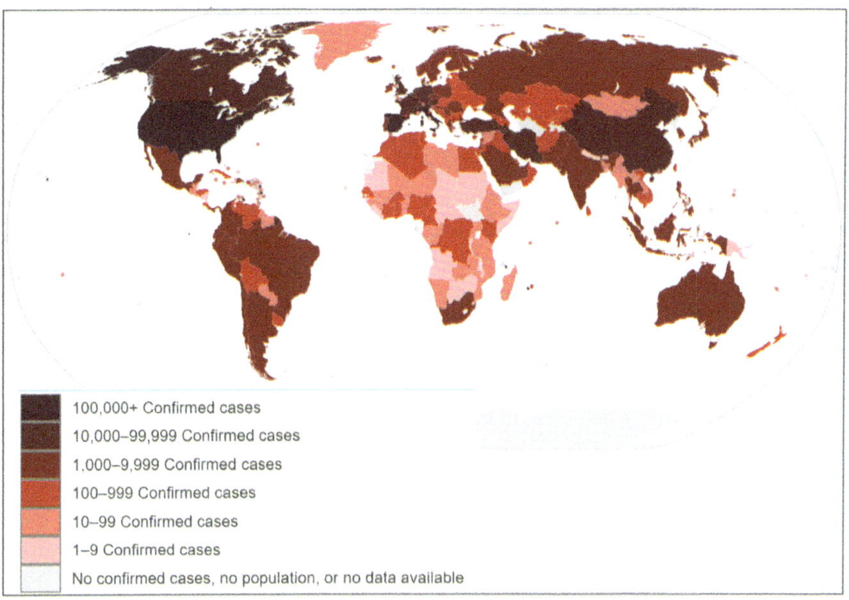

Fig. 1 COVID-19 outbreak world map

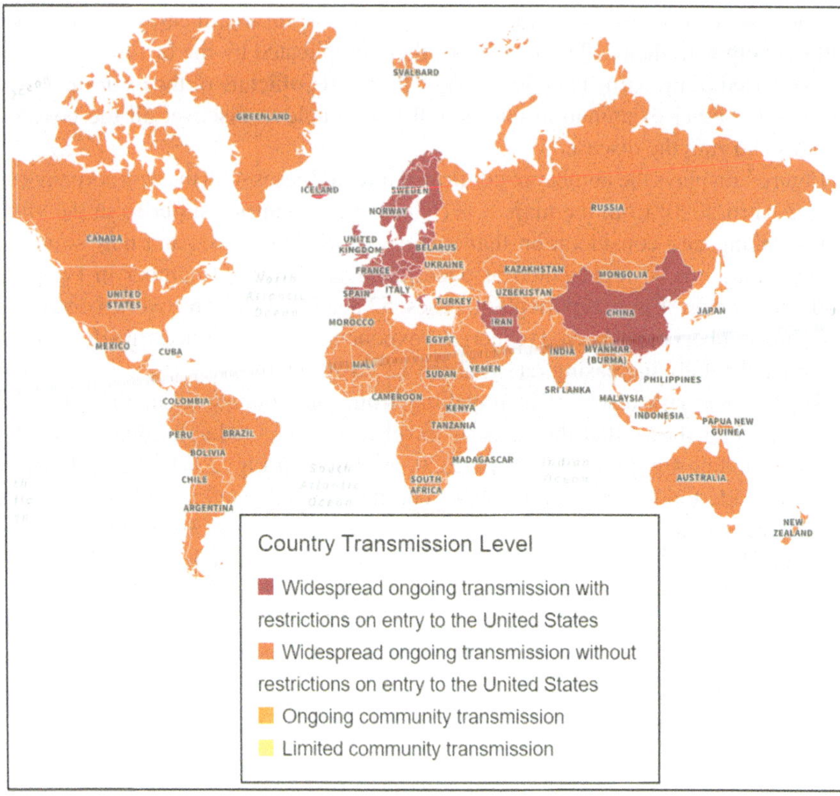

Fig. 2 Geographic risk assessment for COVID-19 transmission

and 4 indicate clearly that the current and the near future situations are not quite right in such a way that foreshadows a catastrophe for most of the countries of the world, including Egypt, if the situation continues as it is now and if strict measures are not taken at the level of governments and peoples, including disinfection of places where large crowds of people gather, including educational institutions.

The rate of the virus spreading affirmed by its reproductive number, represented by the mean number of people for whom one infected person will transmit the disease. It is evaluated in various ranges to be between 1.4 and 5.0 [10].

2 Coronavirus Decontamination Planning Process

It is understood that the disclosure to the severe virus COVID-19 in an education institution like any other firm effects the morale of all concerned people.

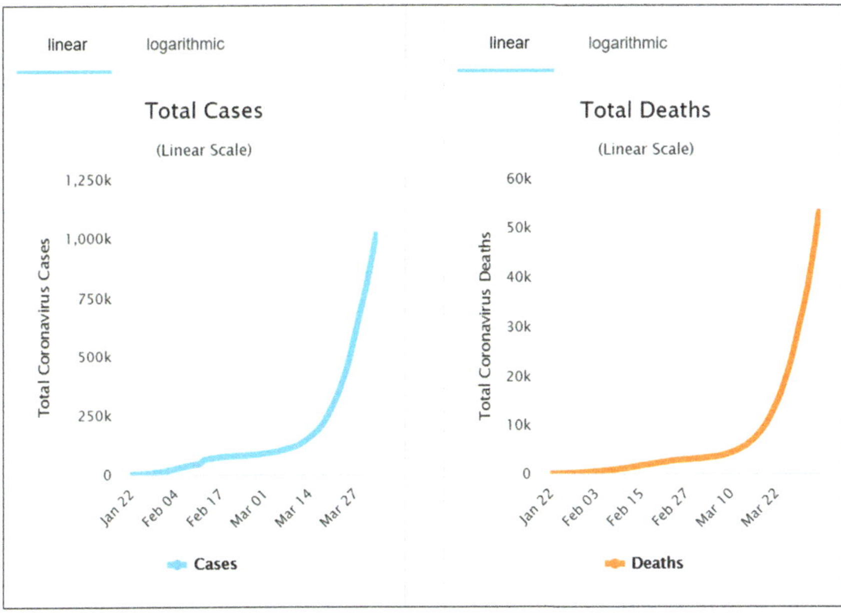

Fig. 3 Total cases and deaths of coronavirus worldwide

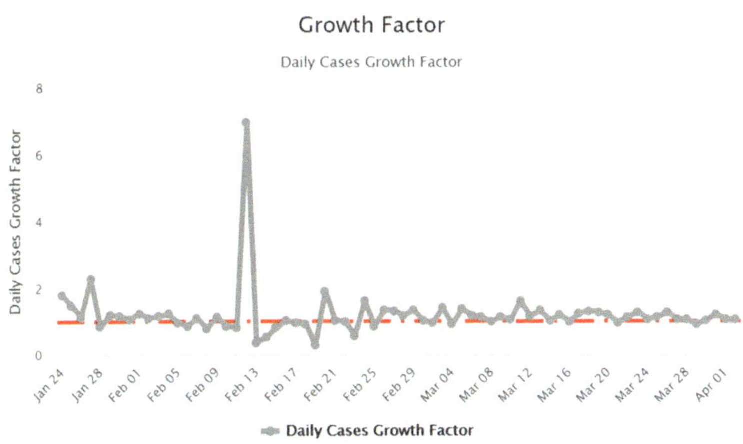

Fig. 4 Growth factor of daily new cases

When anyone is infected with coronavirus, all those in contact with him and his place are fertile to transmit the disease to others. Therefore, disinfection procedures according to the strict procedures announced by the Centres of Disease Control and Prevention website [11] should be taken into consideration wherever the cases of coronavirus infection appear.

An appropriate procedure should be developed, such a protocol involves particular steps to be performed and experts who experience in doing so [12]. The standards of cleaning and disinfection protocols include the thorough cleaning process to remove dirt and impurities including germs and viruses, but this does not kill viruses but removes them and therefore any risk of infection spreading still exists. The cleaning process is followed by disinfection using appropriate chemicals to kill the virus on surfaces that have been exposed to people infected or suspected to be infected with the coronavirus to reduce any risk of spreading the infection. Cleaning the contaminated surfaces in a good way, followed by disinfection, is one of the best practices for preventing from coronavirus. This method aims to reduce the virus's survival in the place where the infection cases appeared.

The disinfection teams consist of specialists and technicians who are well versed in cleaning and disinfection services [13]. Also, each decontamination member of the team has engaged in several specialized training courses in protection and disinfection. The group specialists maintain the World Health Organization (WHO) instructions concerning coronavirus guidance for health workers [13].

Modern cleaning and disinfection equipment and effective materials of international quality are used to ensure the highest levels of decontamination. This is performed according to the latest WHO instructions to combat the coronavirus and limit its spreading.

The decontamination process is to be sure of reducing the possibility of the offices, classrooms, facilities, instruments and equipment from being contaminated. Surfaces and objects that are frequently touched by the staff members, students, employees or visitors at buildings may include: doors and door handles; keyboards and desks; seating areas; sinks and sink handles; handrails; drinking fountains; touch screens; all bathroom surfaces; refrigerators copiers and printers; food service areas; desks; tables and counters and many others [14].

3 Coronavirus Travelling Disinfection-Man Problem (TDP)

A new defined problem which we will call coronavirus travelling disinfection problem (TDP) in network optimization is defined for a cleaning and disinfection group members who want to choose the most effective route for approaching several candidate institutions located in different predetermined places. The group begins in a starting point, say the Egyptian Ministry of Health and Population in Cairo, and next wants to transport to some chosen subset institutions each one quite once during a predetermined time window. The aim of the TDP is to choose precisely a route to maximize the actual working hours in the places (institutions), while in the same time, minimizing the total transportation times between different institutions.

The introduced TDP has a variety of applications in many ministries, government establishments, factories, institutions, places, merchandises, wholesales, stores and many other places. As universities are considered one of the important gathering places that must be cleaned and disinfected perfectly, a number of faculties will be chosen as a real case for application of the suggested TDP.

In education institutions, standard procedures for cleaning and disinfection must be followed, usually, this means sterilizing surfaces and everyday objects that are touched offices, halls, workshops, laboratories, bathrooms, such as work surfaces, stands, doors, computer keyboard, practical training tools, tap handles, phones and other objects. Some institutions may also require more intensive disinfection process according to the standard protocols.

It is the responsibility of the cleaning and disinfection group for education institutions to know what circumstances are in the place that affecting negatively on the staff members, students, employees and even the public. Risk estimation helps defining what is required to be performed in an improved way. The task is to be scheduled and carried out by specialized groups in such a way to do the job technically perfect and in the same time to save unnecessary time and costs.

The definition of the travelling disinfection-man problem (TDP) is somewhat like that of the travelling salesman problem (TSP) and its variants. That proximity is useful for creating the mathematical model for the new proposed problem (TDP). TDP differs from the famous and well-known TSP in these major points:

(1) In the TSP, the time window is open until finishing the visits of all customers, while in the TDP, the available time is bounded by the determined working time window.

(2) In the TSP, the salesman will reach all customers, while in the TDP, the disinfection-man will choose a route composed of some or all the places which improve the utilization of the available predetermined time within the available limits.

(3) In the TSP, the time consumed in customer places is immaterial, while in the TDP, the disinfection time is a basic element influencing the chosen objective functions and the maximum available time condition, so it directly influences the selection of the optimal route for the problem.

(4) In the TSP, the aim is the minimization of the travelling times, while the TDP is aiming at maximizing the utilization of daily available time calculated as the total active disinfection time minus the total wasted travelling time in the chosen route.

4 The Travelling Salesman Problem (TSP) and Its Variations

The travelling salesman problem (TSP) is one of problems that are excessively considered in studying of networks, it possesses broad real-life applications [15]. TSP is summarized as a salesman visiting a number of cities, he begins in his hometown and next wants to visit each place on a collection of places only once. Finally, he returns into hometown. When the number of network nodes increases, the problem will possess a terrible number of possible solutions: finite, but enumeration intractable

[16]. Droste [15] showed that the dimension of different routes is huge, so one cannot solve the problem by simple calculations but needs suitable algorithms to solve such situations.

Better and better algorithms were developed, and the largest solved instance consisted of all 24,978 cities in Sweden [17]. Numerous variants of the TSP are considered in the publications [18] like.

The TSP with priority prizes (TSPPP) [19]; TSP with pickup and delivery or TSP with deliveries and collections (TSPDC)[20]; TSP with backhauls (TSPB) [21–27]; generalized travelling salesman problem (GTSP) [28]; generalized vehicle routing problem (GVRP) [29]; multiple travelling salesman problem (*m*TSP) [30]; multiple depots and *m*TSP with time windows (*m*TSPTW) [31], double travelling salesman problem (*d*TSP) [32]; travelling repairman problem (TRP) [33]. In this kind, customer latency is determined from tour start till the completion of the client's, the *m*TRP [34] and other variations.

Algorithms for solving TSP and its variations are divided into approximate and exact algorithms. An exact algorithm guarantees to find the shortest tour. A heuristic algorithm will find a good tour, but it is not guaranteed that this will be the best tour.

Orman and Williams [35] survey eight models of the TSP as integer programmes (IP). These models are then explained in [36–41] and multi-commodity. Dantzig et.al. [42], Wong [43] and Claus [44] state the TSP conventional formulation.

5 Mathematical Model Formulation for the Travelling Disinfection-Man Problem

The proposed travelling disinfection-man problem (TDP) is designated over a graph G with a n nodes. V denoting the customers and an additional node denotes the place where the disinfection group begins the task, and a set of arcs denoting the transportation times between any two places. The time of inspection in a workplace and the travelling time between two places are specified [45].

While the disinfection group should start the route from the Ministry of Health, they end the route at the last visited workplace, while the driver will return with the vehicle and equipment.

A travelling disinfection-man problem (TDP) is then defined as:

- Each workplace is visited only once by the disinfection group,
- The tour starts at a predetermined position and terminates at the latest visited workplace,
- The overall goal of the problem to be achieved is the best utilization of the available day time, calculated as the total active disinfection time minus the total wasted travelling time in the chosen route.

Mathematical Model:

The mathematical model composed of the design of the decision variables, constraints and objective function are presented in Fig. 5.

The decision variables indicate whether a specific place is approached by the disinfection-man or not.

The positions constraint (I) indicates that each position in the optimum route may be occupied by one place at most. The places constraints (II) indicate that each place can be placed in one position of the disinfection-man route or not visited. The consecutive positions constraints (III) indicate that a position cannot appear in the disinfection-man route unless its previous position appears:

If $\sum_{i=1}^{n} x_i^{m+1} = 1$, then $\sum_{i=1}^{n} x_i^{m} = 1$, $m = 1, 2, \ldots, n-1$,

Design the Decision Variables:

$$x_i^m = \begin{cases} 1, & \text{if place } i \text{ is approached by the Disinfection on position } m \text{ of his route, } i \text{ and } m = 1, 2, \ldots, n. \\ 0, & \text{otherwise.} \end{cases}$$

Formulate the Constraints:

Positions Constraints:

$$\sum_{i=1}^{n} x_i^m \leq 1, m = 1, 2, \ldots, n. \quad \text{(I)}$$

Places Constraints:

$$\sum_{m=1}^{n} x_i^m \leq 1, i = 1, 2, \ldots, n. \quad \text{(II)}$$

Consecutive Positions Constraints:

$$\sum_{i=1}^{n} x_i^{m+1} \leq \sum_{i=1}^{n} x_i^m, m = 1, 2, \ldots, n\text{-}1 \quad \text{(III)}$$

Working Hours / Day Constraints:

$$\sum_{i=1}^{n} t_{0i} x_i^1 + \sum_{m=1}^{n} \sum_{i=1}^{n} (t_i x_i^m) + \sum_{i=1}^{n} \sum_{\substack{j=1 \\ j \neq i}}^{n} t_{ij} . \left(\sum_{m=1}^{n-1} x_i^m . x_j^{m+1}\right) \leq T \quad \text{(IV)}$$

Where:

t_{0i} = Transportation time between headquarter and workplace $\forall i$,

t_{ij} = Transportation time between the two adjacent places $\forall\, i, j$,

t_i = Inspection time for workplace $\forall\, i$.

Binary Constraints:

$$x_i^m = 0 \text{ or } 1, \forall\, i, m. \quad \text{(V)}$$

Create the Objective Function:

Maximize (TDT) – (TTT) =

$$= \left[\sum_{m=1}^{n} \sum_{i=1}^{n} (t_i x_i^m)\right] - \left[\sum_{i=1}^{n} t_{0i} x_i^1 + \sum_{i=1}^{n} \sum_{\substack{j=1 \\ j \neq i}}^{n} t_{ij} . \left(\sum_{m=1}^{n-1} x_i^m . x_j^{m+1}\right)\right] \quad \text{(VI)}$$

Fig. 5 Mathematical model for the problem

If $\sum_{i=1}^{n} x_i^{m+1} = 0$, then there is no restriction on the value of $\sum_{i=1}^{n} x_i^{m}$, $m = 1, 2, \ldots, n-1$.

The working hours/day constraints (IV) indicate that the sum of time duration elapsed by the disinfection-man in transportation and customer disinfection must not exceed the total available working hours/day T. The obtained formula is a quadratic form in two variables, the first term includes the transportation times from the origin to the first position in the route, the second term is the consumed disinfection times at places, and the last term is the transportation times between each two places in the route. Constraints (V) represent the binary constraints for all the used decision variables.

The objective function (VI) indicates that the total disinfection time (TDT) is considered as gain and the total travelling time (TTT) is considered as losses. So, the objective function is formulated as a difference between two terms (TDT)–(TTT).

Finally, we have a suggested a model that contains (n^2) binary variables and ($3n$) constraints.

Any finally obtained optimal solution will lead to twice definite alternatives:

(1) If $\sum_{m=1}^{n} x_i^{m} = 1$, $i = 1, 2, \ldots, n$, then all the n-places are covered by the disinfection group during the first day and the problem is finished.
(2) If $\sum_{m=1}^{n} x_i^{m} = 0$ for any i, then the indicated place i is not covered by the disinfection group in the current day. Then, it is required to discard the covered customers, subjoin other candidate places to be disinfected, add one more day and then recur the process for further one day more.

The solution procedure is presented in Fig. 6.

6 Real Application Case Study Application: Ain Shams University, Cairo

Ain Shams University management and the main two campuses are located in the area of Abbasia, Cairo. It comprises two high institutes and fifteen faculties, and it has seven campuses located in Great Cairo. The administration of the university and three faculties are placed in the major campus. The two institutes, five faculties and one university hospital are placed in the second campus near the previous one. Two faculties and the second hospital are in a third campus at Abassia. The remaining five faculties are each on an independent campus in Shoubra El-Kheima Shoubra El-Kheima, Heliopolis and Abassia, [46]. The proposed travelling disinfection-man problem (TDP) with a group of five-disinfection persons working as one group in each place is applied to the five faculties of Ain Shams University which are located each on a separate campus. Table 1 shows the names and locations (addresses) of each of them. Based on many recorded travels and expert's opinions, Table 2 demonstrates the estimated average travelling and disinfection times, where numbers inside the cells (i, j) represent the travelling times t_{ij} for the problem.

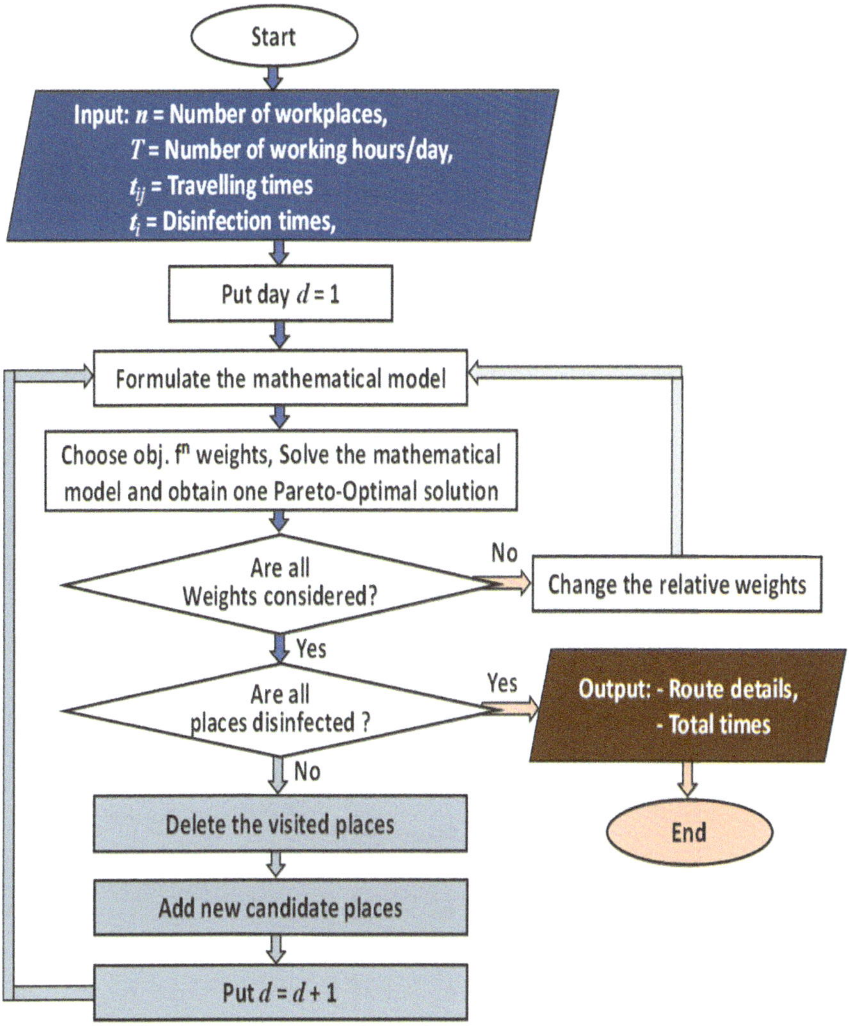

Fig. 6 Steps of the solution procedure of the TDP

The mathematical formulation for the given case is worked out by substituting in the previously described model as follows:

Positions Constraints:

$$x_1^1 + x_2^1 + \ldots + x_5^1 \leq 1 \tag{1}$$

$$x_1^2 + x_2^2 + \ldots + x_5^2 \leq 1 \tag{2}$$

Table 1 Five separate faculty' campuses of Ain Shams university

#	Faculty	Address
0	Ministry of health and population	Parliament of Egypt street, Al Munirah, El-Sayeda Zainab, Cairo
1	Faculty of specific education	Ramsis street, Abassia
2	Faculty of engineering	El-khalifa El Mamoon street, Abassia square, Cairo
3	Faculty of education	Al Maqrizi Strret, Mansheya El-Bakry, Heliopolis, Roxy, Cairo
4	Faculty of women	Asmaa Fahmy street, Nabil El Waqqad street, from Ahmed Tayseer street, Cairo
5	Faculty of agriculture	Shubra Al Kheimah, Al Qalyubia governorate

Table 2 Travelling and disinfection times for the problem

5	4	3	2	1	0	$i\,j$	
1.25	1.25	1.00	0.75	0.50		0	t_i
1.25	0.50	0.25	0.25			1	2.50
1.00	0. 50	0.25				2	2.00
1.25	0.25					3	3.00
1.50						4	1.50
						5	2.25

$$x_1^3 + x_2^3 + \ldots + x_5^3 \leq 1 \tag{3}$$

$$x_1^4 + x_2^4 + \ldots + x_5^4 \leq 1 \tag{4}$$

$$x_1^5 + x_2^5 + \ldots + x_5^5 \leq 1 \tag{5}$$

Places Constraints:

$$x_1^1 + x_1^2 + \ldots + x_1^5 \leq 1 \tag{6}$$

$$x_2^1 + x_2^2 + \ldots + x_2^5 \leq 1 \tag{7}$$

$$x_3^1 + x_3^2 + \ldots + x_3^5 \leq 1 \tag{8}$$

$$x_4^1 + x_4^2 + \ldots + x_4^5 \leq 1 \tag{9}$$

$$x_5^1 + x_5^2 + \ldots + x_5^5 \leq 1 \tag{10}$$

Consecutive Positions Constraints:

$$x_1^1 + x_2^1 + \ldots + x_5^1 - \left(x_1^2 + x_2^2 + \ldots + x_5^2\right) \geq 0 \tag{11}$$

$$x_1^2 + x_2^2 + \ldots + x_5^2 - \left(x_1^3 + x_2^3 + \ldots + x_5^3\right) \geq 0 \tag{12}$$

$$x_1^3 + x_2^3 + \ldots + x_5^3 - \left(x_1^4 + x_2^4 + \ldots + x_5^4\right) \geq 0 \tag{13}$$

$$x_1^4 + x_2^4 + \ldots + x_5^4 - \left(x_1^5 + x_2^5 + \ldots + x_5^5\right) \geq 0 \tag{14}$$

Working Hours/Day Constraint:

$$\begin{aligned}
&0.50x_1^1 + 0.75x_2^1 + 1x_3^1 + 1.25x_4^1 + 1.25x_5^1 \\
&\quad + 2.5x_1^1 + 2x_2^1 + 3x_3^1 + 1.5x_4^1 + 2.25x_5^1 + 2.5x_1^2 + 2x_2^2 + 3x_3^2 \\
&\quad + 1.5x_4^2 + 2.25x_5^2 + 2.5x_1^3 + 2x_2^3 + 3x_3^3 + 1.5x_4^3 + 2.25x_5^3 + 2.5x_1^4 \\
&\quad + 2x_2^4 + 3x_3^4 + 1.5x_4^4 + 2.25x_5^4 + 2.5x_1^5 + 2x_2^5 + 3x_3^5 + 1.5x_4^5 + 2.25x_5^5 \\
&\quad + 0.25\left(x_1^1x_2^2 + x_1^2x_2^3 + x_1^3x_2^4 + x_1^4x_2^5\right) + 0.25\left(x_1^1x_3^2 + x_1^2x_3^3 + x_1^3x_3^4 + x_1^4x_3^5\right) \\
&\quad + 0.5\left(x_1^1x_4^2 + x_1^2x_4^3 + x_1^3x_4^4 + x_1^4x_4^5\right) + 1.25\left(x_1^1x_5^2 + x_1^2x_5^3 + x_1^3x_5^4 + x_1^4x_5^5\right) \\
&\quad + 0.25\left(x_2^1x_1^2 + x_2^2x_1^3 + x_2^3x_1^4 + x_2^4x_1^5\right) + 0.25\left(x_2^1x_3^2 + x_2^2x_3^3 + x_2^3x_3^4 + x_2^4x_3^5\right) \\
&\quad + 0.5\left(x_2^1x_4^2 + x_2^2x_4^3 + x_2^3x_4^4 + x_2^4x_4^5\right) + \left(x_2^1x_5^2 + x_2^2x_5^3 + x_2^3x_5^4 + x_2^4x_5^5\right) \\
&\quad + 0.25\left(x_3^1x_1^2 + x_3^2x_1^3 + x_3^3x_1^4 + x_3^4x_1^5\right) + 0.25\left(x_3^1x_2^2 + x_3^2x_2^3 + x_3^3x_2^4 + x_3^4x_2^5\right) \\
&\quad + 0.25\left(x_3^1x_4^2 + x_3^2x_4^3 + x_3^3x_4^4 + x_3^4x_4^5\right) + 1.25\left(x_3^1x_5^2 + x_3^2x_5^3 + x_3^3x_5^4 + x_3^4x_5^5\right) \\
&\quad + 0.5\left(x_4^1x_1^2 + x_4^2x_1^3 + x_4^3x_1^4 + x_4^4x_1^5\right) + 0.5\left(x_4^1x_2^2 + x_4^2x_2^3 + x_4^3x_2^4 + x_4^4x_2^5\right) \\
&\quad + 0.25\left(x_4^1x_3^2 + x_4^2x_3^3 + x_4^3x_3^4 + x_4^4x_3^5\right) + 1.5\left(x_4^1x_5^2 + x_4^2x_5^3 + x_4^3x_5^4 + x_4^4x_5^5\right) \\
&\quad + 1.25\left(x_5^1x_1^2 + x_5^2x_1^3 + x_5^3x_1^4 + x_5^4x_1^5\right) + \left(x_5^1x_2^2 + x_5^2x_2^3 + x_5^3x_2^4 + x_5^4x_2^5\right) + 1.25 \\
&\quad \left(x_5^1x_3^2 + x_5^2x_3^3 + x_5^3x_3^4 + x_5^4x_3^5\right) + 1.5\left(x_5^1x_4^2 + x_5^2x_4^3 + x_5^3x_4^4 + x_5^4x_4^5\right) \leq 8
\end{aligned} \tag{15}$$

Binary Constraints:

$$x_i^m \in \{0.1\}, i, j = 1, 2, \ldots, n. \tag{16}$$

The Objective Functions:

$$
\begin{aligned}
\text{Maximize (TDT)} - \text{(TTT)} \\
= \big[&2.5x_1^1 + 2x_2^1 + 3x_3^1 + 1.5x_4^1 + 2.25x_5^1 + 2.5x_1^2 + 2x_2^2 \\
&+ 3x_3^2 + 1.5x_4^2 + 2.25x_5^2 + 2.5x_1^3 + 2x_2^3 + 3x_3^3 + 1.5x_4^3 \\
&+ 2.25x_5^3 + 2.5x_1^4 + 2x_2^4 + 3x_3^4 + 1.5x_4^4 + 2.25x_5^4 \\
&+ 2.5x_1^5 + 2x_2^5 + 3x_3^5 + 1.5x_4^5 + 2.25x_5^5 \\
&- \big[0.50x_1^1 + 0.75x_2^1 + 1x_3^1 + 1.25x_4^1 + 1.25x_5^1 \\
&+ 0.25\big(x_1^1x_2^2 + x_1^2x_2^3 + x_1^3x_2^4 + x_1^4x_2^5\big) \\
&+ 0.25\big(x_1^1x_3^2 + x_1^2x_3^3 + x_1^3x_3^4 + x_1^4x_3^5\big) \\
&+ 0.5\big(x_1^1x_4^2 + x_1^2x_4^3 + x_1^3x_4^4 + x_1^4x_4^5\big) \\
&+ 1.25\big(x_1^1x_5^2 + x_1^2x_5^3 + x_1^3x_5^4 + x_1^4x_5^5\big) \\
&+ 0.25\big(x_2^1x_1^2 + x_2^2x_1^3 + x_2^3x_1^4 + x_2^4x_1^5\big) \\
&+ 0.25\big(x_2^1x_3^2 + x_2^2x_3^3 + x_2^3x_3^4 + x_2^4x_3^5\big) \\
&+ 0.5\big(x_2^1x_4^2 + x_2^2x_4^3 + x_2^3x_4^4 + x_2^4x_4^5\big) \\
&+ \big(x_2^1x_5^2 + x_2^2x_5^3 + x_2^3x_5^4 + x_2^4x_5^5\big) \\
&+ 0.25\big(x_3^1x_1^2 + x_3^2x_1^3 + x_3^3x_1^4 + x_3^4x_1^5\big) \\
&+ 0.25\big(x_3^1x_2^2 + x_3^2x_2^3 + x_3^3x_2^4 + x_3^4x_2^5\big) \\
&+ 0.25\big(x_3^1x_4^2 + x_3^2x_4^3 + x_3^3x_4^4 + x_3^4x_4^5\big) \\
&+ 1.25\big(x_3^1x_5^2 + x_3^2x_5^3 + x_3^3x_5^4 + x_3^4x_5^5\big) \\
&+ 0.5\big(x_4^1x_1^2 + x_4^2x_1^3 + x_4^3x_1^4 + x_4^4x_1^5\big) \\
&+ 0.5\big(x_4^1x_2^2 + x_4^2x_2^3 + x_4^3x_2^4 + x_4^4x_2^5\big) \\
&+ 0.25\big(x_4^1x_3^2 + x_4^2x_3^3 + x_4^3x_3^4 + x_4^4x_3^5\big) \\
&+ 1.5\big(x_4^1x_5^2 + x_4^2x_5^3 + x_4^3x_5^4 + x_4^4x_5^5\big) \\
&+ 1.25\big(x_5^1x_1^2 + x_5^2x_1^3 + x_5^3x_1^4 + x_5^4x_1^5\big) \\
&+ \big(x_5^1x_2^2 + x_5^2x_2^3 + x_5^3x_2^4 + x_5^4x_2^5\big) \\
&+ 1.25\big(x_5^1x_3^2 + x_5^2x_3^3 + x_5^3x_3^4 + x_5^4x_3^5\big) \\
&+1.5\big(x_5^1x_4^2 + x_5^2x_4^3 + x_5^3x_4^4 + x_5^4x_4^5\big)\big]
\end{aligned}
\tag{17}
$$

7 Artificial Intelligence Techniques in Optimization

An essential implementation of artificial intelligence (AI) is minimizing the computation burden of optimization. In addition to the gradient-based optimization methods, some new optimization methods have also been proposed that help solve complex problems. In the available classifications, these methods are recognized as "intelligent search" or "intelligent optimization." An advantage of those procedures is that they do not need to perform derivatives or to check convexity, and moreover, they are less likely to fall into local solutions [47]. Optimization procedures are categorized into two types: exact algorithms and approximate algorithms. Exact algorithms are capable of precisely finding optimal solutions, but they are not applicable for complicated optimization problems, and their solution time increases exponentially in such problems. Approximate algorithms can find close-to-optimal solutions for difficult problems in short time [48]. There are different criteria for distinguishing of metaheuristic procedures, among these are nature-inspired vs. non-nature inspiration, memory usage versus memoryless methods, deterministic or stochastic, population-based versus single-point search algorithms and iterative or greedy approach. There are many metaheuristic optimization algorithms, among these are genetic algorithm, simulated annealing, tabu search, ant colony, particle swarm, harmony search, honeybee algorithm, Big Bang-Big Crunch, firefly algorithm, imperialist competitive algorithm, cuckoo search, bat algorithm, charged system search, krill herd algorithm and dolphin echolocation. Among the metaheuristic optimization, algorithms are the new introduced discrete binary gaining-sharing knowledge-based optimization algorithm which will be discussed in the following sections.

8 Proposed Methodology

Metaheuristic approaches are developed for the complex optimization problems. Recently, a human behaviour-related gaining-sharing knowledge-based (GSK) algorithm has been proposed to solve the optimization problems in continuous space [46]. GSK algorithm is based on the acquiring and sharing the knowledge during the human life span. To solve the problems in binary space, a discrete binary variant of GSK algorithm is proposed (DBGSK). DBGSK algorithm is based on the two main stages: binary junior and senior gaining-sharing stage. These stages are introduced to solve the problems in discrete binary space.

Since the proposed problem, i.e., TDP is constrained optimization problem, to solve the constrained optimization problem, there are many constraint handling techniques in the literature [49–51]. In their work, the augmented Lagrangian method is used in which an unconstrained optimization problem is obtained from a constrained optimization one [52–56]. The proposed methodology is described below.

8.1 Overview of Gaining-Sharing Knowledge-Based Optimization Algorithm (GSK)

A mathematical formulation of an optimization problem with constraints is given as:

$$\text{Min} \quad f(X); X = [x_1, x_2, \ldots, x_{Dim}]$$

$$s.to. \quad g_i(X) \leq 0; \quad i = 1, 2, \ldots, m$$

$$X \in [\alpha_p, \beta_p]; \; p = 1, 2, \ldots, Dim$$

where f denotes the objective function; $X = [x_1, x_2, \ldots, x_{Dim}]$ are the decision variables; $g_i(X)$ denotes the inequality constraints and α_p, β_p are the minimum and maximum limits of the decision variables, respectively, and *Dim* is the dimension of an individual. If any optimization problem is of maximization form, then the maximization can be converted into minimization by considering minimization = − maximization.

The basic concept of GSK algorithm is based on sharing the acquired knowledge throughout the human life span. It depends on the stages: first stage is the junior gaining-sharing stage and the other is senior gaining-sharing stage. In junior gaining-sharing stage, the people gain knowledge, ideas or information from their known persons such as family members and relatives. And they wish to share their thoughts with other persons whom they might not familiar. These people have not that much of understanding so that they can choose the bad or good persons. In the senior gaining-sharing stage, people may get information or knowledge through their colleagues, social media friends, etc. And they have some experience with whom they want to share their thoughts or knowledge. Moreover, the people can categorize the others in good or bad category. This concept is explained mathematically in the following steps:

Step 1: Initialize the population: To start the optimization process, an initial population of solutions must be generated in the following way:

$$x_{tp}^0 = \alpha_p + rand_p(\beta_p - \alpha_p) \tag{18}$$

where t denotes the indices for the number of populations; $rand_p$ is the random number that is generated uniformly between *0* and *1*.

Step 2: Calculation of dimensions: At this step, the number of dimensions of junior and senior stages must be calculated using the given formula:

$$Dim_J = Dim \times \left(\frac{Gen^{max} - G}{Gen^{max}}\right)^k \tag{19}$$

$$Dim_S = Dim - Dim_J \tag{20}$$

```
for t=1:NP
  for p=1:Dim
    if rand≤ k_r (knowledge ratio)
      if f(x_t) > f(x_r)
        x_tp^new = (x_t + k_f * ((x_{t-1} − x_{t+1}) + (x_r − x_t)))
      else
        x_tp^new = (x_t + k_f * ((x_{t-1} − x_{t+1}) + (x_t − x_r)))
      end
    else  x_tp^new = x_tp^old
    end
  end
end
```

Fig. 7 Pseudo-code for junior gaining-sharing knowledge stage

where $k(> 0)$ denotes the learning rate that monitors the experience rate. Dim_J and Dim_S denote the number of dimensions for the junior and senior stage, respectively. n^{max} is the maximum count of generations, and G is the count of generation.

Step 3: Junior gaining-sharing knowledge stage: In this stage, the early aged people acquire information through their network and present their knowledge to others who may or may not belong to their group. Therefore, the population of individuals are updated using the following procedure:

The objective function values are calculated, and according to the ascending order of the objective function values, the three individuals are chosen for every individual $x_t(t = 1, 2, \ldots, NP)$.

Select the closest best x_{t-1}; the closest worst x_{t+1} to acquire knowledge, and to share knowledge choose a random vector x_r. Therefore, an individual of population is updated through the pseudo-code which is given in Fig. 7.where $k_f(> 0)$ is the knowledge factor.

Step 4: Senior gaining-sharing knowledge stage: It contains the impact and effect of other persons (good or bad) on the individual. The individual are updated by classifying the individuals in three categories as best, middle and worst.

The three categories are based on the obtained objective values. The objectives values are put in ascending order and then each category is evaluated as:

Best individual = $100p\ \%\ (x_{\text{best}})$, middle individual = $Dim - 2 * 100\ p\ \%\ (x_{\text{middle}})$, worst individual = $100p\ \%(x_{\text{worst}})$.

For every individual x_t, choose the top and bottom $100p\ \%$ individuals to gain the information, the third one (middle individual) is chosen to share the acquired knowledge. Therefore, a new individual is modified using the pseudo-code that is dictated in Fig. 8. In the pseudo-code, $p \in [0, 1]$ is the percentage of best and worst classes.

```
for t=1:NP
    for p=1:Dim
        if rand≤ k_r (knowledge ratio)
            if f(x_t) > f(x_r)
                x_tp^new = (x_t + k_f * ((x_{t-1} - x_{t+1}) + (x_r - x_t)))
            else
                x_tp^new = (x_t + k_f * ((x_{t-1} - x_{t+1}) + (x_t - x_r)))
            end
        else  x_tp^new = x_tp^old
        end
    end
end
```

Fig. 8 Pseudo-code of senior gaining-sharing knowledge stage

8.2 Discrete Binary Gaining-Sharing Knowledge-Based Optimization Algorithm (DBGSK)

The proposed case study is based on the binary search space; therefore, to obtain the solution of the same, a novel discrete binary gaining-sharing knowledge-based optimization algorithm (DBGSK) is suggested. The modification is made in three stages of GSK algorithm to develop the DBGSK algorithm. To start the optimization process, the generation of initial population is the first step. The initial population is generated over discrete binary space, and after that, binary junior and senior stages are introduced.

The following subsections represent the working mechanism of DBGSK algorithm:

First Step: Generate Discrete Binary Population

The optimization process is initiated with the generation of population of solutions. Therefore, to initialize the population, a discrete binary population must be generated using Eq. (21):

$$x_{tp}^{0} = round(rand(0, 1)) \tag{21}$$

To obtain the number into binary form, round operator is used which changes the decimal number into its nearest integer.

Second Step: Modify the Junior Gaining-Sharing Stage

In the second step, the original junior gaining-sharing stage will be modified using the pseudo-code (Fig. 6). The new discrete binary junior stage is introduced with $k_f = 1$. The original junior stage contains two cases and, in each case, $k_f = 1$ is

Table 3 Results of the discrete binary junior gaining and sharing stage of case 1

	x_{t-1}	x_{t+1}	x_r	Results	Modified results
(i)	0	0	0	0	0
	0	0	1	1	1
	1	1	0	0	0
	1	1	1	1	1
(ii)	1	0	0	1	1
	1	0	1	2	1
	0	1	0	−1	0
	0	1	1	0	0

substituted due to the generation of binary junior and senior gaining and sharing stage. The cases are following described:

Case 1. When $f(\boldsymbol{x}_r) < f(\boldsymbol{x}_t)$: x_{t-1}, x_{t+1}, x_r are three binary vectors i.e. $x_{t-1}, x_{t+1}, x_r \in \{0, 1\}$ which implies that total of 8 (2^3) combinations are possible that are elaborated in Table 3. The eight possibilities of binary vectors are divided into two subcases [(i) and (ii)] and each subcase contains four combinations and the corresponding results are also shown in Table 3.

(i) If x_{t-1} and x_{t+1} are equal then the resulting vector is x_r.

(ii) If x_{t-1} and x_{t+1} are not equal then the resulting vector is equal to x_{t-1} in which −1 is taken as 0 and 2 is taken as 1.

The case 1 is mathematically formulated as:

Case 2. When $f(\boldsymbol{x}_r) \geq f(\boldsymbol{x}_t)$: This case contains four binary vectors $x_{t-1}, x_t, x_{t+1}, x_r$ i.e., $x_{t-1}, x_t, x_{t+1}, x_r \in \{0, 1\}$. Since $k_f = 1$ is considered with original GSK algorithm, then the resulting case is constructed total of 16 (2^4) combinations. All possible combinations are categorized into two subcases [(iii) and (iv)] in which subcase (iii) contains four combinations and subcase (iv) contains twelve combinations. The total possible combinations are listed in Table 4.

(iii) If x_{t-1} and x_{t+1} are not equal, but x_{t+1} and x_r are equal, then the resulting vector will be x_{t-1}.

(iv) If any of the possibilities arises other than subcase (iii), then the resulting vector will be x_t by taking -1 and -2 as 0, and 2 and 3 as 1.

The case 2 can be formulated mathematically as:

$$x_{tp}^{\text{new}} = \begin{cases} x_{t-1}; \ if \ x_{t-1} \neq x_{t+1} = x_r \\ x_t; \qquad \text{Otherwise} \end{cases}$$

Third Step: Modify the senior gaining-sharing stage

The third step of DBGSK algorithm is similar to the second step of DBGSK algorithm. The senior gaining-sharing stage of original GSK algorithm is modified using

Table 4 Results of the discrete binary junior gaining and sharing stage of case 2

	x_{t-1}	x_t	x_{t+1}	x_r	Results	Modified results
(iii)	1	1	0	0	3	1
	1	0	0	0	1	1
	0	1	1	1	0	0
	0	0	1	1	−2	0
(iv)	0	0	0	0	0	0
	0	1	0	0	2	1
	0	0	1	0	−1	0
	0	0	0	1	−1	0
	1	0	1	0	0	0
	1	0	0	1	0	0
	0	1	1	0	1	1
	0	1	0	1	1	1
	1	1	1	0	2	1
	1	0	1	1	−1	0
	1	1	0	1	2	1
	1	1	1	1	1	1

$k_f = 1$. In the pseudo-code of senior gaining-sharing stage, there are two cases and these two cases are further modified.

Case 1. $f(\boldsymbol{x}_{\text{middle}}) < f(\boldsymbol{x}_t)$: $x_{\text{best}}, x_{\text{middle}}, x_{\text{worst}}$ are three different binary vectors which takes only 0 and 1 values. Therefore, only eight different combinations are obtained, and these eight combinations are further divided into two subcases [(i) and (ii)]. The subcases (i) and (ii) has four combinations, respectively. The list of combinations is shown in Table 5.

Table 5 Results of discrete binary senior gaining and sharing stage of case 1

	x_{best}	x_{worst}	x_{middle}	Results	Modified results
(i)	0	0	0	0	0
	0	0	1	1	1
	1	1	0	0	0
	1	1	1	1	1
(ii)	1	0	0	1	1
	1	0	1	2	1
	0	1	0	−1	0
	0	1	1	0	0

Table 6 Results of discrete binary senior gaining and sharing stage of case 2 with $k_f = 1$

	x_{best}	x_t	x_{worst}	x_{middle}	Results	Modified results
(iii)	1	1	0	0	3	1
	1	0	0	0	1	1
	0	1	1	1	0	0
	0	0	1	1	−2	0
(iv)	0	0	0	0	0	0
	0	1	0	0	2	1
	0	0	1	0	−1	0
	0	0	0	1	−1	0
	1	0	1	0	0	0
	1	0	0	1	0	0
	0	1	1	0	1	1
	0	1	0	1	1	1
	1	1	1	0	2	1
	1	0	1	1	−1	0
	1	1	0	1	2	1

(i) If x_{best} and x_{worst} are equal then the result will be equal to x_{middle}.

(ii) Contrarily, if x_{best} and x_{worst} are not equal then the resulting vector will be x_{best} by using −1 as 0 or 2 as 1.

The mathematical formulation of case 1 is as:

Case 2. $f(\boldsymbol{x}_{\text{middle}}) > f(\boldsymbol{x}_t)$: In this case, $x_{\text{best}}, x_{\text{middle}}, x_{\text{worst}}, x_t$ are four different binary vectors this implies that total 16 combinations are possible. The all possible combinations are presented in Table 6. The total 16 combinations are further divided into two subcases [(iii) and (iv)]. The subcase (iii) contains four and the subcase (iv) contains twelve combinations.

(iii) x_{best} and x_{worst} are not equal and x_{worst} and x_{middle} are equal, then the resulting vector will be x_{best}.

(iv) If any condition is obtained other than (iii), then the resulting vector will be x_t by using −2 and −1 as 0 and 2 and 3 as 1.

The case 2 is formulated mathematically as:

$$x_{tp}^{\text{new}} = \begin{cases} x_{\text{best}}; & if\ x_{\text{best}} \neq x_{\text{worst}} = x_{\text{middle}} \\ x_t; & \text{Otherwise} \end{cases}$$

The pseudo-code of DBGSK is presented in Fig. 9.

```
Start
    Initialize the value of parameters (Gen^max, NP, k_r, k, p)
    Initialize the generation (G = 0)
    Create discrete binary population using equation (21)
    Evaluate f(x_t).
    For G = 1 to Gen^max
        Compute the dimensions of both stages (Discrete Binary junior
        and senior gaining sharing stage)
        Apply Discrete Binary Junior gaining sharing stage
        Apply Discrete Binary Senior gaining sharing stage
        Update the population
        Select the global best solution
    End
End
```

Fig. 9 Pseudo-code for DBGSK

9 Experimental Results

The TDP is handled by using the proposed novel DBGSK algorithm, and the used parameters are presented in Table 7. DBGSK runs over personal computer Intel® CoreTM i5-7200U CPU@ 2.50 GHz and 4 GB RAM and coded on MATLAB R2015a30 independent runs are compiled to get the optimal solutions, and the obtained statistics are provided in Table 8, including the best, median, average, worst solutions and the DBGSK standard deviations. Moreover, Fig. 10 shows the convergence graph of the solutions of TDP using DBGSK. From the figure, it can be observed that after the 24th iteration, it converges to the global optimal solution (6.00), which shows the robustness of the DBGSK.

Table 7 Numerical values of parameters

Parameters of DBGSK	Considered values
NP	500
k	10
k_r	0.9
p	0.1
k_f	1
Max number of iterations	200

Table 8 Statistical results of TDP using DBGSK

Algorithm	Best (maximum)	Median	Average	Worst (minimum)	Standard deviation
DBGSK	6.00	6.00	6.00	6.00	0.00

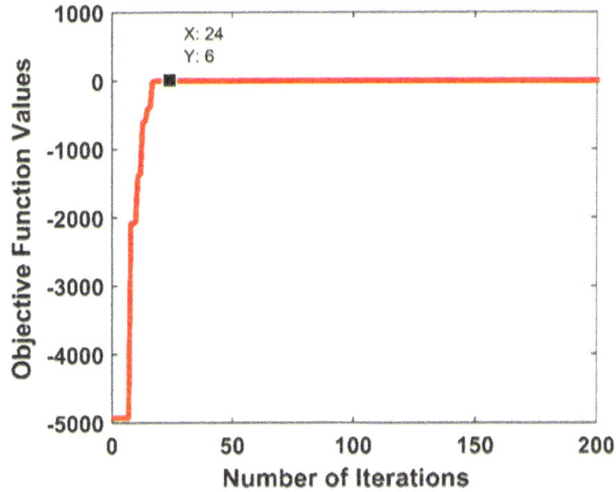

Fig. 10 Convergence graph of DBGSK

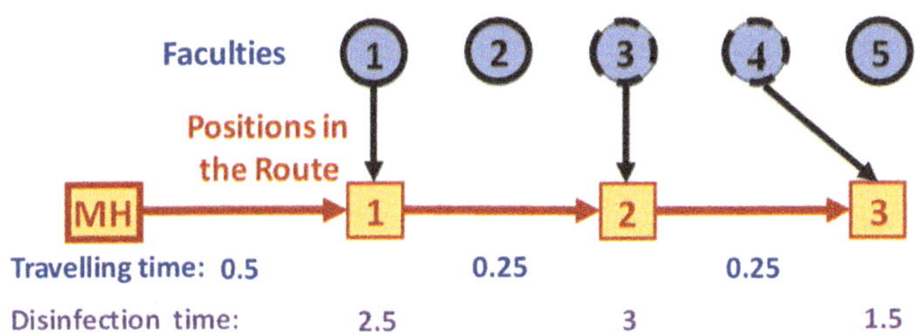

Fig. 11 Optimum solution for the case study example

The route provided by the optimum solution can be seen in Fig. 11. The route begins in the Ministry of Health (MH) and then is composed of three faculties numbers 1, 3 and 4: Faculty of Specific Education, Faculty of Education and Faculty of Women, respectively. The corresponding route length is 8 h, which means that all the available working daytime is utilized completely without any slack. The total disinfection time is 7 h and the total travelling time is only 1 h.

The remaining two faculties numbers 2 and 5 can be treated in another day, and the optimum solution for such a case is very simple and can be calculated directly since there are only two possibilities: either to go first to faculty number 2 then 5, or to start from 5 then 2, the judgement will depend upon the shorter travelling time between the starting position and both faculties 2 and 5.

10 Conclusions

1. An improved scheduling of the disinfection process of the new COVID-19 which recently placed humans in all countries in front of a huge hazard. The scheduling is aiming at achieving the best utilization of the available day time, which is calculated as the total disinfection time minus the total loss travelling time.
2. A new application problem is presented, which is called a travelling disinfection-man problem (TDP) dealing with improving scheduling of the disinfection process of the new coronavirus.
3. Travelling disinfection-man problem (TDP) is similar to the travelling salesman problems with major differences, where a disinfection group is likely to select a route of a subset of nodes (places) so that to reach the most utilization of the available time for disinfection of contaminated places.
4. A nonlinear binary constrained model is designed for the proposed problem. The designed binary decision variables indicate the placing of chosen infected places in the positions of the chosen route of the disinfection group.
5. The mathematical model is used to formulate a real application case study for disinfecting five faculties in Ain Shams University in Cairo. The detailed mathematical model and the solution procedure are exhaustively explained.
6. The proposed problem TDP is solved by a novel discrete binary gaining-sharing knowledge-based optimization algorithm (DBGSK), which involves two main stages: discrete binary junior and senior gaining and sharing stages with a knowledge factor $k_f = 1$. DBGSK is discrete binary variant of GSK that solves the problem with binary decision variables.
7. DBGSK shows that it has the ability of finding the solutions of TDP, and the obtained results demonstrate the robustness and convergence of DBGSK towards the optimal solutions.

11 Points for Future Researches

1. To use other mathematical formulations for the introduced problem comprising the decision variables, the objective function, and the constraints, and then comparing the between these models.
2. To enhance the problem to cover travelling disinfection-man problem (TDP) variations like: TDP with time window (TDPTW), TDP with multiple disinfection groups (mTDP), stochastic travelling disinfection-man problem (STDP), multi-objective stochastic multiple travelling disinfection-man problem (MOSmTDP) and other versions.
3. To utilize the same formulation to other application fields like: business, industry, agriculture, education, social and community services, telecommunications, quality assurance, investing, pollution, medical, tourism, sales,

marketing, sports, advertising, arts, cooking and others. The only difference is the actual working time of the group in the considered field of study.
4. To evaluate the effectiveness of the DBGSK approach for various complex problems, and to extend the DBGSK with different kinds of constraint handling methods.

References

1. Cleemput, S., Dumon, W., Fonseca, V., Abdool Karim, W., Giovanetti, M., Alcantara, L. C., Deforche, K., & de Oliveira, T. (2020, 28 February). Genome detective coronavirus typing tool for rapid identification and characterization of novel coronavirus genomes. *Bioinformatics*, btaa145. Retrieved at: https://doi.org/10.1093/bioinformatics/btaa145
2. The Lancet website (2020). A novel coronavirus outbreak of global health concern, retrieved on March 30, 2020. https://www.thelancet.com/journals/lancet/article/PIIS0140-6736(20)30185-9/fulltext
3. World Health Organization (WHO) website. (2020a). Novel coronavirus (2019-nCoV) situation report–7, Data as reported by 27 January 2020.
4. Guan, W., Ni, Z., Hu, Y., Liang, W., Ou, C., He, J., Liu, L., Shan, H., Lei, C., Hui, D. S. C., Du, B., & Li, L. (2020, February 28) Clinical characteristics of coronavirus disease 2019 in China. *The New England Journal of Medicine*. https://doi.org/10.1056/NEJMoa2002032. https://doi.org/10.1056/NEJMoa200203
5. Wikimedia Commons website. (2020). Retrieved on April 3, 2020. https://commons.wikimedia.org/wiki/File:COVID-19_Outbreak_World_Map.svg
6. Ministry of Health and Population (Egypt). (2020). Retrieved on 31 March 2020. https://m.facebook.com/story.php?story_fbid=146349830248971&id=113432613540693
7. Centers for Decease Control and Prevention (CDC) website. (2020a). COVID-19 travel recommendations by country. Retrieved on April 3, 2020. https://www.cdc.gov/coronavirus/2019-ncov/travelers/map-and-travel-notices.html
8. Worldometer website. (2020a). COVID-19 Coronavirus pandemic. Retrieved on April 3, 2020. https://www.worldometers.info/coronavirus/#ref-13
9. Worldometer website (2020b). Coronavirus cases. Retrieved on April 1, 2020. https://www.worldometers.info/coronavirus/coronavirus-cases/#total-cases
10. Zhao, S., Lin, Q., Ran, J., Musa, S. S., Yang, G., Wang, W., Lou, Y., Gao, D., Yang, L., He, D., & Wang, M. H. (2020 March). Preliminary estimation of the basic reproduction number of novel coronavirus (2019-nCoV) in China, from 2019 to 2020: A data-driven analysis in the early phase of the outbreak. *International Journal of Infectious Diseases*, *92*, 214–217. https://doi.org/10.1016/j.ijid.2020.01.050
11. Centers of Disease Control and Prevention (CDC) website. (2020b). Coronavirus disease 2019. Retrieved on March 31, 2020. https://www.cdc.gov/
12. ServiceMaster DSI website. (2020). Preventive cleaning and decontamination, COVID-19 coronavirus disinfection. Retrieved on March 30, 2020. https://servicemasterdsi.com/coronavirus-decontamination/
13. Sentrex website. (2020). UK coronavirus infection control & fogging. Retrieved on March 28, 2020. https://sentrex.co.uk/service/coronavirus-infection-control/
14. World Health Organization (WHO) website. (2020b). Guidance for health workers. Retrieved on March 29, 2020. https://www.who.int/emergencies/diseases/novel-coronavirus-2019/technical-guidance/health-workers
15. Applegate, D. L., Bixby, R. E., Chvatal, V., & Cook, W. J. (2006). *The traveling salesman problem: A computational study*. Princeton University Press.

16. Environmental Consultants Inc. APEX. (2020). General guidance for building managers regarding novel coronavirus. Retrieved. https://www.smrecover.com/wp-content/uploads/2020/03/COVID-19-General-Guideline-for-Building-Managers-Final.pdf
17. Gleixner, A. M. (2014, April 10–11). Introduction to constraint integer programming, 5th. Porto meeting on mathematics for industry, Porto, Zuse Institute Berlin, Matheon, Berlin mathematical school.
18. Droste, I. (2017). *Algorithms for the travelling salesman problem.* Bachelor thesis, mathematics. Utrecht University.
19. Applegate, D. L., Bixby, R. E., Chvátal, V., Cook, W., Espinoza, D. G., Goycoolea, M., & Helsgaun, K. (2009). Certification of an optimal TSP tour through 85,900 cities. *Operations Research Letters, 37*(1), 11–15.
20. Sarubbi, J. F. M., & Luna, H. P. L. (2007). *The multi-commodity traveling salesman problem.* INOC—International Network Optimization Conference, April 2007. https://www.poms.ucl.ac.be/inoc2007/Papers/author.68/paper/paper.68.pdf
21. Pureza, V., Morabito, R., & Luna, H. P. (2018). Modelling and solving the traveling salesman problem with priority prizes. *Pesquisa Operacional, 38*(3), 499–522. Brazilian Operations Research Society Printed version ISSN 0101-7438/Online version ISSN 1678-5142 www.scielo.br/pope. https://doi.org/10.1590/0101-7438.2018.038.03.0499
22. Baldacci, R., Hadjiconstantinou, E., & Mingozzi, A. (2003). An exact algorithm for the traveling salesman problem with deliveries and collections. *Networks, 42*(1), 26–41, Wiley Periodicals, Inc.
23. Gendreau, M., Hertz, A., & Laporte, G. (1996). The travelling salesman problem with backhauls. *Computers and Operations Research, 23*(1996), 501–508
24. Aramgiatisiris, T. (2004, April–June). An exact decomposition algorithm for the traveling salesman problem with backhauls, operations research and management science units, department of industrial engineering, Kasetsart university, Bangkok, Thailand. *Journal of Research in Engineering and Technology, 1*(2).
25. Mosheiov, G. (1994). The travelling salesman problem with pick-up and delivery. *European Journal of Operational Research, 79*(1994), 299–310
26. Anily, S., & Mosheiov, G. (1994). The traveling salesman problem with delivery and backhauls. *Operations Research Letter, 16*(1994), 11–18
27. Gendreau, M., Laporte, G., & Vigo, D. (1999). Heuristics for the traveling salesman problem with pickup and delivery. *Computers and Operations Research, 26*(1999), 699–714
28. Halse, K. (1992). Modelling and solving complex vehicle routing problems, Ph.D. thesis, IMSOR, Technical University of Denmark.
29. Dumitrescu, I., Ropke, S., Cordeau, J., & Laporte, G. (2010, February). The traveling salesman problem with pickup and delivery: polyhedral results and a branch-and-cut algorithm. *Mathematical Programming, 121*, 269.
30. Pop, P. C. (2007). New integer programming formulations of the generalized travelling salesman problem. *American Journal of Applied Sciences, 4*(11), 932–937. Science Publications. ISSN 1546-9239.
31. Kara, I., & Bektas, T. (2003, July 6–10). Integer linear programming formulation of the generalized vehicle routing problem, presented in 5th EURO/INFORMS Joint international meeting.
32. Bektas, T. (2006). The multiple traveling salesman problem: An overview of formulations and solution procedures. *OMEGA: The International Journal of Management Science, 34*(3), 209–219.
33. Oberlin, P., Rathinam, S., & Darbha, S. (2009, June 10–12). A transformation for a heterogeneous, multi-depot, multiple traveling salesman problem. In *Proceedings of the American control conference*, (pp. 1292–1297), St. Louis.
34. Demiral, M. F., & Şen, H. (2016, May–August). Integer programming model for two-centered double traveling salesman problem. *European Journal of Economics and Business Studies, 2*(2). ISSN 2411-9571.

35. Silva, M. M., Subramanian, A., Vidal, T., & Ochi, L. S. (2012). A simple and effective metaheuristic for the minimum latency problem. *European Journal of Operational Research, 221*, 513–520
36. Onder, G., Kara, I., & Derya, T. (2016). New integer programming formulation for multiple traveling repairmen problem, 19th. EURO Working group on transportation my assays Ltd., My Curve Fit software, online curve fitting. Retrieved. https://mycurvefit.com/
37. Orman, A. J., & Williams, H. P. (2005). A survey of different integer programming formulations of the travelling salesman problem. Operational research working papers, LSEOR 04.67. Department of operational research, London school of economics and political science. Revised July 2005.
38. Fox, K. R., Gavish, B., & Graves, S. C. (1980). An n-constraint formulation of the (time dependent) travelling salesman problem. *Operations Research, 28*, 1018–1021
39. Vajda, S. (1961). *Mathematical programming*. Addison-Wesley.
40. Miller, C. E., Tucker, A. W., & Zemlin, R. A. (1960). Integer programming formulation of travelling salesman problems. *Journal of the ACM, 3*, 326–329
41. Sawik, T. (2016). A note on the Miller-Tucker-Zemlin model for the asymmetric traveling salesman problem. *Bulletin of the Polish Academy of Sciences Technical Sciences, 64*(3), 2016. https://doi.org/10.1515/bpasts-2016-0057
42. Gavish, B., & Graves, S. C. (1978). *The travelling salesman problem and related problems*. Working Paper OR-078-78, Operations research center, MIT.
43. Finke, G., Claus, A., & Gunn, E. (1983). A two-commodity network flow approach to the travelling salesman problem, Combinatorics, Graph theory and computing, Proceedings 14th South Eastern conference. Atlantic University.
44. Dantzig, G. B., Fulkerson, D. R., & Johnson, S. M. (1954). Solutions of a large scale travelling salesman problem. *Operations Research, 2*, 393–410
45. Wong, R. T. (1980). *Integer programming formulations of the travelling salesman problem*. Proceedings IEEE conference on circuits and computers, (pp. 149–152). https://www.who.int/docs/default-source/coronaviruse/situation-reports/20200127-sitrep-7-2019--ncov.pdf
46. Ain Shams University official web site. (2020). *History*. Retrieved. https://www.asu.edu.eg/
47. Claus, A. (1984). A new formulation for the travelling salesman problem. *SIAM Journal Algebraic and Discrete Mathods, 5*, 21–25
48. Pinter, C. C., (2014). *A book of set theory*. Dover Publications Inc. ISBN10 0486497089, ISBN13 9780486497082.
49. Koopialipoor, M., & Noorbakhsh, A. (2020). Applications of artificial intelligence techniques in optimizing drilling, Chapter 6. In: A. Azizi, (Ed.), *Emerging trends in mechatronics*, InTechOpen. https://doi.org/10.5772/intechopen.85398
50. Azizi, A. (2017). Introducing a novel hybrid artificial intelligence algorithm to optimize network of industrial applications in modern manufacturing. *Complexity, 18*. https://doi.org/10.1155/2017/8728209
51. Mohamed, A. W., Hadi, A. A., & Mohamed, A. K. (2020). Gaining-sharing knowledge-based algorithm for solving optimization problems: A novel nature-inspired algorithm. *International Journal of Machine Learning and Cybernetics, 11*, 1501–1529
52. Deb, K. (2000). An efficient constraint handling method for genetic algorithms. *Computer Methods in Applied Mechanics and Engineering, 186*(2–4), 311–338
53. Coello, C. A. C. (2002). Theoretical and numerical constraint-handling techniques used with evolutionary algorithms: A survey of the state of the art. *Computer Methods in Applied Mechanics and Engineering, 191*(11–12), 1245–1287
54. Muangkote, N., Photong, L., & Sukprasert, A. (2019). Effectiveness of constrained handling techniques of improved constrained differential evolution algorithm applied to constrained optimization problems in mechanical engineering.

55. Long, W., Liang, X., Huang, Y., & Chen, Y. (2013). A hybrid differential evolution augmented Lagrangian method for constrained numerical and engineering optimization. *Computer-Aided Design, 45*(12), 1562–1574
56. Bahreininejad, A. (2019). Improving the performance of water cycle algorithm using augmented Lagrangian method. *Advances in Engineering Software, 132*, 55–64

COVID-19 Lock Down Impact on Mental Health: A Cross-Sectional Online Survey from Kerala, India

C. B. Rajesh, Nafih Cherappurath, V. Vinod, Masilamani Elayaraja, Sakeer Hussain, and N. Sreelekha

Abbreviations

2019-nCoV	Novel Corona Virus 2019
AYUSH	Ayurveda, Yoga and Naturopathy, Unani, Siddha and Homeopathy
CDC	Centres of Disease Control and Prevention
ICTV	International Committee on Taxonomy of Viruses
PG	Postgraduate
SARS-CoV-2	Severe Acute Respiratory Syndrome Coronavirus 2
UG	Undergraduate
WHO	World Health Organisation

C. B. Rajesh
Department of Physical Education, NSS College of Engineering, Palakkad, Kerala, India
e-mail: rajeshcb@nssce.ac.in

N. Cherappurath (✉) · S. Hussain
Department of Physical Education, University of Calicut, Calicut, Kerala, India

V. Vinod
Department of Mechanical Engineering, NSS College of Engineering, Palakkad, Kerala, India

M. Elayaraja
Department of Physical Education & Sports, Pondicherry University, Pondicherry, India

N. Sreelekha
Department of Applied Psychology, Pondicherry University, Pondicherry, India

M. Niranjanamurthy et al. (eds.), *Intelligent Data Analysis for COVID-19 Pandemic*,
Algorithms for Intelligent Systems, https://doi.org/10.1007/978-981-16-1574-0_14

1 Introduction

The coronavirus disease, also known as COVID-19, is an infectious respiratory disease that was once epidemic to the Wuhan province in China, but has now become a pandemic with around 31,343,430 confirmed cases and 965,294 deaths (as on 22 September 2020). It must also be noted that 21,518,790 individuals have recovered from the disease (as on 22 September 2020) [7]. China reported a cluster of cases in Wuhan, Hubei Province in Dec 2019 and then it spread across the world. The outbreak was declared a Public Health Emergency of International Concern on 30 January 2020 [8]. The coronavirus is a member of the family of coronaviruses—*Coronaviridae*. They are named based on the crown-shaped structure that the virus possesses when viewed under a microscope [4]. Some coronaviruses affect human beings and cause illness ranging from the common cold to mild/moderate respiratory illnesses. Other kinds of coronaviruses affect animals. At some instances, it is observed that certain coronaviruses jump from the animal species to the human population.

The Novel Coronavirus 2019 is getting so much attention because it has a new kind of viral strain that the world has not seen before. It was named 2019-nCoV by the WHO and was later changed to SARS-CoV-2 by the International Committee on Taxonomy of Viruses (ICTV). The virus is very much similar to the bat coronavirus. The pandemic has urged countries to make travel restrictions and implement nationwide lockdowns. Lockdown due to COVID-19 was announced in India from midnight of 24 March 2020 onwards, when the number of confirmed positive coronavirus cases was approximately 500. Several restrictions were imposed from that date. It included total shutdown of public transport, road, rail and air, all educational institutions including schools, colleges and professional institutions, lockdown of all industries, shopping malls, theatres, amusement parks, etc. Services such as food shops, banks and ATMs, petrol pumps, other essentials and their manufacturing were exempted. Citizens were allowed to travel only for very essential services with restrictions. As a result of such strict measures, India was able to confine the spread of disease to a large extend. India has a population of 1.35 billion, there are only 0.1 million COVID-19 cases. The recovery rate is above 40% and doubling rate is 13 days.

1.1 Motivation for Doing the Research

The COVID-19 pandemic is a reminder to us that, mental health is just as important as physical health. As the economic and social conditions worsen due to the pandemic, we can expect to see a rise in mental health conditions like anxiety, depression and substance use disorder. Frontline health workers with huge workloads, life or death decision-making situations and risk of infections are mainly affected. Our children and adolescence whose daily life has been disrupted are also at risk of serious mental conditions. Elderly people who live alone are at risk of social isolation.

As the countries around the world are taking measures to restrict movement and isolate people socially in order to combat the pandemic, people are making major changes in their daily life and routine. Working from home, unemployment, fear of contracting the disease, reduced physical contact with family and friends are some of the new realities which take some time to get adapted to. Concern about people who are close to us and having other diseases, adapting to lifestyle changes, etc., can be very challenging to all of us. For people who like to get socialized, this could drain their mood due to lack of interaction with other humans, and other problems relating to disrupted daily activities, exercises, programmes and businesses are also raised. A long-time quarantine life may lead to stress, anxiety, frustration, boredom and depression, and even induce suicidal tendency and attempts.

Kerala had a Nipah outbreak in 2018, which has taught its people some hard lessons on how to manage a health crisis. The death rate in the state due to COVID-19 is 0.56. The nationwide lockdown helped to contain cases. Kerala was managing this pandemic through its quick, decisive moves of government, commitment of people, efficient healthcare systems and decentralization policies of local body systems. Kerala is also incorporating the AYUSH sector by developing indigenous Ayurveda medicines. Ayurveda, homeopathy and other AYUSH sectors work in conjunction with modern medicine to combat the pandemic.

The study is carried out to understand how people are coping with the lifestyle changes due to the COVID-19 lockdown and whether they are mentally affected by it. A questionnaire was circulated online among various individuals of age between 19 and 65 years in the last week of April, 2020 and the survey ended in the third week of May, 2020. The survey was largely conducted within the State of Kerala, India. Nearly 85% of the respondents were staying at their own homes, the remaining stayed in apartments and rented houses.

2 Review of Literature

Isolation is an act of being separated from the people and environment. Loneliness is the outcome of isolation. It can be thought of as a feeling of sadness about being disconnected and socially isolated from the world around you. Living alone, feeling of loss, depression, fear of rejection, lack of purpose in life, linguistic, cultural and geographical barriers, etc., can be considered as some of the reasons why a person would feel lonely. Adapting to lifestyle changes, managing the fear of contracting the virus and worry about people close to us who are particularly vulnerable are challenging for all of us [3]. They can be particularly difficult for people with mental health conditions. A person who is lonely is at risk of depression, anxiety, panic attacks, etc. It can also lead to severe physical health issues as well, including body aches and pains, headaches and worsening of prevailing health conditions.

Each individual responds differently to stressful situations. According to the Centres of Disease Control and Prevention (CDC), how a person responds to a certain situation, particularly an outbreak, depends mostly on the person's background and his/her way of life [1]. People with mental health issues, doctors, healthcare workers, children and teens, older people with chronic illnesses, etc., may respond more strongly to the stress of the crisis. Fear of contracting the virus and the stereotypic behaviour towards the infected individuals are a major cause of concern [2]. There is separation of families, increasing unemployment and other major changes in the way we live that have the potential to cause depression and anxiety. Repeatedly watching the news and other media reports about COVID-19 may cause stress in individuals' especially older people. The immune response is essential to control and eliminate coronavirus infections; people will panic thinking about their immune system. Deeper understanding of the interaction between coronaviruses and the innate immune systems of the hosts may reduce the risk of lung inflammation caused by the virus and bring out positive results [5].

The WHO has warned all countries to be prepared for a massive increase in mental health issues arising from the pandemic among its citizens. During any outbreak of an infectious disease, the population's psychological reactions play a critical role in shaping both spread of the disease and the occurrence of emotional distress and social disorder both during and after the outbreak [9]. It has urged countries to conduct rapid and rigorous research on the impact of COVID-19 on mental health, so that, the impact of the pandemic can be limited. Health experts have observed an increase in the feeling of frustration, depression, anger and helplessness. They say the lockdown could result in major long-term impacts on mental health.

3 Methods

The study focused on collecting information regarding how people belonging to different age groups were coping with various situations that came up during the lockdown was conducted. A questionnaire was circulated to collect information from about sample of 9852 individuals who belong to the categories like professionals, engineering (UG & PG) and medical students (UG & PG) and others, etc. Data were collected regarding the various activities performed by the individual to utilize their available time. With all the fake news, false notions and stereotypes circulating around the world through social media and other modes of communication, it was necessary to know whether people were aware about the mental and psychological effects that the lockdown could have on individuals. Thus, a few questions where devoted to gathering information on whether the individual was aware of the various health conditions that could arise due to the lockdown and the steps taken by them to control and manage such situations.

4 Results and Discussions

The data collected from various individuals like professionals, engineering and medical students and others were tabulated based on various parameters.

4.1 Types of Activities

Graphs were plotted and comparisons were made between professionals, engineering and medical students.

From the data collected from professionals, it could be concluded that a larger proportion of the respondents, nearly 88%, engaged themselves in exercises and physical workout. The professionals may have considered the COVID-19 lockdown as an opportunity to return to their healthy habits. But then, only a smaller percentage was observed to engage themselves in productive activities like gardening, reading, academic pursuits, etc. After 'exercise' most of them spend their time in social media and watching television. It was also observed that only 37% of the professionals were engaged in academic pursuits.

On comparing undergraduate (UG) and postgraduate (PG) engineering students, it was observed that a larger percentage of the PG students, approximately 75%, focused on engaging themselves in academic pursuits. This was in stark contrast to the 23% of the UG students who did the same. Another observation was that the percentage of students who spent time with their families and engaged in household activities was higher than the percentage of professionals who did the same. Some of the respondents were engaging in more than one kind of activity and marked their interest in more activities. Educational institutions were shut down much earlier than the professional work places and companies. Professionals, who were working in COVID-affected places, became anxious of being put to quarantine/isolation centre. This prompted them to stay at their own work place rather than return to their homes. This could have resulted in the above-mentioned observation.

The percentage of PG medical students who focused on academic pursuits were lower compared to engineering PG students. From Fig. 4 it can be observed that the percentage of PG medical students who engaged themselves in household activities, family time and physical exercise was much lower compared to professionals and engineering students. This could be because, postgraduate medical students were directed to stay back in their medical colleges and engage themselves in treating COVID-19 patients.

From both Figs. 1 and 2, it can be observed that the number of PG students engaged in academic pursuits is more than the UG students. This is because the postgraduate course is more of a self-learning course compared to the undergraduate courses. It has a shorter span of 2 years compared to the 3/4 years UG programmes. PG students are expected to learn more by themselves, and therefore, the lockdown has given them an opportunity to pursue more in their academics.

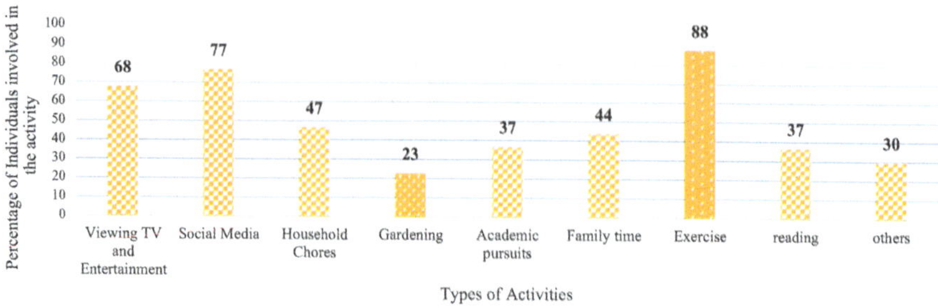

Fig. 1 Activities performed by professionals

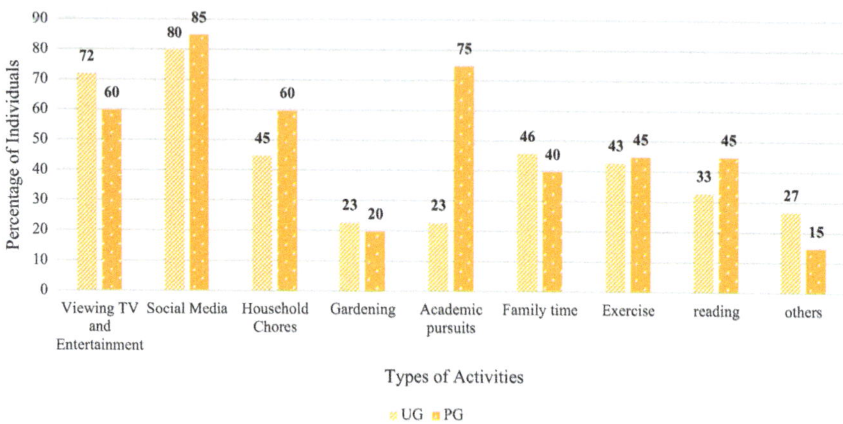

Fig. 2 Activities performed by UG and PG engineering students

Unlike engineering colleges, medical colleges were shutdown only much later. During the initial days, medical students were instructed to stay back in their respective medical colleges and assist doctors in treating COVID-19 patients. It was only much later that the government intervened to send back the UG students to their respective homes. UG medical students were also asked to study and complete online courses on COVID-19 treatment. This could be reason why the percentage of UG medical students who engaged themselves in academic pursuits is almost twice as that of the UG engineering students.

From the above graph (Figs. 3 and 4), it can be observed that there is significant improvement in the percentage in professionals who engaged themselves in exercises and physical workouts compared to students. A general observation can be made that, the percentage of individuals engaged in productive work like gardening and reading was comparatively less. They spend most of their time engaging themselves in social media and other entertainment with the UG students topping the chart. Less than 50% of the responded individuals were observed to spend quality time with their family.

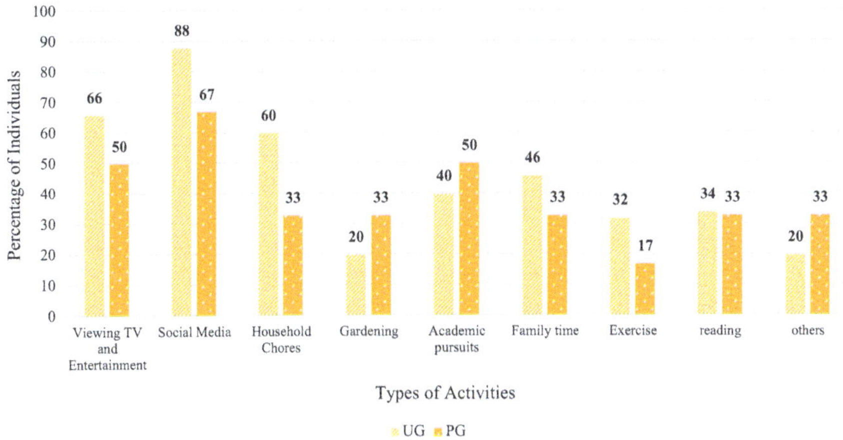

Fig. 3 Activities performed by UG and PG medical students

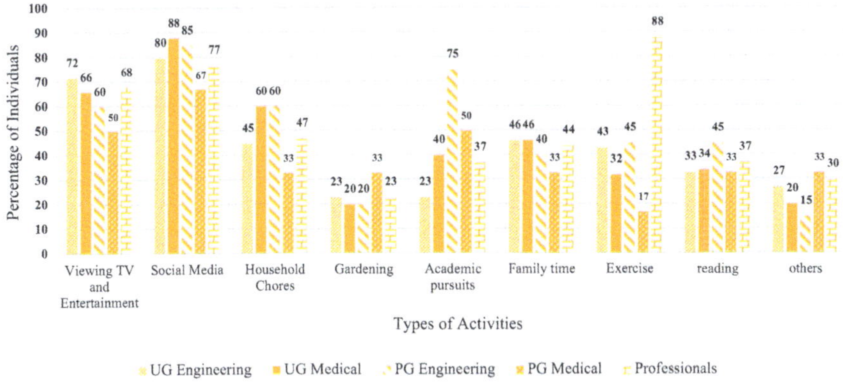

Fig. 4 Comparison of the various activities performed by professionals, UG and PG engineering and medical students

It can also be observed that the UG students were comparatively more engaged with their family.

4.2 *Mental Health Issues and Eating Behaviour*

When it comes to increased anxiety, most of the respondents were observed to have not experienced any sort of issue with anxiety. But this was not true throughout. In the case of PG medical students, the percentage of those who experienced or occasionally experienced anxiety was 55%. But when it comes to the professionals it was no surprise to observe that only 17% of the respondents reported issues with anxiety and mental stress. This can very well be attributed to their increased engagement in physical exercise and fitness routine as observed from Fig. 1.

It can be observed from the graph that more than 50% of all students, both UG and PG, have reported mental stress issues. This was very much expected since there was always an uncertainty as to how and when the educational institutions would reopen and carry on with their regular activities. Most students did not expect the lockdown to extend for such a long period of time. This feeling of uncertainty could have resulted in a greater number of students reporting mental stress issues.

More than 60% of all individuals belonging to each category were observed to have experienced changes in their sleeping behaviour. Although professionals experienced less mental stress and anxiety, even they experienced changes in their sleeping pattern. It is to be noted that PG medical students who may take up duties in hospitals are experiencing changes in their seeping pattern due to the overtime shifts and other COVID duties.

Anxiety and mental stress may negatively affect a person's eating behaviour. Figure 8 confirms this statement. Most professionals reported that they had not experienced any changes in the eating behaviour while more than 50% of both engineering and medical students felt that their eating behaviour had changed.

The observations from Figs. 5, 6, 7 and 8 could be used to conclude that even healthy individuals who experience less mental stress and anxiety and who have a healthy diet could experience sleeping disorders.

In some individuals, a sudden change in the daily routine activities due to the lockdown and change in pattern of physical activities could have resulted in change in eating and sleeping behaviour. The mental stress was also analysed in the present study. It was observed that 52% of the respondents mostly or occasionally experienced mental stress and 42% experienced increased anxiety. Isolation, loneliness and fear of disease could have resulted in this increased mental stress. This observation is in agreement with the various studies conducted by the World Health Organization on 'Depression and Mental Disorders' [6].

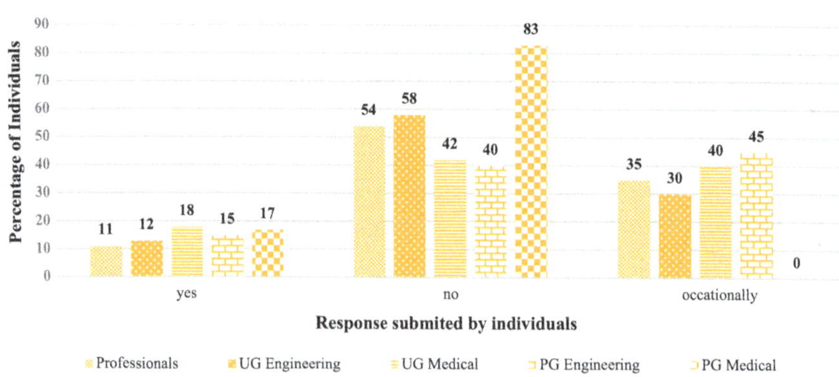

Fig. 5 Comparison between various individuals on whether they experience increased anxiety

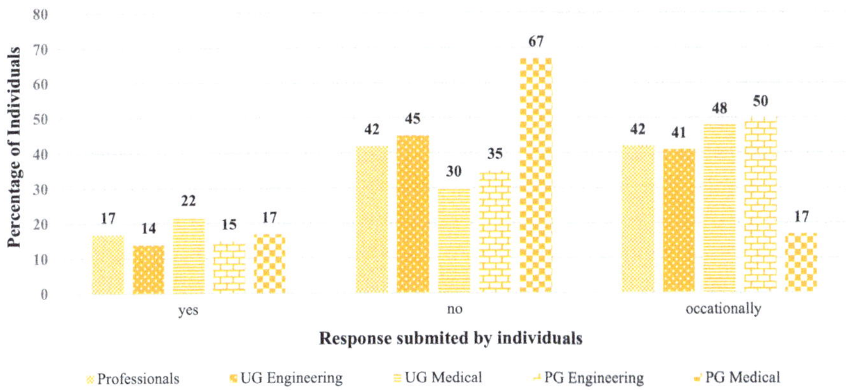

Fig. 6 Comparison between various individuals on whether they experience mental stress

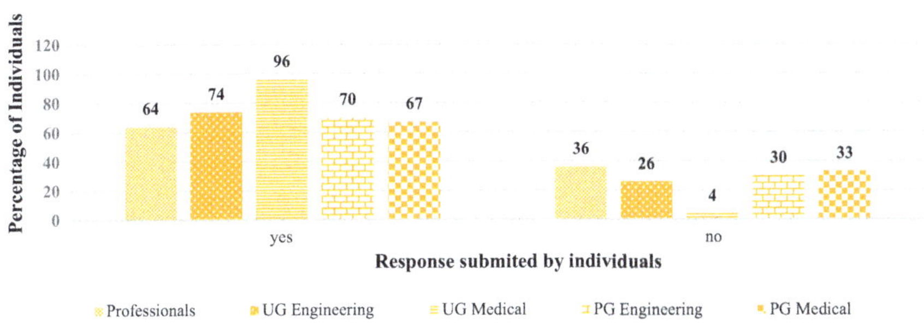

Fig. 7 Comparison between various individuals on whether they experienced any changes in sleeping pattern

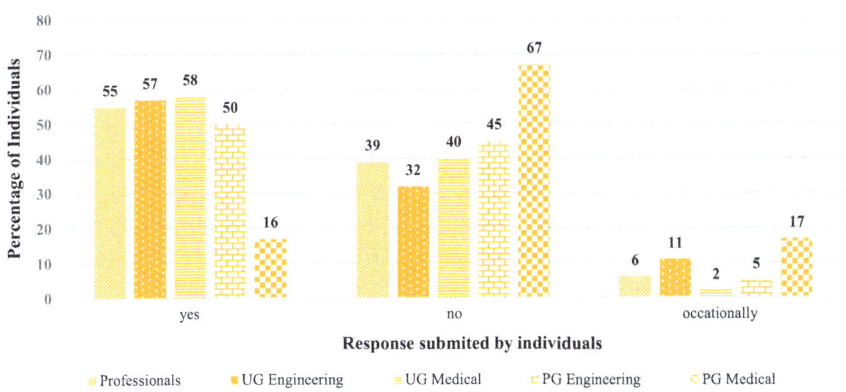

Fig. 8 Comparison between various individuals on whether they experienced any changes in eating behaviour

4.3 Awareness Among People

The COVID-19 lockdown was something that was absolutely necessary in order to maintain public health and social order. Through the survey, it was analysed whether the respondents were aware that the lockdown had the potential to cause mental health issues in people. It was no surprise that nearly 83% of our respondents knew about the various mental issues like depression and anxiety that the lockdown could cause. Would not we then expect the people to maintain themselves in good health? Both emotionally and physically? The survey observations prove otherwise. This would have been due to the sudden introduction of the lockdown without any prior notice or preparation. People were uncertain about what the future holds. The fear of an uncertain future makes people very uncomfortable and put themselves in a situation where they have no idea as to; what to do next. This may be why most people are observed to indulge themselves more on social media and other entertainment platforms than focus on useful and productive work.

5 Conclusion

From the data collected from 9852 individuals and tabulated, it was concluded that the COVID-19 lockdown, though it caused less anxiety, did cause mental stress issues particularly among the student community. The manner in which the entire pandemic was managed by the governments and the global organizations is the major reason for controlling the rapid spread of the disease. At the same time, it was observed that 52% of the respondents mostly or occasionally experienced mental stress and 42% experienced increased anxiety. More than 60% of all individuals belonging to various categories were observed to have experienced changes in their sleeping behaviour. It was found that a larger percentage of the PG students, approximately 75%, focused on engaging themselves in academic pursuits. Most students did not expect the lockdown to extend for such a long period of time. The feeling of uncertainty in academic activities could have resulted in a greater number of students reporting mental stress issues. A sudden change in the daily routine activities due to the lockdown and lesser time spend for physical activities could have had resulted in this change in eating and sleeping behaviour. It was observed that medical professionals and students were experiencing changes in their seeping pattern due to the overtime shifts and other COVID-related duties.

More than 65% of individuals belonging to all categories were observed to engage in social media platforms. It should also be noted that the social media is clogged with news, both real and fake, regarding the pandemic. This could be a major cause of concern to all countries trying to cope with the crisis. International organizations like the WHO and the governments should focus a little more on the mental and psychological issues that could be caused due to the lockdown and take all necessary steps and measures to make people comfortable. The graphs and charts depicted above show major changes in the sleeping pattern and eating behaviour among the student community. This is bound to result in major health issues in the near future. Governments should take care that the measures taken to contain the outbreak should not impact the citizens in a manner that it leads to another health crisis.

References

1. Centres for Disease Control and Prevention. (2020, August 29). *Coronavirus disease 2019 (COVID-19)—Coping with stress*. Retrieved from the Centres for Disease Control and Prevention website. https://www.cdc.gov/coronavirus/2019-ncov/daily-life-coping/managing-stress-anxiety.html
2. Cullen, W., Gulati, G., & Kelly, B. D. (2020). Mental health in the COVID-19 pandemic. *QJM: Monthly Journal of the Association of Physicians, 113*(5), 311–312. https://doi.org/10.1093/qjmed/hcaa110
3. Li, G., Fan, Y., Lai, Y., Han, T., Li, Z., Zhou, P., Pan, P., Wang, W., Hu, D., Liu, X., Zhang, Q., & Wu, J. (2020). Coronavirus infections and immune responses. *Journal of Medical Virology, 92*(4), 424–432. https://doi.org/10.1002/jmv.25685
4. Ministry of Health and Family Welfare. (2020, August 22). *Minding our minds during the COVID-19*. Retrieved from the Ministry of Health and Family Welfare website. https://www.mohfw.gov.in/pdf/MindingourmindsduringCoronaeditedat.pdf
5. Tufan, A., Güler, A. A., & Matucci-Cerinic, M. (2020). Covid-19, immune system response, hyperinflammation and repurposinantirheumatic drugs. *Turkish Journal of Medical Sciences, 50*(SI-1), 620–632. https://doi.org/10.3906/sag-2004-168
6. Wikipedia. (2020, September 21). *COVID-19 pandemic*. Retrieved from the Wikipedia website. https://en.wikipedia.org/wiki/COVID-19_pandemic
7. Worldometer. (2020, September 23). *Coronavirus update*. Retrieved from the Worldometer website. https://www.worldometers.info/coronavirus/
8. World Health Organization. (2020a, April 13). *Mental health & COVID-19*. Retrieved from the World Health Organization website. https://www.who.int/teams/mental-health-and-substance-use/covid-19
9. World Health Organization. (2020b, September 11). *Healthy at home-mental health*. Retrieved from the World Health Organization website. https://www.who.int/news-room/campaigns/connecting-the-world-to-combat-coronavirus/healthyathome/healthyathome---mental-health

Analysis, Modelling and Prediction of COVID-19 Outbreaks Using Machine Learning Algorithms

V. Ajantha Devi

1 Introduction

COVID-19 is a rising sickness responsible for contaminating great many individuals and killing thousands worldwide since the principal notice until these days, as indicated by the World Health Organization (WHO) [1, 2]. Due to the effects of the COVID-19 pandemic in individuals' lives and the world's economy, the administrations and populace are generally worried about (i) when the COVID-19 flare-up will top; (ii) how long the episode will last and (iii) the number of individuals will inevitably be tainted [3]. Further, [4] have recognized in any event three established researchers that may collaborate in the push to manage the flow pandemic: (i) the network of applied mathematicians, virologists and disease transmission specialists, creating advanced dispersion models to the particular properties of a given microorganism; (ii) the network of complex frameworks researchers who study the spread of contaminations utilizing compartmental models, utilizing strategies and standards from measurable mechanics and non-direct elements; and (iii) the network of researchers who join man-made consciousness (AI) and most explicitly profound learning ways to deal with produce precise prescient models.

Additionally, various examinations are assessing the effects of COVID-19 on society, regardless of whether through expectations of future cases, just as factors fit for assisting with understanding the spread of this illness [5–9]. Additionally, epidemiological time arrangement estimating assumes a significant function in well-being public framework, when it permits the chiefs to create key intending to keep away from potential pandemics. Estimating maladies as precise as conceivable is significant because of their effect on the general well-being framework. To guarantee this exactness, AI models have been generally used to estimate epidemiological time arrangement throughout the years [10–12]. In addition, in the AI setting, Vaishya et al. [13] introduced an audit of patterns in COVID-19 information investigation.

V. Ajantha Devi (✉)
Research Head, AP3 Solutions, Chennai, India

M. Niranjanamurthy et al. (eds.), *Intelligent Data Analysis for COVID-19 Pandemic*, Algorithms for Intelligent Systems, https://doi.org/10.1007/978-981-16-1574-0_15

The COVID-19 confirmed cases in India are 1,637, and the death toll is 38 by 1 April 2020, as per the world metre data. With this record, we attempt to make available numerous huge open-information assets on COVID-19 for mainstream researchers. Much of the time, recognizing satisfactory sources is troublesome, particularly for non-master information researchers. For instance, GitHub store contains numerous significant data sets worldwide also, territorial degree, however it may be trying to find them without sufficient direction. In addition, the unwavering quality of the information source supplier can be a worry. Hence, this chapter is planned for giving a large image of the accessible information source suppliers for breaking down COVID-19 engendering and control.

2 COVID-19 Around the Global

To screen the spread of COVID-19, the unmistakable commonplace foundations are assessing the amount of confirmed, death, recovered, hospitalized, crisis unit cases, etc. Considering the agonizing time span [8], all of these elements are associated with the amount of spoiled cases in a conceded manner. One of the central focuses of those establishments is to evaluate the fundamental conceptive number R0, which serves to portray the spread of the contamination [10]. A couple of works have decided R0 for specific scenes of unequivocal regions. The evaluated characteristics are going from 2 to 3 [11]. Nevertheless, simply limited data has been used in numerous works. On the other hand, achieving an exact model of the disease engendering is a trying undertaking, which incorporates various elements and endorsement steps. Unfortunately, the data sets available before long are secretly accumulated, free with different models, clashing with data models and deficient.

3 Machine Learning and Its Types

Machine learning is created on sets of numerical and statistical equations that figure out how to discover examples and settle on choices based on past experience. Consequently, machine learning strategies are utilized to perform investigative assignments, for example, classification and regression.

Further, there are two principle machine learning draws near: supervised learning and unsupervised learning [14–16]. Supervised learning is the assignment of gathering a capacity from named preparing information. Inside supervised learning, prescient modellers are given a set of highlight occurrences along with comparing right outputs. These models conjecture future yields dependent on earlier information by being prepared on preparing information and assessed on testing information.

When managing unlabelled information, unsupervised learning is utilized. All the perceptions are thought to be brought about by inert factors. Consequently, the objective of unsupervised learning is to portray information's structure by sorting out it, for instance, by gathering the information into cluster.

A supervised learning approach is the point at which the information comprises both the input and output factors. By computing the mistake from the contrast between the model's anticipated worth and the real output value, it is conceivable to change the model's loads and inclinations to limit this mistake [17]. Supervised learning tackles relapse and order issues. By utilizing grouping, information can be sorted into a class, for instance, red or vehicle. By utilizing relapse, it is possible to appraise a mathematical output value, for instance, the quantity of treats that will get sold.

Unsupervised learning is utilized when there is no output information. Rather, the calculation attempts to discover designs in the information all alone. Unsupervised learning is utilized to discover groups and put inconspicuous information in a reasonable neighbourhood [17].

With the information data set utilized in this postulation and its mathematical output esteem, plainly this is a relapse issue. As there are more than one time subordinate factors in the picked information, it is viewed as multi-variate time arrangement, and the supervised learning technique is favoured over a unsupervised learning strategy because of the accessibility of the information.

3.1 Supervised Learning

Supervised learning has two fundamental methodologies: classification and regression. In the event that the ideal output comprises at least one constant factors, at that point it is known as a regression issue. A supervised learning methodology is worked to make a forecast at the point when it is given an unknown information occurrence. The trained model at that point produces an expectation for the provided unexpected factor information or testing data [18]. This learning technique may utilize regression procedures and classification algorithms for prescient models' turn of events.

Three regression models have been utilized for this investigation of COVID-19 forecasting.

Artificial Neural Network.

The most extreme broadly artificial neural network [19] used in the estimation issue is multilayer perceptions, which utilizes the single levels feed forward system [20]. This strategy is arranged by an arrangement of three layers. The hubs in a few levels are also distinguished as adjusting basics.

Support Vector Machine.

Support vector machine (SVM) is a supervised learning model with related learning calculation that research data used for classification and regression analysis [20, 21]. An SVM is a discriminative classifier authoritatively portrayed by a secluding hyperplane. Thusly, given named preparing information, the algorithm outputs a perfect hyperplane which arranges new models. An SVM model is a depiction of the models as centres in space, arranged with the objective that the cases of the various classes [20] are divided by a sensible gap that is as wide as could be normal in the light of the current situation. Despite performing linear classification, SVMs can gainfully play out a nonlinear classification, certainly arranging their commitments to high-dimensional part spaces.

Linear Regression.

In regression model [21], a target feature is predicated on the free features. This procedure can be, therefore, used to find the association among autonomous and subordinate elements and besides for deciding. Linear regression [21–24] is the principle thought for the use depending on the straightforwardness, notoriety, and adequacy of this technique for request forecasting. Basic linear regression is an essential yet successful and helpful technique in insights. In this technique, the best-fitted straight line is utilized as the linear regression line. The line condition can be utilized to anticipate the future estimations of dependent variables. The amount of the blunders ought to be zero because of the meaning of this strategy, and in view of that in residual plot we should search for the horizontal-fitted line.

4 Implementation

The COVID-19 has demonstrated a current potential danger to human life, which is causing a huge number of death what is more, the passing rate is expanding step by step all through the global.

Added to this pandemic condition control, this examination tries to perform future assessing on the end rate, the amount of step-by-step affirmed cases and the quantity of recovery cases in the exceptional 10 days. The assessing has been done by using two machine learning gravitates towards that are fitting to this particular circumstance. The data set used in this examination contains step-by-step time course of action diagram tables, including the amount of affirmed, recoveries and deaths cases in the past number of days from which the pandemic started. From the start, the data set has been pre-processed for this examination to find the overall estimations of the step-by-step number of affirmed, recoveries and deaths cases.

4.1 Evaluation Metrics

Before a machine learning model can be utilized, it must be tried and assessed for exactness on test (information that the model is not prepared on). This should regularly be possible by picking fitting measurements for assessing the exhibition. The objective of learning is to foresee the yields comparable to conceivable. To know how effectively a learning calculation has performed, expectation made by a classifier can be contrasted and known names. The initial step parcels a data set into a preparation and testing data, where the preparation data set is utilized to assemble the underlying model, furthermore, the testing data set (or assessment data set) is utilized to assess the learning model.

Testing data set should be pre-processed through indistinguishable strides as the preparing data set. To get a well-performing model, the preparing data set needs to cover the full scope of qualities for all highlights the model may experience. To accomplish this, there is a usually utilized dividing strategies. Dividing a data set is by haphazardly examining 80% of the data set as preparing information, and the left 20% of the data set is utilized as testing information.

5 Time Series Data set

This part used three sorts of data sets, the basic educational assortment is the 2019 Novel Coronavirus COVID-19 (2019-nCoV) Data Repository by Johns Hopkins CSSE (https://github.com/CSSEGISandData/COVID-19), the second data set is used from world metres site (https://www.worldometers.info/), and third is from Kaggle. Data set records are contained in the coordinator on the GitHub store named (csse_covid_19_time_series). The coordinator contains each day time arrangement outline tables, including the amount of confirmed, deaths and recovered. The data set is taken from Kaggle which contains four sections which are new active cases, current deaths, total active cases and all out number of deaths. The data set contains the nation wise data portraying the above segments for every nation on an ordinary premise. The data is accessible from 1 April 2020 to 20 July 2020. After the fundamental data pre-processing step, the data set has been apportioned into two subsets: a training set and testing set. The learning models, for instance, ANN, SVM, LR have been used in this investigation. These models have been set up on the days and as of late attested cases, recovery, and downfall plans.

This examination proposes a machine learning structure for COVID-19 time arrangement determining. Two profound learning models LR and SVM have been applied to estimate every day confirmed and recuperated cases. The overall system of the determining proposed procedures is represented in Fig. 1. The COVID-19 gauging has been done on two fundamental stages: preparing and testing. In the principal stage, the crude information is pre-processed and normalized, and afterwards it is utilized to build the profound learning model. The estimations of boundaries of profound learning models are chosen with the end goal that the misfortune work is limited during the preparation. Here, Adam enhancer is utilized for this reason. From that point forward, in the testing stage, the recently developed models with the chose boundaries are utilized to conjecture the quantity of COVID cases. The exactness of the model will be checked by contrasting the deliberate information and genuine information by means of various factual pointers.

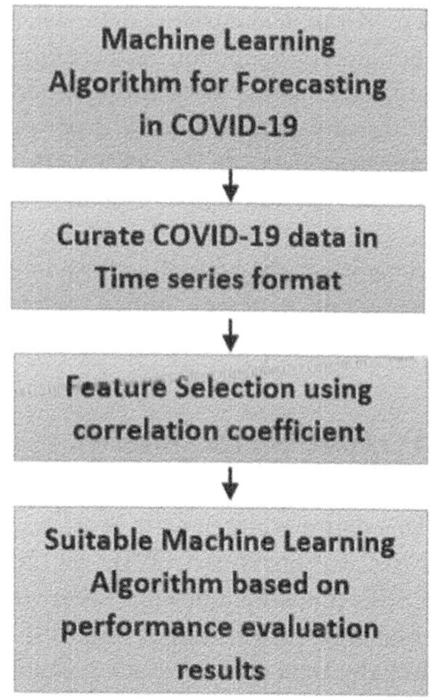

Fig. 1 Data flow of forecasting in COVID-19

5.1 Analysis, Modelling and Prediction of COVID-19

Day of the week affect number of daily cases:

- Pre-processing: Get separate data frames for each day of the week. We can do this easily with the dates as datetime objects
- Drop unnecessary columns
- Use pandas function 'diff' to get differences between previous column
- Sum up all rows for each date
- Convert dates to datetime objects
- Drop lat, long and province/state
- Aggregate data using group by based on day of the week each row belongs to
- Day of the week can be retrieved by accessing a member of the datetimes.

Analysis:

Compare statistics of the data frames such as mean, median, max and min. You can use pandas to describe function to do this easily. Plot each data frame using COVID-19 Daily State Cases Visualizer as shown below.

- Figure 2 plots the number of COVID-19 confirmed cases on every Monday
- Figure 3 plots the number of COVID-19 confirmed cases on every Tuesday
- Figure 4 plots the number of COVID-19 confirmed cases on every Wednesday
- Figure 5 plots the number of COVID-19 confirmed cases on every Thursday
- Figure 6 plots the number of COVID-19 confirmed cases on every Friday

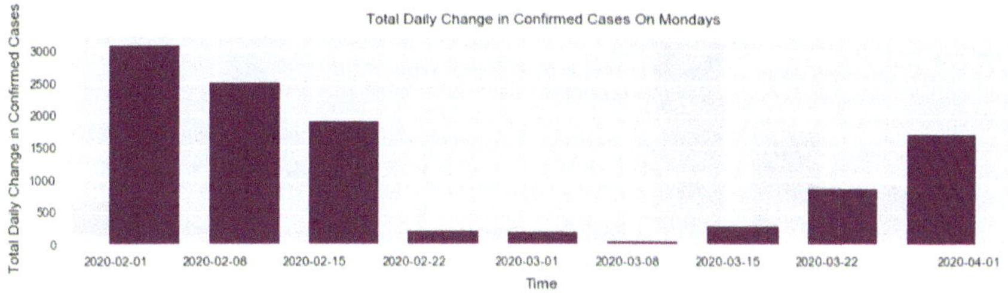

Fig. 2 Confirmed cases on Monday

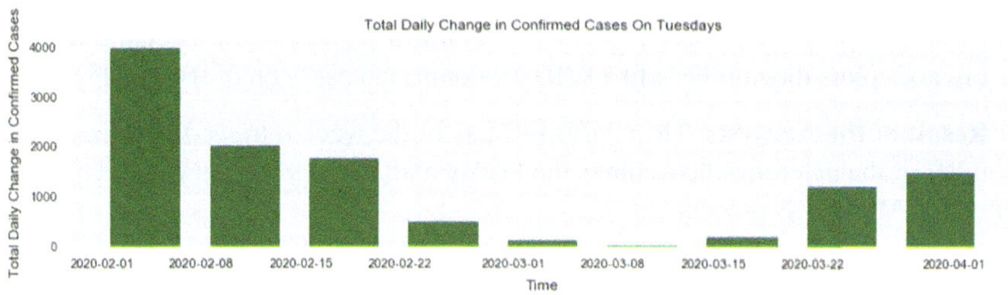

Fig. 3 Confirmed cases on Tuesday

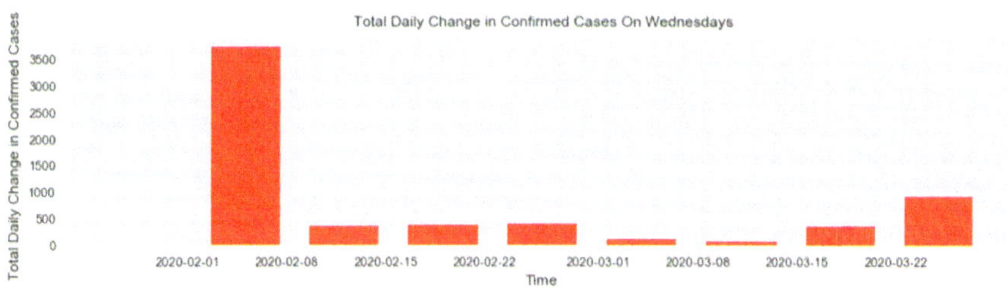

Fig. 4 Confirmed cases on Wednesday

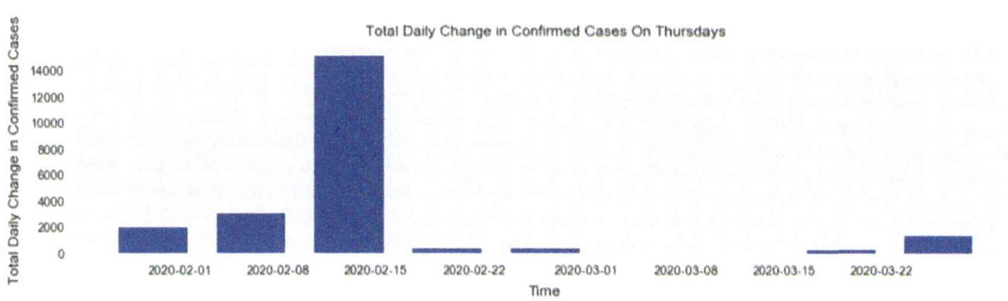

Fig. 5 Confirmed cases on Thursday

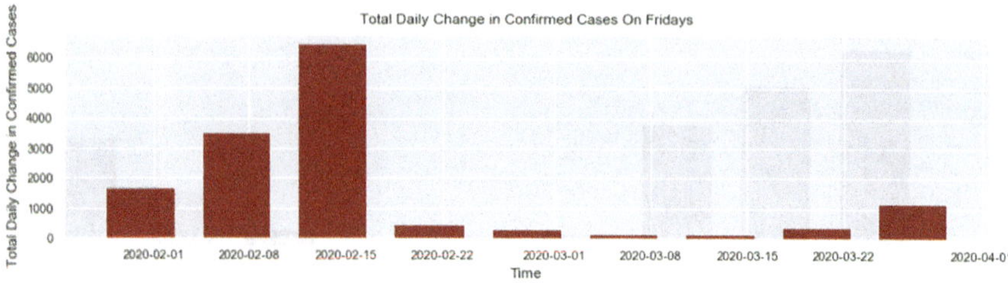

Fig. 6 Confirmed cases on Friday

- Figure 7 plots the number of COVID-19 confirmed cases on every Saturday
- Figure 8 plots the number of COVID-19 confirmed cases on every Sunday.

Result of the Analysis: The analysis of day of the week retrieved by accessing a member of the datetimes determines the Friday and seems to be the worst day to go out while Monday is the safest.

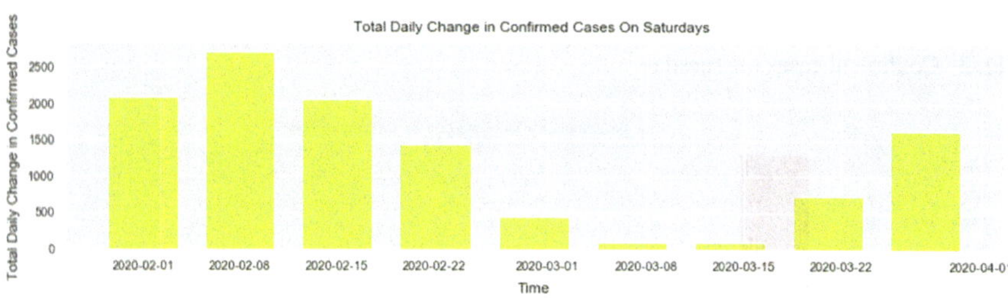

Fig. 7 Confirmed cases on Saturday

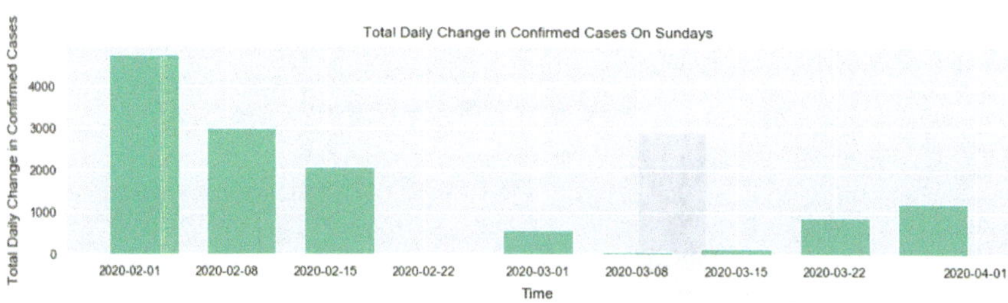

Fig. 8 Confirmed cases on Sunday

5.2 *Confirmed Cases and Death Cases as on 20 July 2020—World*

After the analysis of day of the week retrieved by accessing a number of the datetimes, Fig. 9 plots the daily increases in cases as confirmed, recovered and death cases.

With the above analysis, the average increase in no. of cases every day is shown in Table 1, and total number of confirmed and death as on 20 July 2020 is shown in Table 2.

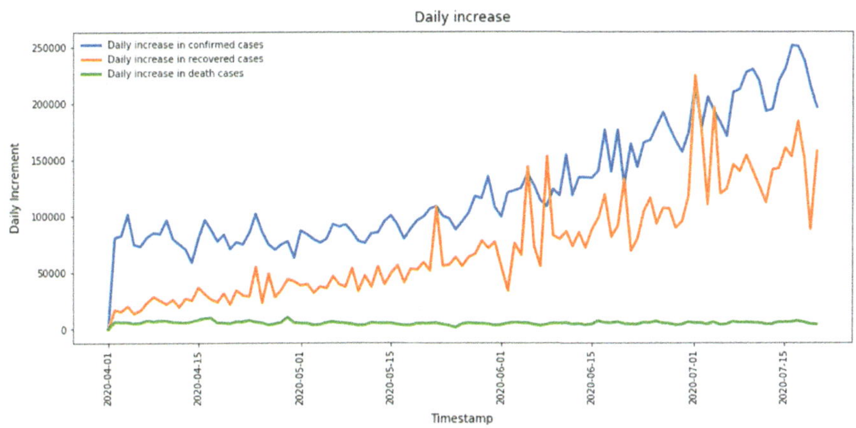

Fig. 9 Daily increases in cases

Table 1 Average increase in number of everyday

Sl. No.	Category	Average increase in No. of everyday
1	No. of confirmed	124,060
2	No. of recovered	72,948
3	No. of deaths	5073

Table 2 Total no. of confirmed and death as on 20 July 2020

Sl. No.	Category	Total number–around the world
1	Confirmed cases	14,703,293
2	Recovered cases	8,290,431
3	Deaths cases	609,887
4	Active cases	5,802,975
5	Closed cases	8,900,318

Table 3 Total number–India as on 20 July 2020

Sl. No.	Category	Total number–India as on 20 July 2020
1	Confirmed	1,155,338
2	Recovered	724,578
3	Deaths	28,082
4	Active cases	402,678
5	Closed cases	752,660

5.3 Confirmed Cases and Death Cases as on 20th July 2020–India

The outbreak of COVID-19 has now spread to several nations and territories. It is hugely expanding day by day. While a lot is still unknown about the virus that causes COVID-19, it continues to spread so it is essential that communities take action to prevent in addition transmission, minimize the impacts of the outbreak and assist control measures (Table 3).

Summarization of the Analysis.

- It took 111 days in India to reach 1,155,338 confirmed cases.
- It took 111 days in Italy to reach no. of confirmed cases to India.
- It took 32 days in the USA to reach no. of confirmed cases to India.
- It took 111 days in Spain to reach no. of confirmed cases to India.
- It took 111 days in China to reach no. of confirmed cases to India.

5.4 Model of Machine Learning Algorithm

For examination and making prediction model, for different nations additionally, we have checked number of cases on 28th day like India and remembering it, prepared data utilizing SVM and linear regression. The same model is appropriate for all the nations. Be that as it may, just to demonstrate the rightness of model of SVM and LR about India as a contextual analysis appeared in Fig. 10 shows the expansion in number of cases for COVID-19 step by step for next 10 days. For preparing reason, 80% information is considered for preparing and staying 20% information is utilized for forecast model (Figs. 11 and 12).

5.5 Predicting the Outgrowth in the Next 3 Months–India

This strategy may really prompt marginally overestimated values in the event that we think about the whole world in general. At the point when the pandemic had just barely begun in certain nations, in certain others it was at its pinnacle. In certain nations, the

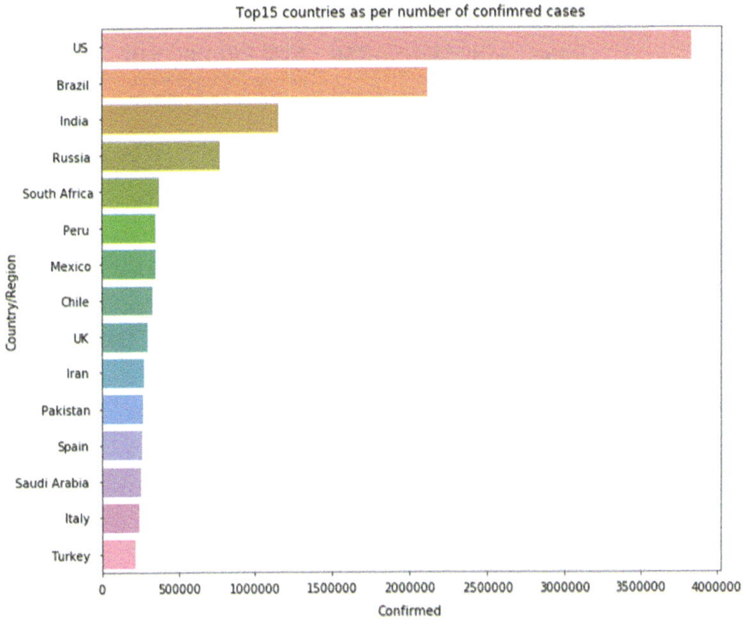

Fig. 10 Top 15 countries—confirmed cases as on 20 July 2020

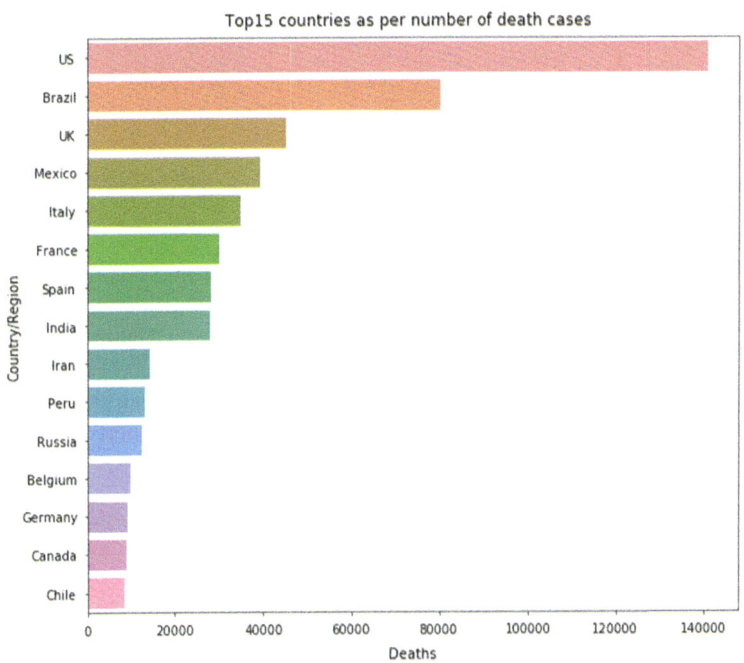

Fig. 11 Top 15 countries—death cases as on 20 July 2020

	Dates	LINEAR REGRSN	SVM PREDICTION
0	2020-07-21	12140766	24410379
1	2020-07-22	12247697	25518089
2	2020-07-23	12354629	26676371
3	2020-07-24	12461560	27887053
4	2020-07-25	12568491	29152017
5	2020-07-26	12675422	30473190
6	2020-07-27	12782353	31852555
7	2020-07-28	12889284	33292144
8	2020-07-29	12996215	34794042
9	2020-07-30	13103146	36360388
10	2020-07-31	13210077	37993376
11	2020-08-01	13317008	39695256
12	2020-08-02	13423939	41468332
13	2020-08-03	13530870	43314969
14	2020-08-04	13637801	45237587
15	2020-08-05	13744733	47238667
16	2020-08-06	13851664	49320750

Fig. 12 LR and SVM model prediction

development has begun to impede now while in some others it is as yet developing at a disturbing rate. For this heterogeneity, this technique for anticipating of the spread accepting the whole world in general may not give wonderful figures, yet it would surely give some functional transient gauges that would be slight overestimates. In any nation, heterogeneity may not be excessively high, and thus for a particular nation a particularly mathematical methodology would be valuable for short-term forecasts as shown in Figs. 13 and 14.

6 Conclusion

As indicated by the specialists, infectious ailments are not certain how long they will continue in the environment. Furthermore, COVID-19,, which has made destruction around the world, is found to have higher irresistible rate and lower however unsure

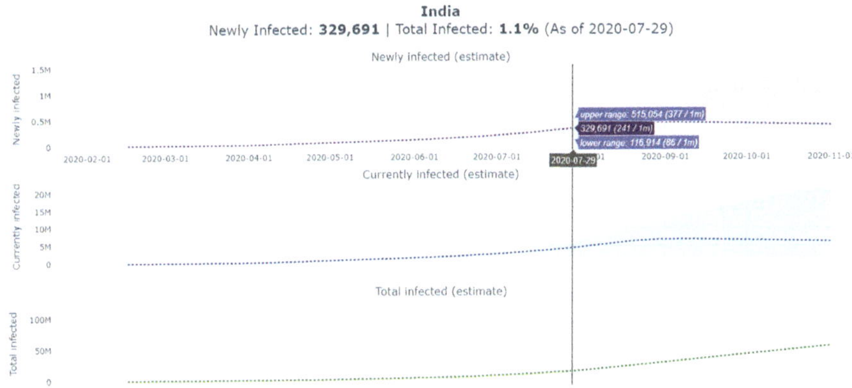

Fig. 13 On the basis of death cases, predicting the outgrowth in the next 3 months

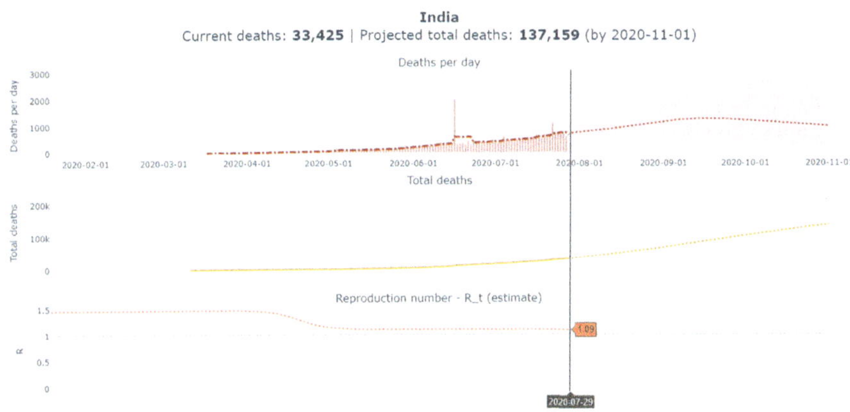

Fig. 14 On the basis of confirmed cases, predicting the outgrowth in the next 3 months

death rate. The quantity of confirmed novel coronavirus cases in India has arrived at near 1250 cases as of 31 March 2020. As per the Indian well-being service, COVID-19 has overall contaminated over 1.5 lakh individuals, and it is probably going to cause more terminations over the nation.

In the event that legitimate preventive measures are not followed, the quantity of cases will shoot up in the coming days. Being the second most populated nation on the planet, India will need to confront a great deal of moves identified with giving satisfactory treatment and clinical offices to tainted individuals. The forecasts were shown from 1 April 2020 to 20 July 2020, and it included the expectation of the quantity of cases considering the quantity of cases that would recover and impact of the lockdown. This information will help in guaranteeing the nation's readiness towards confronting the future difficulties and arranging the exercises appropriately.

Preventive measures regarding social removing are, therefore, at present a need of great importance as it will help in decreasing the quantity of cases and diminish the weight on India's economy.

References

1. Sohrabi, C., Alsafi, Z., O'Neill, N., Khan, M., Kerwan, A., Al-Jabir, A., Losifidis, C., Agha, R. (2020). World health organization declares global emergency: A review of the 2019 novel coronavirus (COVID-19). *International Journal Surgery*, https://doi.org/10.1016/j.ijsu.2020.02.034
2. WHO: World Health Organization. (2020). Coronavirus disease (COVID-2019) situation Reports. https://www.who.int/emergencies/diseases/novelcoronavirus-2019/situation-reports/. Accessed 9 June, 2020.
3. JHU: John Hopkins University. (2020). COVID-19 dashboard by the center for systems science and engineering (CSSE) at Johns Hopkins University (JHU). https://www.coronavirus.jhu.edu/map.html. Accessed 9 June, 2020.
4. Davenport, T., & Kalakota, R. (2019). The potential for artificial intelligence in healthcare. *Future Healthcare Journal, 6*(2), 94–98. https://doi.org/10.7861/futurehosp.6-2-94
5. Bai, Y., Yao, L., Wei, T., Tian, F., Jin, D. Y., Chen, L., Wang, M. (2020). Presumed asymptomatic carrier transmission Of COVID-19. *Research Letter, 323*, 1406–1407. Available online: https://jamanetwork.com/journals/jama/articleabstract/2762028. Accessed 10 April, 2020.
6. Ferretti, L., Wymant, C., Kendall, M., Zhao, L., Nurtay, A., Abeler-Dörner, L., Parker, M., Bonsall, D., Fraser, C. (2020). Quantifying SARS-CoV-2 transmission suggests epidemic control with digital contact tracing. *Science*, eabb6936. [CrossRef] [PubMed].
7. Ismail, B. M., Reddy, B. E., Reddy, B. T. (2018). "Cuckoo inspired fast search algorithm for fractal image encoding." *Journal of King Saud University Computer and Information Sciences, 30*(4), 462–469 https://doi.org/10.1016/j.jksuci.2016.11.003
8. Lauer, S. A., Grantz, K. H., Bi, Q., Jones, F. K., Zheng, Q., Meredith, H. R., Azman, A. S., Reich, N. G., & Lessler, J. (2020). The incubation period of coronavirus disease 2019 (COVID-19) from publicly reported confirmed cases: Estimation and application. *Annals of International Medicine*, [CrossRef].
9. Mohammed Ismail, B. B., & Eswara Reddy, T. (2015). "Improved fractal image compression using range block size" IEEE Proc (CGVIS) pp. 284–289. https://doi.org/10.1109/CGVIS.2015.7449938
10. Hellewell, J., Abbott, S., Gimma, A., Bosse, N. I., Jarvis, C. I., Russell, T. W., Munday, J. D., Kucharski, A. J., Edmunds, W. J., Sun, F., & Flasche, S. et al. (2020) Feasibility of controlling COVID-19 outbreaks by isolation of cases and contacts. *Lancet Global Health, 8*, e488–e496. [CrossRef].
11. Liu, Y., Gayle, A.A., Wilder-Smith, A., & Rocklöv, J. (2020). The reproductive number of COVID-19 is higher compared to SARS coronavirus. *Journal of Travel Medicine, 27*, taaa021. [CrossRef].
12. Makridakis, S., Spiliotis, E., & Assimakopoulos, V. (2018). "Statistical and machine learning forecasting methods: Concerns and ways forward." *PloS one, 13*(3).
13. Bontempi, G., Taieb, S. B., Le Borgne, Y.-A. (2012). "Machine learning strategies for time series forecasting." In *European business intelligence summer school*, (pp. 62–77). Springer.
14. Ajantha Devi, V. (2018). "Supervised learning approach to object identification and recognition." *International Journal of Pure and Applied Mathematics, 119*(10), 463–470.
15. Bishop, C. (2007). Pattern recognition and machine learning (information science and statistics), (1st edn., 2006. corr. 2nd printing edn). Springer.
16. Mohri, M., Rostamizadeh, A., & Talwalkar, A. (2012). *Foundations of machine learning (adaptive computation and machine learning series)*. MIT Press.

17. Jain, A. K., Murty, M. N., & Flynn, P. J. (1999). Data clustering: A review. *ACM computing surveys (CSUR), 31*(3), 264–323.
18. Talabis, M. R. M., McPherson, R., Miyamoto, I., Martin, J. L., & Kaye, D. (2015). "Chapter 1—Analytics defined." In *Information security analytics, syngress*, (pp. 1–12). [Online]. Available: https://www.sciencedirect.com/science/article/pii/B9780128002070000010
19. Lapuerta, P., Azen, S. P., & LaBree, L. (1995). Use of neural networks in predicting the risk of coronary artery disease. *Computers and Biomedical Research, 28*(1), 38–52.
20. Adhikari, R., & Agrawal, R. K. (2012). Forecasting strong seasonal time series with artificial neural networks. *Journal of Scientific and Industrial Research, 10*, 657–666.
21. Shanthi, S., & Kumar, D. (2012). Prediction of blood glucose concentration ahead of time with feature based neural network. *Malaysian Journal of Computer Science, 25*, 136–148.
22. Barrow, D. K., Crone, S. F., & Kourentzes, N. (2010). An evaluation of neural network ensembles and model selection for time series prediction. *The 2010 International Joint Conference on Neural Networks* (IJCNN), (pp. 1–8).
23. Science, C. (2003). Dimensionality reduction for indexing time series based on the minimum distance. *Work, 711*, 697–711.
24. Yang, S. H., Liang, C. K., & Hsieh, C. Y. (2005). Watermarking MPEG-4 2D mesh animation with time-series analysis. *Journal of Information Science and Engineering, 21*, 341–359.

Tracking and Analysis of Corona Disease Using Intelligent Data Analysis

M. P. Amulya, M. Niranjanamurthy, H. K. Yogish, and G. K. Ravikumar

1 Introduction

Artificial intelligence refers to the recreation of human knowledge in personalized machines to think like people and copy their activities. The term can also be applied to any machine that displays qualities related to the human psyche, for example, learning and critical thinking. Man-made reasoning advancements are rapidly developing, fundamentally in light of the fact that AI measures a lot of information a lot quicker and makes expectations more precisely than humanly conceivable. In this global wellness emergency, the clinical sector is looking for new advances to detect and control the spread of the COVID-19 pandemic. Computerized intelligence is one of those innovations that can undoubtedly track the spread of this infection, distinguish high-risk patients, and is valuable in gradually controlling this contamination. You can also predict mortality risk by sufficiently analyzing information from previous patients. It plans to survey the part of AI as an unequivocal innovation to investigate and set us up for counteraction and battle against COVID-19 and different pandemics.

Man-made reasoning is the recreation of human insight measures by machines. Man-made reasoning advancements are rapidly developing, fundamentally on the grounds that AI measures a lot of information a lot quicker and makes forecasts more precisely than humanly conceivable. As the pandemic has moved around the planet, nations are thinking of uses of artificial intelligence to come up which new and imaginative plans to fight against it. Artificial intelligence offers several preferences

M. P. Amulya (✉)
Department of Computer Science and Engineering, Adichunchanagiri University, B G Nagar, Mandya 571448, India

M. Niranjanamurthy · H. K. Yogish
Department of Master of Computer Applications, M S Ramaiah Institute of Technology, Bangalore 560054, India

G. K. Ravikumar
Adichunchanagiri University, B G Nagar, Mandya 571448, India

M. Niranjanamurthy et al. (eds.), *Intelligent Data Analysis for COVID-19 Pandemic*, Algorithms for Intelligent Systems, https://doi.org/10.1007/978-981-16-1574-0_16

over routine investigations and dynamic clinical methods. Learning calculations can be more accurate and precise when connected to information preparation, allowing people to gain extraordinary experiences in diagnosis, measures of care, fluctuation in treatment, and patient outcomes.

There is a critical need for dynamic innovations in health associations to address this infection and help them continually obtain adequate proposals to prevent its spread. Artificial intelligence works in a way capable of emulating human knowledge. It could also take on an essential task in organizing and recommending the progress of a COVID-19 vaccination. This results-driven innovation is used for legitimate screening, research, expectation, and follow-up of current and prospective future patients. Huge applications are applied to track information of confirmed, recovered, and approved cases. Emergency clinics, general well-being organizations, and business well-being organizations are looking for open approaches to screen patients, for example, online side-effect checkers, which could permit them to screen themselves for indications of COVID-19.

An application can provide an early discovery and determination of contamination. This will help to give a faster dynamic that is smart. Artificial intelligence is useful in determining contaminated cases using advances in clinical imaging such as computed tomography (CT) and the production of magnetic reverberation images (MRI) of parts of the human body.

One step can be worked on for scheduled observation and prediction of the spread of infection. It will include an aid for fair and comprehensive examinations for infectious diseases and, in addition, it helps to recognize problem areas. This innovation can track and measure the idea of infection from accessible information, online media and media stages, about the dangers of contamination and its likely spread. Also, you can anticipate the number of positive and approved cases in any district. Computerized intelligence can help recognize weaker areas, individuals, and nations and take gauges in the same way. Computerized intelligence is used for drug research by finding accessible information on COVID-19. It can help to recognize useful drugs for the treatment of patients with COVID-19. It has become a useful asset for symptomatic testing plans and advancing inoculation. Artificial intelligence helps create antibodies and drugs at a somewhat faster rate than expected and is also useful for clinical foreplay as vaccination progresses.

With the help of a constant informative survey, AI can provide up-to-date data, which is helpful in the fight against this disease. It is often used to predict potential destinations for contamination, convergence of infection, need for beds, and expert medical care during this emergency. Simulated intelligence is useful in fighting future infections and diseases, with the help of past information guided through predominant information at different times. It distinguishes the qualities, causes, and purposes of the spread of the disease. In the future, this will turn out to be a major innovation in fighting various pests and pandemics. It can take a preventative measure and fight many different infections. In the future, AI will take on the critical job of providing more premonitory and preventive medical services.

Computerized reasoning is a valuable and proximate tool to recognize early diseases due to covid and also helps to observe the condition of infected patients.

Basically, you can improve the consistency and dynamics of processing by creating valuable stones. Artificial intelligence is not only useful in the treatment of patients infected with COVID-19, but also for their adequate control of well-being. You can follow the emergence of COVID-19 at different scales, for example, clinical, atomic, and epidemiological applications.

2 AI Versus COVID-19

Covid, COVID-19, has been all the rage for weeks, if not months. The bad dream of the pandemic continues to threaten the world. It is unusual to accept that malls that claim to host entire PVR lanes, the cluster at Starbucks Stadium in Mexican ghost towns.

As of March 23, 2020, more than 349,000 people had obtained the covid novel, and in any case, 15,308 had kicked the bucket, according to a tally by Johns Hopkins University. Despite the fact that the cases registered with respect to the total recovery are 100,165, the number of casualties due to the coronavirus is greater than the SARS (2002–20,040) and the avian influenza of 2013, and gradually closes with the complete disappearance of the swine flu (2009–2010), for example, 18,036.

So with lives, a shrinking economy, the travel industry in question, the tech giants must make a dangerous bet on artificial intelligence. Artificial intelligence anticipated the possibility of a pandemic long before the World Health Organization (WHO) and the Centers for Disease Control and Prevention (CDC) in the USA. Let us do a quick survey on how AI has changed thanks to its battle with SARS-COV-2 infection and how the Indian government can take notes.

2.1 Prediction and Data Sharing

BlueDot, a Toronto-based well-being reconnaissance organization dispatched in 2014, had cautioned its customers not to go to Wuhan China when it found puzzling pneumonia influencing the individuals here. It utilized AI calculations to examine the accessible information which included carrier flight courses, animals well-being, reports from well-being associations, and so forth and discovered likenesses to the SARS episode.

"InferVISION" is another AI-based programming that professes to give indications of infection caused pneumonia in speculated patients. It is controlled by NVIDIA's Clara SDKs.

Analysts at Harvard University's School of Public Health and the National Tsing Hua University, in Taiwan, are working with Facebook to follow the movement history of the influenced individuals.

2.2 R&D Sector

Finding a remedy for an infection is a brain numbingly extensive methodology. Other than this, it additionally imprints the monetary assets.

On account of AI, it can

- Progress antibodies and immunizations.
- Check-through drug history for a current medication.
- Design medications to battle the current strain or upcoming plagues.

Be that as it may, on a silver coating, Google's DeepMind's AlphaFold System delivered structure expectations of a few proteins related with the infection. This is accepted to manage logical personalities in understanding the infection.

DeepMind's specialists composed on the AI lab's site. "We affirmed that our framework gave an exact forecast to the tentatively decided SARS-CoV-2 spike protein structure partook in the Protein Data Bank, and this gave us certainty that our model expectations on different proteins might be valuable."

In another piece of the world, British startup Exscienta turned into the primary organization to put an AI-planned medication particle to human preliminaries recently.

2.3 Deception

The greater part of the informal communication destinations and Web crawlers are attempting to limit the dissemination of falsehood, paranoid fears, phishing, and so forth.

All the stages currently have a spring up connection that guides clients to true pages containing data and preventive measures to be taken.

2.4 Monitoring

Did you also were pointed a firearm like gadget, set on your temple at a public spot by security work force just to know whether you are in danger. Indeed, you are in good company. As of now, the majority of the urban communities around the world are utilizing conventional strategies like thermometer weapons, which utilizes an infrared sensor to quantify either your frontal or body heat. All things considered, we can utilize progressed scanner like Badu's AI-fueled, non-contact sensor framework. This framework can do a speedy multifilter in open regions, recognizing clients with fever. This takes away the danger of cross-disease and deals with the group successfully while giving precise outcomes. It is right now being used at Beijing's Qinghe Railway Station, where it checks 200 individuals for each moment and banners individuals with temperature over 37.3 °C. SenseTime is a man-made reasoning SaaS organization and examines individuals to check in the event that they are wearing veils. Because of its infectious nature, the greater part of the clinical group is under consistent openness to the infection. Man-made intelligence turns a legend here. China is utilizing robots to give quicker analytic checks. In Hangzhou, city ambulances are helped by AI to speed through traffic.

Jack Ma's Alibaba new AI framework can recognize covid in CT outputs of patients' chests with 96% exactness inside 20 s. It can separate between a COVID-19 infection and standard viral pneumonia.

2.5 Data Overload

Since the infection turned out to be truly newsworthy in December 2019, more than 3000 articles and review articles have been distributed on the Web. Taking advantage of experiences on the Web can be overwhelming and time consuming, especially when we are in a race with time as an adversary. The White House Office of Science and Technology Policy has reported on a company called COVID-19 Open Research Dataset, also known as CORD-19. In this activity, he collaborated with Microsoft Research, National Library of Medicine, Kaggle, Allen Institute for AI's Semantic Scholar project (AI2), Chan Zuckerberg Initiative and others. They used normal language management to collect and filter more than 29,000 articles identified with the new infection and the covid family in general, including 13,000 of them prepared for PCs to see hidden information, in addition to data on the creators and their affiliations. This progression will strengthen the match between groups and help examine hidden infection history, risk factors, and create a potential bulk drug or antibody option.

2.6 Arrangement of Automated Vehicles

Admittance to medical services and assets is critical to battle the spread of the covid. While drones are utilized to guarantee inhabitants are avoiding potential risk, in pieces of the world, they have been relegated to lead warm imaging, dispatch help like testing packs, food, meds to the poor. It lessens individual-to-individual contact and blocks a lack of clinical staff.

Additionally, the Guangdong Provincial People's Hospital in Guangzhou City is likewise utilizing independent conveyance robots to move drugs around the clinic.

This fortifies contactless observing of the episode as well.

Denmark-based UVD Robots' are ending up being helpful by sanitizing patients without human impedance. These bots transmit UV light to clean the objective zone and slaughter infections.

Table 1 Variances between the AI learning techniques

	Supervised learning	Unsupervised learning	Reinforcement learning
Definition	It learns by utilizing labeled data	It is trained on unlabeled data	The practitioner interacts with its environments, whereas performing actions and leaning from the rewards or errors
Problem type	Classification and regression	Clustering and association	Based on rewards
Data type	Labeled data	Unlabeled data	Absent of predefined data
Training	External supervision	No supervision	No supervision
Approach	Inputs being labeled are mapped to the known output	Patterns are being understood and output is discovered	Trial and error are being implemented
Operation	ML	ML	ML
Exploration	No exploration	No exploration	Adapts through exploration
Strategy	Learning algorithm and data-dependent	Classification and data-dependent	Learns from experience

Despite the fact that AI is yet to resemble human intelligence, they are ending up being exceptionally useful in following the flare-up, diagnosing patients, sterilizing regions, and accelerating the way toward finding a solution for COVID-19. While the frenzy and rise of new problem areas proceeds, this advancement by AI has demonstrated to be motivating and earth shattering (Table 1).

2.7 *Variances Between the AI Techniques [1]*

See Table 1.

3 Using AI to Detect, Respond, and Recover from COVID-19

Before the world was even aware of the danger it posed (COVID-19), artificial reasoning (AI) executives had identified the episode of an obscure type of pneumonia in the People's Republic of China (as of this time), China. As the episode now has a global pandemic, the devices and advances in AI can be used to help the efforts of policymakers, the clinical network, and society around the world to cope with each phase of the disease, emergence and its consequences: localization, avoidance, reaction, recovery, and accelerating the investigation (Fig. 1).

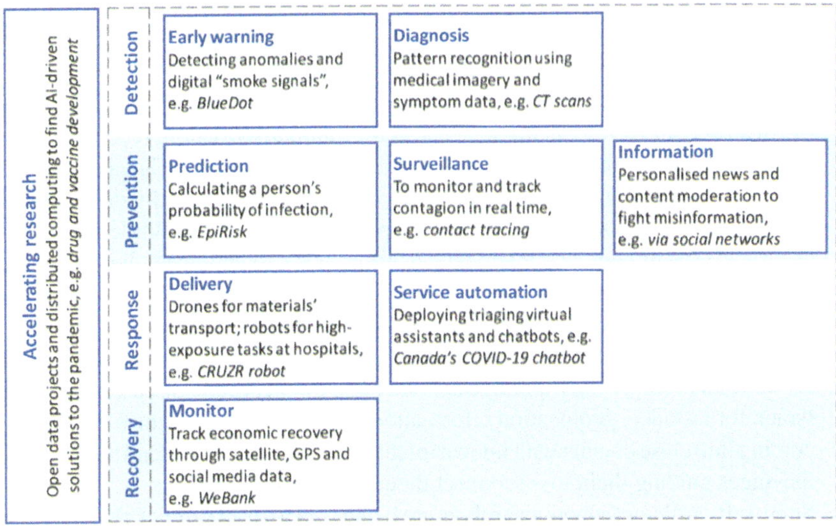

Fig. 1 Examples of A-I applications at diverse stages of the COVID-19 disaster

(Resource https://www.oecd.org/coronavirus/policy-responses/using-artificial-intelligence-to-help-combat-covid-19-ae4c5c21/).

Utilizing AI to help distinguish, analyze, and forestall the spread of the covid.

Computer-based intelligence can likewise be utilized to help distinguish, analyze, and forestall the spread of the infection. Calculations that distinguish examples and oddities are as of now attempting to identify and foresee the spread of COVID-19, while picture acknowledgment frameworks are accelerating clinical determination. For instance:

- AI-powered early warning frameworks can help distinguish epidemiological examples by exploiting standard news, online substances, and other data hijacks in various dialects to give early warnings, which can complement syndromic observation and other medical and service organizations information flows (e.g., the WHO Early Warning System, BlueDot).
- AI devices can help distinguish infection transmission chains and detect broader financial effects. In some cases, advances in AI have demonstrated its ability to obtain epidemiological information faster than the usual announcement of welfare information. Foundations, for example, Johns Hopkins University and the OECD (oecd.ai) have also made intuitive dashboards available that allow live infection tracking and ongoing information on confirmed covid cases, recoveries, and deaths.
- Rapid analysis is vital to restrict infection and comprehend the sickness spread. Applied to pictures and side-effect information, AI could help to quickly analyze COVID-19 cases. Consideration should be given to gathering information illustrative of the entire populace to guarantee versatility and exactness.

Restricting infection is a need in all nations and AI applications are forestalling the infection's spread.

- A number of nations are utilizing populace observation to screen COVID-19 cases (for instance, in Korea calculations use geolocation information, reconnaissance camera film and charge card records to follow covid patients). China appoints a danger level (shading code—red, yellow, or green) to every individual demonstrating infection hazard utilizing mobile phone programming. While AI models use travel, installment, and interchanges information to anticipate the area of the following flare-up, and illuminate line checks, Web indexes, and Web-based media are likewise assisting with following the sickness continuously.
- Many nations, including Austria, China, Israel, Poland, Singapore, and Korea have set up contact following frameworks to recognize conceivable disease courses. In Israel, for instance, geolocation information was utilized to recognize individuals coming into close contact with known infection transporters, and send them instant messages guiding them to disconnect themselves right away.
- Semi-self-sufficient robots and robots are being sent to react to quick requirements in emergency clinics, for example, conveying food and drugs, cleaning and sanitization, helping specialists and medical attendants, and performing conveyances of hardware.

Figure 2 shows the covid confirmed, dead, and active state of July 13, 2020. It represents the day-by-day covid patients ratio increasing [2].

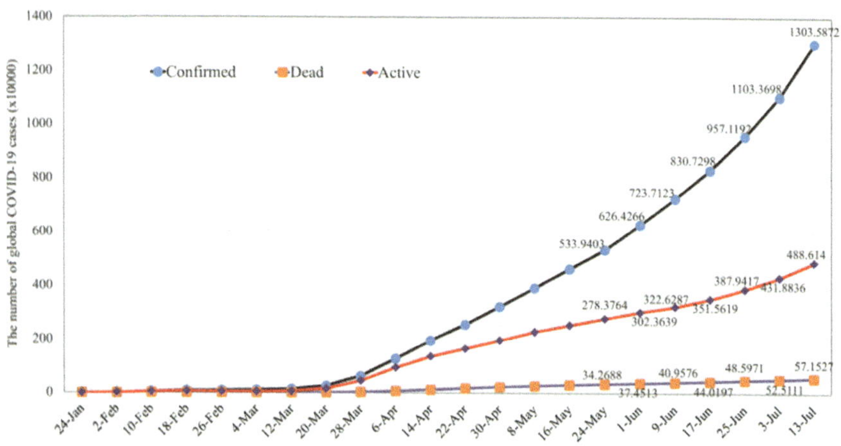

Fig. 2 Global COVID-19 trend. *Source* CoronaBoard. Data accurate as of July 13, 2020

3.1 *Computer-Based Intelligence for COVID-19 Medical Response*

A portion of the AI frameworks made to help COVID-19 clinical reaction help analyze and identify COVID-19 through essential Web-based screening or investigating chest pictures. Others, for example, the approaching form of eCART can help anticipate COVID-explicit results and advise clinical choices. This is especially valuable for clinical volunteers without aspiratory preparing, who should survey patients' conditions and choose who needs assistance first. Artificial intelligence tech may likewise demonstrate supportive in the quest for a COVID-19 immunization and different treatments.

In any case, the information holes we referenced before have significant ramifications for clinical AI frameworks and AI-improved immunization preliminaries. Individuals respond diversely to infections, antibodies, and medicines, as past flare-ups like SARS and Ebola have shown. Information accessible on COVID-19 external the USA, for instance, shows that people face distinctive casualty rates, and a new exploration paper found that ladies patients admitted to the Wuhan Union Hospital had more significant levels of COVID-19 antibodies than men. Given foundational imbalances demolish well-being results for certain racial and ethnic gatherings, and it is similarly critical to comprehend COVID-19 well-being results for various personalities, just as the intersectional suggestions.

Calculations do not represent existing disparities hazard making mistaken forecasts—or more awful. In 2019, an investigation found that the broadly utilized Optum calculation, which utilized medical care spending as an intermediary to quantify need, was one-sided against dark Americans. It did not represent segregation or absence of access, the two of which lead to bring down spending on medical care by dark Americans. In the midst of the COVID-19 emergency, AI frameworks that advise restricted asset allotments, (e.g., who to put on a ventilator) should be mindful so as not to incidentally organize certain characters over others. While designers intend to make calculations race-dazzle by barring race as a measurement, this can overlook or stow away—as opposed to forestall—separation. For instance, calculations that advise clinical choices may utilize intermediaries, for example, prior conditions. Diabetes is a prior condition connected to higher paces of COVID-19, and it has a higher occurrence for dark Americans. In the event that a calculation utilizes previous conditions yet is oblivious in regard to race, it can result in excessively organizing white Americans over dark Americans.

While a few firms cling to thorough testing—leading huge approval concentrates preceding delivering items, for instance—not all organizations are careful. Further, the dynamic cycles of most AI calculations are not straightforward. This makes the way for erroneous or unfair forecasts for specific socioeconomics, and accordingly presents massive dangers to the people and specialists utilizing them.

4 AI for COVID-19 Social Control

Another new use of AI is contact following, or following individuals who have come into contact with the infection to help contain it. By following client data, for example, well-being and area, and utilizing AI-fueled facial acknowledgment, these instruments can authorize social separating and advise residents regarding contact with positive cases. In China, clients are relegated a covid score, which impacts their admittance to public transportation, work, and school. What is more, US government authorities have started raising the chance of mass reconnaissance, gathering "anonymized, total" client area information from tech goliaths like Facebook and Google to plan the spread of COVID-19.

However, reconnaissance instruments have moral ramifications—once more, especially for underestimated populaces. Utilizing AI to choose who leaves their home could prompt a type of COVID-19 redlining, exposing certain networks to more noteworthy implementations. This brings to mind another AI model that outcomes in higher reconnaissance of helpless networks of shading: prescient policing. In the USA, hazard appraisal calculations utilize criminal history data, however do not consider profound established racial inclination in the policing framework, that dark Americans are captured all the more regularly for more modest wrongdoings and that neighborhoods with high grouping of dark Americans are all the more intensely watched. Dark Americans end up overrepresented in the information, which at that point connects to racially one-sided policing results. Essentially, people group affected by proposed observation frameworks would probably be more unfortunate networks of shading harder hit by COVID-19 for an assortment of reasons connected to chronicled disparities and separation.

It is not clear how or how long government organizations or different substances will utilize these sorts of AI instruments. In China, following could stay after the emergency, permitting Beijing specialists to screen strict minorities, political nonconformists, and other minimized networks with a background marked by being oversurveilled. Also, in spite of the fact that information assortment in the USA will at first be anonymized and accumulated, there is potential for abuse and deanonymization later on.

4.1 Man-Made Reasoning in the Battle Against COVID-19

Man-made reasoning can help battle the covid through applications including populace screening, warnings of when to look for clinical assistance and following how disease spreads. The COVID-19 flare-up has set off extreme work on such applications, yet it will require some investment before results become obvious.

Even with the covid, computerized advances are fundamental for both social well-being and financial execution. An advanced reaction to the COVID-19 pandemic can take various structures and bring huge worth. One significant region in which there have been fast improvements over the most recent couple of weeks is new uses of man-made reasoning (AI) and AI (ML) for screening of the populace and surveying disease chances.

Screening the populace to distinguish who is conceivably sick is vital for containing COVID-19. In China, which was hit first, customary infrared imaging scanners and handheld thermometers were presented in various public areas, particularly in Beijing. Chinese AI champion firms have now presented further developed AI-fueled temperature screening frameworks in spots including metro and railroad stations. The upside of these frameworks is that they can screen individuals from a good ways and inside the space of minutes can test many people for fever.

In China and somewhere else, new AI-controlled cell phone applications are being created to screen person's well-being and track the topographical spread of the infection. Such applications expect to foresee which populaces and networks are generally vulnerable to the antagonistic effects of a covid episode, to empower patients to get constant holding up time data from their clinical suppliers, to furnish individuals with exhortation and updates about their ailment without them visiting a medical clinic face to face, and to tell people of potential disease hotspots progressively so those zones can be dodged.

4.2 Information Access

These advances for the most part need admittance to information communicated by cell phones, including locational information. While the instruments are being created, it is critical to likewise build up a system so they can be as compelling as conceivable by and by. For this, nearby coordination between specialists, telecoms administrators, innovative industry, and examination establishments is required. Innovative firms and driving colleges can give the apparatuses, telecoms firms can give admittance to people's information, and specialists ought to guarantee that information sharing adjusts with security runs and does not make chances the information of people will be abused [3]. Dissimilar steps in the presentation of AI-based approaches employed to overcome COVID-19 challenges [4].

For instance, in Belgium, datasets from telecoms administrators are joined with well-being information under the oversight of the Belgian Data Protection Authority to produce total and anonymized local-level datasets that can be utilized to survey how the infection spreads and which territories are high danger. Comparative activities are in progress in different nations. The genuine estimation of these endeavors is that computerized advances can offer observing continuously, empowering specialists to be more proactive.

In Austria, the biggest telecom administrator agreed with the specialists to give anonymized information, while a comparable anonymized client information sharing component has been set up to follow and investigate populace developments in Italy's hard-hit Lombardy locale.

4.3 Security Ensuring Applications

Scholarly examination can likewise be useful in representing how data sharing can be planned while dodging protection chances. The Human Dynamics Group at MIT Media Lab for instance has worked widely with cell phone information to dissect the conduct of people while regarding high protection norms. It prescribes secure multiparty calculation to save clients' protection.

MIT's security amicable information instruments could be a reason for planning an information sharing model to restrict the spread of COVID-19. A consortium of disease transmission specialists, engineers, information researchers, protection activists, teachers, and scientists from various pieces of the world are chipping away at an open-source cell phone application to forestall the spread of the infection without building a reconnaissance state. The application checks for covers of clients' GPS trails with the path of every tainted patient (whose anonymized information is given by well-being specialists), while cryptographic techniques are utilized and there is no sharing of crude information (individual information does not leave the gadget). This framework gives early cautions and customized data that permit people who joined to the application to comprehend their own openness and dangers, in light of prior contact with tainted patients. Such administrations must be viable if an extraordinary number of patients and others buy in.

With so much data as an info, research on (informal communities) is attempting to gauge how and how much the infection will spread, given a bunch of predecided boundaries and qualities. Specialists can utilize these situations to set up their alternate courses of action as expected.

Utilizing data on the time people spend in a specific area and on the quantity of diseases that happen there, researchers make spatial models that portray the advancement of contacts between tainted individuals, to catch how transmission advances. One of the primer discoveries of such endeavors is that anticipating the transmission of COVID-19 is trickier than for past infections since people can convey the infection without indicating side effects, and their diseases are hence hard to distinguish. An enormous number of the contaminations in Wuhan appear to have been communicated through such asymptomatic transporters (Stanford's Lin Lab gauges that half of tainted people are asymptomatic). In this way, escalated COVID-19 testing programs (like that executed in South Korea) can be useful by giving information to the better exhibition of these models.

Man-made intelligence can likewise be applied to the programmed discovery and expulsion of falsehood identified with the infection posted on informal organizations; delivering profoundly exact and opportune CT filters for the location of infection actuated pneumonia; 3D printing to create the apparatuses required for concentrated medical care; advancement of clinical preliminaries of medications and possible antibodies; improvement of mechanical frameworks to clean tainted zones; and online frameworks for the clinical assessment of people.

Timing is obviously basic (an investigation on the 1918 flu pandemic shows that US urban areas that received non-drug measures at a beginning stage had top demise rates half lower than those that did not). Governments have been condemned for neglecting to comprehend the seriousness of the covid circumstance and not overwhelming composed measures as expected.

While the AI people group is working seriously on conveying applications that can assist with containing the infection, AI frameworks are still at a starter stage and it will require some investment before the consequences of such AI measures are obvious.

5 How Artificial Intelligence Applications can Contain Coronavirus COVID-19

Another new use of AI is contact following, or following individuals who have come into contact with the infection to help contain it. By following client data, for example, well-being and area, and utilizing AI-fueled facial acknowledgment, these instruments can authorize social separating and advise residents regarding contact with positive cases. In China, clients are relegated a covid score, which impacts their admittance to public transportation, work, and school. What is more, US government authorities have started raising the chance of mass reconnaissance, gathering "anonymized, total" client area information from tech goliaths like Facebook and Google to plan the spread of COVID-19.

However, reconnaissance instruments have moral ramifications—once more, especially for underestimated populaces. Utilizing AI to choose who leaves their home could prompt a type of COVID-19 redlining, exposing certain networks to more noteworthy implementations. This brings to mind another AI model that outcomes in higher reconnaissance of helpless networks of shading: prescient policing. In the USA, hazard appraisal calculations utilize criminal history data, however do not consider profound established racial inclination in the policing framework, that dark Americans are captured all the more regularly for more modest wrongdoings and that neighborhoods with high grouping of dark Americans are all the more intensely watched. Dark Americans end up overrepresented in the information, which at that point connects to racially one-sided policing results. Essentially, people group affected by proposed observation frameworks would probably be more unfortunate networks of shading harder hit by COVID-19 for an assortment of reasons connected to chronicled disparities and separation [5, 6].

It is not clear how or how long government organizations or different substances will utilize these sorts of AI instruments. In China, following could stay after the emergency, permitting Beijing specialists to screen strict minorities, political nonconformists, and other minimized networks with a background marked by being oversurveilled. Also, in spite of the fact that information assortment in the USA will at first be anonymized and accumulated, there is potential for abuse and deanonymization later on [7, 8].

5.1 Man-Made Reasoning in the Battle Against COVID-19

Man-made reasoning can help battle the covid through applications including populace screening, warnings of when to look for clinical assistance and following how disease spreads. The COVID-19 flare-up has set off extreme work on such applications, yet it will require some investment before results become obvious [9].

Even with the covid, computerized advances are fundamental for both social well-being and financial execution. An advanced reaction to the COVID-19 pandemic can take various structures and bring huge worth. One significant region in which there have been fast improvements over the most recent couple of weeks is new uses of man-made reasoning (AI) and AI (ML) for screening of the populace and surveying disease chances.

Screening the populace to distinguish who is conceivably sick is vital for containing COVID-19. In China, which was hit first, customary infrared imaging scanners and handheld thermometers were presented in various public areas, particularly in Beijing. Chinese AI champion firms have now presented further developed AI-fueled temperature screening frameworks in spots including metro and railroad stations. The upside of these frameworks is that they can screen individuals from a good ways and inside the space of minutes can test many people for fever.

In China and somewhere else, new AI-controlled cell phone applications are being created to screen person's well-being and track the topographical spread of the infection. Such applications expect to foresee which populaces and networks are generally vulnerable to the antagonistic effects of a covid episode, to empower patients to get constant holding up time data from their clinical suppliers, to furnish individuals with exhortation and updates about their ailment without them visiting a medical clinic face to face, and to tell people of potential disease hotspots progressively so those zones can be dodged.

5.2 Information Access

These advances for the most part need admittance to information communicated by cell phones, including locational information. While the instruments are being created, it is critical to likewise build up a system so they can be as compelling as conceivable by and by. For this, nearby coordination between specialists, telecoms administrators, innovative industry, and examination establishments is required. Innovative firms and driving colleges can give the apparatuses, telecoms firms can give admittance to people's information, and specialists ought to guarantee that information sharing adjusts with security runs and does not make chances the information of people will be abused.

For instance, in Belgium, datasets from telecoms administrators are joined with well-being information under the oversight of the Belgian Data Protection Authority to produce total and anonymized local-level datasets that can be utilized to survey how the infection spreads and which territories are high danger. Comparative activities are in progress in different nations. The genuine estimation of these endeavors is that computerized advances can offer observing continuously, empowering specialists to be more proactive.

In Austria, the biggest telecom administrator agreed with the specialists to give anonymized information, while, a comparable anonymized client information sharing component has been set up to follow and investigate populace developments in Italy's hard-hit Lombardy locale.

5.3 Security Ensuring Applications

Scholarly examination can likewise be useful in representing how data sharing can be planned while dodging protection chances. The Human Dynamics Group at MIT Media Lab for instance, has worked widely with cell phone information to dissect the conduct of people while regarding high protection norms. It prescribes secure multiparty calculation to save clients' protection.

MIT's security amicable information instruments could be a reason for planning an information sharing model to restrict the spread of COVID-19. A consortium of disease transmission specialists, engineers, information researchers, protection activists, teachers, and scientists from various pieces of the world are chipping away at an open-source cell phone application to forestall the spread of the infection without building a reconnaissance state. The application checks for covers of clients' GPS trails with the path of every tainted patient (whose anonymized information is given by well-being specialists), while cryptographic techniques are utilized and there is no sharing of crude information (individual information does not leave the gadget). This framework gives early cautions and customized data that permit people who joined to the application to comprehend their own openness and dangers, in light of prior contact with tainted patients. Such administrations must be viable if an extraordinary number of patients and others buy in.

With so much data as an info, research on (informal communities) is attempting to gauge how and how much the infection will spread, given a bunch of prede-cided boundaries and qualities. Specialists can utilize these situations to set up their alternate courses of action as expected.

Utilizing data on the time people spend in a specific area and on the quantity of diseases that happen there, researchers make spatial models that portray the advancement of contacts between tainted individuals, to catch how transmission advances. One of the primer discoveries of such endeavors is that anticipating the transmission of COVID-19 is trickier than for past infections since people can convey the infection without indicating side effects, and their diseases are hence hard to distinguish. An enormous number of the contaminations in Wuhan appear to have been communicated through such asymptomatic transporters (Stanford's Lin Lab gauges that half of tainted people are asymptomatic). In this way, escalated COVID-19 testing programs (like that executed in South Korea) can be useful by giving information to the better exhibition of these models.

Man-made intelligence can likewise be applied to the programmed discovery and expulsion of falsehood identified with the infection posted on informal organizations; delivering profoundly exact and opportune CT filters for the location of infection actuated pneumonia; 3D printing to create the apparatuses required for concentrated medical care; advancement of clinical preliminaries of medications and possible antibodies; improvement of mechanical frameworks to clean tainted zones; and online frameworks for the clinical assessment of people.

Timing is obviously basic (an investigation on the 1918 flu pandemic shows that US urban areas that received non-drug measures at a beginning stage had top demise rates half lower than those that did not). Governments have been condemned for neglecting to comprehend the seriousness of the covid circumstance and not overwhelming composed measures as expected.

Ved Parkash Pati discussed while the AI people group is working seriously on conveying applications that can assist with containing the infection, AI frameworks are still at a starter stage and it will require some investment before the consequences of such AI measures are obvious.

Since December 2019, when the unrelenting coronavirus disease, or COVID-19, was identified in China, artificial intelligence (AI), machine learning, data and analytics, and natural language processing, have been clamored about as a few potent solutions we have to fight the disease and bring about sustainable development.

And rightly so, on December 31, 2019, the Canadian AI company BlueDot rose to fame when it alarmed its customers about the pneumonia cases that had surfaced a few days back in Wuhan, China. This was nine days before the World Health Organization confirmed the finding of the coronavirus.

Therefore, AI, with its combined might of machine learning, natural language processing, and computer vision had announced its potency right since the advent of the disease. AI models have the potential to contribute toward the combined fight through each step of the "containment chain" namely—TRACK, TREAT, ANALYZE, PREDICT, and DEVELOP (Fig. 3).

- Track: Video Surveillance—CCTV monitoring of people's behaviour.
  Remote biosignal measurement—face heartbeat, selfie video measurement wearable data—record heart rate fluctuations.
- Treat: Machine learning diagnostics—powered by computer vision that is "fatigue-proof" and helps in reducing the number of "false negative."
- Analyze: Grassroots analysis—powered by chat bots and social media.

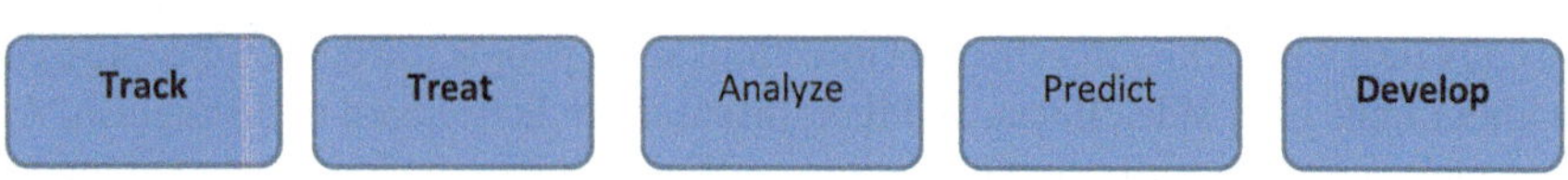

Fig. 3 AI capabilities across the pandemic containment spectrum

- Predict: Mathematical modeling—based on the historical data of other similar infectious diseases and past pandemic evolution data.
- Development: AI-based protein analysis—creation and molecule creation.

Treatment verification: AI can fabricate a revealing step for scheduled observation and prediction of the spread of this infection. A neural organization can also be created to separate the visual highlights of this disease, which would help in the proper observation and treatment of those affected [10].

Personality contact tracing: AI can help to examine the degree of contamination with this infection by recognizing groups and "problem areas" and can effectively track and assess people's contacts. You can predict the future course of this infection and a likely return.

6 Conclusion

Computerized reasoning is an imminent and valuable tool to recognize early contamination due to covid and also helps to observe the condition of infected patients. You can completely improve the consistency and dynamics of your processing by creating valuable calculations. Artificial intelligence is not only useful in the treatment of patients infected by COVID-19, but also for the correct observation of their well-being. Intelligent data analysis used for early detection and diagnosis of infections, treatment monitoring, individual contact follow-up, case and mortality projection, drug and vaccine development, health worker workload reduction, and disease prevention. You can track the COVID-19 emergency at different scales, for example, clinical, subatomic, and epidemiological applications. It is also helpful to promote examination of this infection by dissecting accessible information. Artificial intelligence can help create legitimate treatment regimens, anticipation techniques, drugs, and antibody enhancement. Artificial intelligence works in a way that can masquerade as human knowledge. It could also play a critical role in agreeing and recommending advancement of a COVID-19 vaccine. This results-driven innovation is used for legitimate screening, ventilation, expectation, and follow-up of current and prospective future patients.

References

1. Hussain, A. A., Bouachir, O., Al-Turjman, F., & Aloqaily, M. (2020). AI techniques for COVID-19. *IEEE Access, 8*, 128776–128795. https://doi.org/10.1109/ACCESS.2020.3007939
2. Pham, Q., Nguyen, D. C., Huynh-The, T., Hwang, W., & Pathirana, P. N. (2020). Artificial Intelligence (AI) and big data for coronavirus (COVID-19) pandemic: A survey on the state-of-the-arts. *IEEE Access, 8*, 130820–130839. https://doi.org/10.1109/ACCESS.2020.3009328
3. Zheng, N., et al. (2020, July). Predicting COVID-19 in China using hybrid AI model. *IEEE Transactions on Cybernetics, 50*(7), 2891–2904. https://doi.org/10.1109/TCYB.2020.2990162

4. Jamshidi, M., et al. (2020). Artificial Intelligence and COVID-19: Deep learning approaches for diagnosis and treatment. *IEEE Access, 8*, 109581–109595. https://doi.org/10.1109/ACCESS.2020.3001973
5. Mertz, L. (2020, July-August). AI-Driven COVID-19 tools to interpret, quantify lung images. *IEEE Pulse, 11*(4), 2–7. https://doi.org/10.1109/MPULS.2020.3008354
6. Chowdhury, M. E. H., et al. (2020). Can AI help in screening viral and COVID-19 pneumonia? *IEEE Access, 8*, 132665–132676. https://doi.org/10.1109/ACCESS.2020.3010287
7. Bekhet, S., Hassaballah, M., Kenk, M. A., & Hameed, M. A. (2020). An artificial intelligence based technique for COVID-19 diagnosis from chest X-Ray, In *2020 2nd Novel Intelligent and Leading Emerging Sciences Conference (NILES)*, Giza, Egypt (pp. 191–195). https://doi.org/10.1109/NILES50944.2020.9257930
8. Ulhaq, A., Born, J., Khan, A., Gomes, D. P. S., Chakraborty, S., & Paul, M. (2020). COVID-19 control by computer vision approaches: A survey. *IEEE Access, 8*, 179437–179456. https://doi.org/10.1109/ACCESS.2020.3027685
9. Tseng, V. S., Ying, J. J. C., Wong, S. T. C., Cook, D. J., & Liu, J. (2020, November). Computational intelligence techniques for combating COVID-19: A survey. *IEEE Computational Intelligence Magazine, 15*(4), 10–22. https://doi.org/10.1109/MCI.2020.3019873
10. Vaishya, R., Javaid, M., Khan, I. H., & Haleem, A. (2020). Artificial Intelligence (AI) applications for COVID-19 pandemic.*Diabetes & Metabolic Syndrome: Clinical Research & Reviews, 14*(4), 337–339, ISSN 1871-4021. https://doi.org/10.1016/j.dsx.2020.04.012

Index

M. Niranjanamurthy et al. (eds.), *Intelligent Data Analysis for COVID-19 Pandemic*, Algorithms for Intelligent Systems, https://doi.org/10.1007/978-981-16-1574-0

The manufacturer's authorised representative in the EU is Springer Nature Customer Service Centre GmbH, Europaplatz 3, 69115 Heidelberg, Germany. If you have any concerns regarding our products, please contact ProductSafety@springernature.com

Printed and bound by CPI Group (UK) Ltd, Croydon, CR0 4YY
30/09/2026
02225330-0012